BASIC
GERIATRIC
NURSING

Visit our website at www.mosby.com

BASIC GERIATRIC NURSING

GLORIA HOFFMANN WOLD, RN, BSN, MS

Nursing Instructor
Milwaukee Area Technical College
Milwaukee, Wisconsin

SECOND EDITION

Illustrated

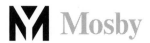

St. Louis   Baltimore   Boston   Carlsbad   Chicago   Minneapolis   New York   Philadelphia   Portland
London   Milan   Sydney   Tokyo   Toronto

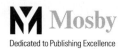

A Times Mirror
Company

Publisher: Sally Schrefer
Editor: Yvonne Alexopoulos
Developmental Editor: Laurie K. Muench
Project Manager: David Orzechowski
Production Editor: Susie Coladonato
Designer: Renée Duenow
Manager of Manufacturing and
Production-Philadelphia: William A. Winneberger, Jr.

SECOND EDITION

Composition by Graphic Composition, Inc.
Printing/binding by R.R. Donnelley & Sons
Lithography by Trinity Graphics

Mosby, Inc.
11830 Westline Industrial Drive
St. Louis, Missouri 63146

Library of Congress Cataloging-in-Publication Data

Wold, Gloria.
   Basic geriatric nursing / Gloria Hoffman Wold.--2nd ed.,
illustrated.
     p. cm.
   Includes bibliographical references and index.
   ISBN 0-8151-8392-5
   1. Geriatric nursing. I. Title.
   [DNLM: 1. Geriatric Nursing--methods. 2. Aging nurses'
instruction. WY 152W852b 1999]
RC954.W58 1999
610.73'65--dc21
DNLM/DLC
for Library of Congress
                                   98-27917
                                      CIP

98 99 00 01 02 / 9 8 7 6 5 4 3 2 1

Reviewers

Linda M. Cater, RN, BSN
Division Chair for Nursing and Allied Health
Harry M. Ayers State Technical College
Anniston, Alabama

Mary Ann Cosgarea, RN, BA, BSN
Coordinator, Nurse Administrator
Portage Lakes Career Center—W. Howard Nicol School of Practical Nursing
Green, Ohio

PREFACE

Aging is neither good nor bad—it is a fact of life. Aging begins the day we are born and ends the day we die. We all have a different view of what getting old means. Children and adolescents rarely consider what it means to get old; old age is too far away and they are too busy living each day to worry about it. Young adults are too caught up in the fight for survival and success to pay attention to old age. Middle age brings a new awareness of the passing of time, particularly when one's parents slip into old age and then die. The reality of aging can no longer be denied when one becomes part of the oldest living generation of a family.

Since the publication of the first edition of this textbook, I have done some soul searching. I have begun to come to grips with the fact that getting older, like all other stages of life, has its ups and downs. I have spent less time voicing unhappiness about getting older and tried to live each day as fully as possible. I have spent more time looking at aging role models than at young fashion models. For inspiration I look at 65-year-old retirees going back to college or starting new careers, a 70-plus-year-old former president going skydiving, a 95-year-old senator insisting that he'll serve in Congress until he's 100, and a 77-year-old former astronaut planning to go into space again. These people, and others like them, give me hope.

I hope that the second edition of *Basic Geriatric Nursing* will give the beginning nursing student a balanced perspective on the realities of aging. I hope that information gained by using this text will broaden the neophyte nurse's viewpoint regarding aging people so that their needs can be met in a compassionate, caring, and appropriate manner.

Part I presents an overview of aging. This section (I) examines the trends and issues affecting the older adult—including demographic factors, and economic, social, cultural, and family influences; (2) explores various theories and myths associated with aging; and (3) reviews the physiologic changes that occur with aging.

Part II includes a wide range of information related to modifying basic nursing skills to be more appropriate to the aging population. This section (1) focuses on health promotion and health maintenance for the elderly; (2) explores age-appropriate verbal and nonverbal communication; (3) reviews age-appropriate nutritional needs; (4) discusses alterations in pharmacodynamics and concerns related to medication administration for older adults; and (5) reviews age-appropriate health assessment techniques and methods.

Part III addresses the physical needs of the elderly using the nursing process. Areas of content include: (1) safety; (2) nutrition and fluid; (3) hygiene and skin care; (4) elimination; (5) activity and exercise; and (6) sleep and rest.

Part IV addresses the psychosocial needs of the elderly using the nursing process. Areas of content include: (1) cognition problems; (2) self-perception and self-concept; (3) changing roles and relationships; (4) coping and stress management; (5) values and beliefs; and (6) sexuality. Parts III and IV provide assessment questions, nursing diagnoses, and nursing approaches suitable for institutional and home settings. Key information is highlighted in easy-to-read boxes, tables, and sample care plans to assist the learner. A study guide is provided for reinforcement of learning and review.

Gloria Hoffmann Wold

CONTENTS

BASIC
GERIATRIC
NURSING

I

OVERVIEW OF AGING

OVERVIEW OF AGING

The objectives of this textbook:

1. Examine some of the trends and issues that affect the elderly person's ability to remain healthy.
2. Explore the theories and myths of aging.
3. Study the normal changes that occur with aging.
4. Review the pathologic conditions that are commonly observed in elderly people.
5. Emphasize the importance of effective communication in working with older adults.
6. Explore the general methods used to assess the health status of older adults.
7. Describe the specific methods of assessing functional needs.
8. Identify the most common nursing diagnoses associated with older adults and discuss the nursing interventions related to these diagnoses.
9. Explore the impact of medication and medication administration on older adults.

INTRODUCTION TO GERIATRIC NURSING

Historical Perspective on the Study of Aging

Until the middle of the 19th century, only two stages of human growth and development were identified: childhood and adulthood. In many ways, children were treated like small adults. No special attention was given to them or to their needs. Families had to produce many children to ensure that a few would survive and reach adulthood. In turn, children were expected to contribute to the family's survival. Little or no concern was given to those characteristics and behaviors that set one child apart from another.

As time passed, society began to view children differently. People learned that there were significant differences between children of different ages and that children's needs changed as they developed. Childhood is now divided into substages (e.g., infant, toddler, preschool, school-age, adolescence). Each stage is associated with unique challenges related to the individual child's stage of growth and development. Because the substages are related to obvious physical changes or to significant life events, this classification method is now accepted as logical and necessary.

Until recently, society also viewed adults of all ages interchangeably. Once you became an adult, you remained an adult. Perhaps society perceived dimly that older adults were different from younger adults, but it was not greatly concerned with theses differences because few people lived to old age. In addition, the physical and developmental changes during adult-

hood are more subtle than those during childhood; therefore, these changes received little attention.

Until the 1960s, sociologists, psychologists, and health care providers focused their attention on meeting the needs of the typical or average adult: people between 20 and 65 years of age. This group was the largest and most economically productive segment of the population; they were raising families, working, and contributing to the growth of the economy. Only a small percentage of the population lived beyond 65 years of age. Disability, illness, and early death were accepted as natural and unavoidable.

In the late 1960s, research began to indicate that adults of all ages are not the same. At the same time, the focus of health care shifted from illness to wellness. Disability and disease were no longer considered to be unavoidable parts of aging. Increased medical knowledge, improved preventive health practices, and technologic advances helped more people live longer, healthier lives.

Older adults now constitute a significant group in society, and interest in the study of aging is increasing. The study of aging is expected to be a major area of attention for years to come.

What's in a Name: Geriatrics, Gerontology, and Gerontics

The term **geriatric** comes from the Greek words "geras," meaning old age, and "iatro," meaning relating to medical treatment. Thus *geriatrics* is the medical specialty that deals with the physiology of aging, and with the diagnosis and treatment of diseases affecting the aged. Geriatrics, by definition, focuses on abnormal conditions and the medical treatment of these conditions.

The term **gerontology** comes from the Greek words "gero," meaning related to old age, and "ology," meaning the study of. Thus *gerontology* is the study of all aspects of the aging process, including the clinical, psychological, economic, and sociological problems of the elderly, and the consequences of these problems for the elderly and society. Gerontology affects nursing, health care, and all areas of our society—including housing, education, business, and politics.

The term **gerontics**, or gerontic nursing, was coined by Gunter and Estes in 1979 to define the nursing care and the service provided to the elderly. The aim of gerontic nursing is "to safeguard and increase health to the extent possible, and to provide comfort and care to the extent necessary."

This textbook focuses on gerontic nursing. It addresses ways to promote high-level functioning and ways to provide care and comfort for the elderly.

TRENDS AND ISSUES

LEARNING OBJECTIVES

1. Describe the subjective and objective ways that aging is defined.
2. Identify personal and societal attitudes toward aging.
3. Define *ageism*.
4. Discuss the myths that exist with regard to aging.
5. Identify recent demographic trends and their impact on society.
6. Describe the effects of recent legislation on the economic status of the elderly.
7. Identify the political interest groups that work as advocates for the elderly.
8. Identify the major economic concerns of the elderly.
9. Describe the housing options that are available to the elderly.
10. Discuss the health care implications of an increase in the population of older adults.
11. Describe the changes in family dynamics that occur as family members become older.
12. Examine the role of nurses in dealing with an aging family.
13. Identify the different forms of elder abuse.
14. Recognize the most common signs of abuse.
15. Describe methods that are effective in preventing elder abuse.

WHO IS "OLD"

The dictionary defines *old* as "having lived or existed for a long time." The meaning of *old* is highly subjective; to a great degree it depends on how old we ourselves are. Few people like to consider themselves old. Old age seems to come later as we become older. A recent study reveals that people under 30 years of age view those over 63 as "getting older." People 65 years of age and older don't think people are "getting older" until they are 75.

Aging is a complex process that can be described chronologically, physiologically, and functionally. **Chronologic age,** the number of years a person has lived, is most often used when we speak of aging because it is the easiest to identify and measure. Unfortunately, chronologic age is probably the least meaningful measurement of aging. Many people who have lived a long time remain functionally and *physiologically* young. These individuals remain physically fit, stay mentally active, and are productive members of society. Others are chronologically young but physically or functionally old.

Categorizing the Aging Population

Even when we use chronologic age as our measure, authorities use various systems to categorize the aging population (Box 1-1).

To many people 65 is a magic number in terms of aging. The wide acceptance of age 65 as a landmark of aging is interesting. Since the 1930s, the age of 65 has come to be accepted as the age of retirement, when it is expected that a person willingly or unwillingly stops paid employment. Before the 1930s, however, most people worked until they decided to stop working, until they became too ill to work, or until they died. When the New Deal politicians established the Social Security program, they set 65 the age at which benefits could be collected; and the average life expectancy of the time was 63. The Social Security program was designed as a fairly low-cost way to win votes

BOX 1-1	
Categorizing the Aging Population	
55 to 64—	older
65 to 74—	elderly
75 to 84—	aged
85 and older—	extremely aged
	or
60 to 74—	young-old
75 to 84—	middle-old
85 and older—	old-old

because most people would not live long enough to collect the benefits. If 65 was considered old then, it certainly is not now. If the same standards were applied today, the retirement age would be 77. For various reasons, however, society clings to 65 as "retirement age" and resists political proposals designed to move the start of social security benefits to a later age.

ATTITUDES TOWARD AGING AND THE ELDERLY

Before we look at the attitudes of others, it is important to examine our own attitudes, values, and knowledge about aging. The four critical thinking boxes that follow are designed to help us assess how we feel about aging.

Our attitudes are the product of our knowledge and values. Our life experiences and our current age strongly influence our views about aging and old people. Most of us have a rather narrow perspective, and our attitudes may reflect this: We tend to project our personal experiences onto the rest of the world. Because most of us have a somewhat limited exposure to aging, we are likely to believe quite a bit of inaccurate information. When dealing with the elderly, our limited understanding and vision can lead to serious errors and mistaken conclusions. If we view old age as a time of physical decay, mental confusion, and social boredom, we are likely to have very negative feelings toward aging. Conversely, if we see old age as a time for sustained physical vigor, renewed mental challenges, and social usefulness, our perspective on aging will be quite different.

It is important to separate fact from myth when examining our attitudes about aging. The single most important factor that influences how poorly or how well a person will age is *attitude*. This statement is true not only for others but also for ourselves.

AGEISM AND THE MYTHS RELATED TO AGING

Throughout time, youth and beauty have been desired (or at least viewed as desirable) and old age and physical infirmity have been loathed and feared. Greek statues portray youths of physical perfection. Artists' works throughout history have shown heroes and heroines as young and beautiful, and evildoers as old and ugly. Little has changed to this day. Few cultures cherish their elderly members and view them as the keepers of wisdom (Fig. 1-1). Even in the Orient, where tradition demands respect for the elderly, societal changes are destroying this venerable mindset.

Mainstream American society does not, by and

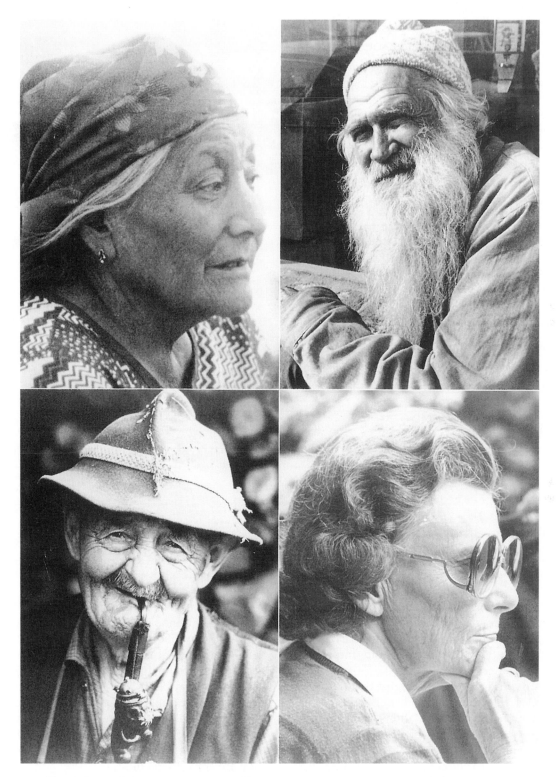

FIG. 1-1 The faces of aging. (Courtesy of American Society on Aging. **Top left,** photograph by Patricia Lee Chorazy; **top right,** photograph by Richard L. Obering; **bottom left,** photographer unknown; **bottom right,** photograph by John C. Kramer.)

CRITICAL THINKING • YOUR VIEWS ABOUT AGING

1. How many "old people" do you know personally?
2. Do *you* think they are "old," or do *they* think they are "old"?
3. How do you personally define "old"?
4. Why is "getting old" an issue today?
5. Should Social Security laws be changed to reflect today's longer life expectancy?

CRITICAL THINKING • YOUR ATTITUDES ABOUT AGING

Please complete the following statements. Write as many applicable comments as you can. *There are no right or wrong answers.*

A person can be considered old when _____

_____ .

When I think about getting old, I _____

_____ .

Growing old means _____

_____ .

When I get old I will lose my _____

_____ .

Seeing an old person makes me feel _____

_____ .

Old people always _____

_____ .

Old people never _____

_____ .

The best thing about getting old is _____

_____ .

The worst thing about getting old is _____

_____ .

Looking back at my responses, I feel that aging is _____

_____ .

---

large, value its elders. The United States tends to be a youth-oriented society where people are judged by age, appearance, and wealth. Young, attractive, and wealthy people are viewed positively; old, imperfect, and poor people are not.

It is hard for young people to imagine that they will ever be old. Despite some cultural changes, becoming old retains many negative connotations. Many people continue to do everything they can to fool the clock. Wrinkles, gray hair, and other physical changes related to aging are actively confronted with makeup, hair dye and cosmetic surgery. Until recently, advertising seldom portrayed people over 50 years of age except to sell eyeglasses, hearing aids, hair dye, laxatives, and other rather unappealing products. The message seemed to be, "Young is good, old is bad;

therefore, everyone should fight getting old." It is significant that trends in advertising appear to be changing. As the number of healthier, dynamic "senior citizens" with significant spending power has increased, advertising campaigns have become increasingly likely to portray older adults as the consumers of their products, including exercise equipment, health beverages, and cruises. Despite these societal improvements, however, many people do not know enough about the realities of aging and because of ignorance they are *afraid* to get old.

This fear of aging and the refusal to accept the elderly into the mainstream of society is known as **gerontophobia.** Both senior citizens and younger persons can fall prey to such irrational fears.

Gerontophobia sometimes results in very strange

behavior. Teenagers buy anti-wrinkle creams. Thirty-year-olds consider facelifts. Forty-year-olds have hair transplants. Long-term marriages dissolve so that one spouse can pursue someone younger. All of these behaviors result from the fear of growing older.

The extreme forms of gerontophobia are ageism and age discrimination. **Ageism** is the disliking of aging and older people based on the belief that aging makes people unattractive, unintelligent, and unproductive. It is an emotional prejudice or discrimination against people solely on the basis of age. Ageism allows the young to separate themselves physically and emotionally from the old and to view the elderly as somehow having less human value. Like sexism or racism, ageism is a negative belief pattern that can result in irrational thoughts and destructive behaviors such as intergenerational conflict and name calling. Like other forms of prejudice, ageism occurs because of myths and stereotypes about a group of people who are different from ourselves.

Health care providers are not immune to ageism. Few of the "best and brightest" nurses and physicians seek careers in geriatrics in spite of the increasing need for these services.

Ageism can have a negative effect on the way health care providers relate to elderly clients, which in turn can result in poor health care outcomes in these individuals.

Research by the National Institute on Aging reports that (1) older patients receive less information than do younger patients with regard to resources, health management, and illness management; (2) less information is provided to elders on lifestyle changes such as weight reduction and smoking cessation; (3) limited rehabilitation is available for elders with chronic disease despite studies demonstrating that individuals over 85 years of age do benefit from rehabilitation programs; and (4) only 47% of physicians feel that the elderly should receive the same evaluation and treatment for acute illness as their younger counterparts.

CRITICAL THINKING • YOUR VALUES ABOUT AGING

Quickly name three elderly people who have had an impact on your life. List five characteristics that you associate with each person. *There are no right or wrong answers.*

Person 1	Person 2	Person 3
Name _____	Name _____	Name _____
Relationship _____	Relationship _____	Relationship _____

CHARACTERISTICS:

1. _____	1. _____	1. _____
2. _____	2. _____	2. _____
3. _____	3. _____	3. _____
4. _____	4. _____	4. _____
5. _____	5. _____	5. _____

Look at the characteristics you described and think about the feelings you experienced as you considered these individuals. Do your feelings correspond to your attitudes about aging? Were these three people's characteristics similar or different? What do these characteristics say about *your* values?

CRITICAL THINKING • YOUR CURRENT KNOWLEDGE ABOUT AGING

Respond to the following questions to the best of your knowledge.
1. You are old at age _____ .
2. There are _____ elderly in the United States.
3. Most elderly people live in _____ .
4. Economically, older people are _____ .
5. With regard to health, older people are _____ .
6. Mentally, older people are _____ .

Because the elderly comprise an increasing portion of the population, health care providers need to do some soul searching with regard to their own attitudes. Further, they must confront signs of ageism whenever and wherever they appear. Activities such as increased positive interactions with the elderly and improved professional training designed to address misconceptions regarding aging are two ways of fighting ageism.

Age discrimination reaches beyond emotions and leads to actions. Age discrimination results in different treatment of older people simply because of their age. Refusing to hire older persons, barring them from approval for home loans, and limiting the types or amount of health care they can receive are all examples of discrimination that occur despite laws prohibiting them. Some older individuals respond to age discrimination with passive acceptance, whereas others are banding together to speak up for their rights.

PREPARING FOR OLD AGE

The reality of getting old is that no one knows what it will be like until it happens. But that is the nature of life—growing older is just the continuation of a process that started at birth. Elderly people are no different from the people they were when they were younger. Physical, financial, social, and political conditions may change, but the person remains the same. Old age has been described as the "more-so" stage of life.

Aging can be a freeing experience. Aging seems to decrease the need to maintain pretenses, and the elderly person may finally be comfortable enough to reveal the real person that existed beneath the facade. If a person has been essentially kind and caring throughout life, he or she will generally reveal more of these positive personal characteristics as time marches on. Likewise, if they were miserly or unkind, often people will reveal more of these negative personal characteristics as they grow older. The more successful a person has been at meeting the developmental tasks of life, the more likely he or she will be to face aging successfully.

Perhaps the best advice to all who are preparing for old age is contained in the Serenity prayer:

O God, give us the serenity to accept what cannot be changed; courage to change what should be changed; and wisdom to distinguish one from the other. *Reinhold Niebuhr*

DEMOGRAPHICS

Demographics is the statistical study of human populations. Demographers are concerned with a population's size, distribution, and vital statistics. **Vital statis-** tics include birth, death, age at death, marriage(s), race, and many other variables. The collection of demographic information is an ongoing process. The most inclusive demographic research in the United States is done every 10 years by the Bureau of the Census. The most recent census was completed in 1990.

Demographic research is important to many groups. Demographic information is used by the government as a basis for granting aid to cities and states, by cities to project their budget needs for schools, by hospitals to determine the number of beds needed, by public health agencies to determine the immunization needs of a community, and by marketers to sell products. The politicians of the 1930s used demographics to formulate plans for the Social Security program. Demographic studies provide information about the present that allows projections into the future.

One very important piece of demographic information is life expectancy. **Life expectancy** is the number of years an average person can expect to live. Projected from the time of birth, life expectancy is based on the ages of all people who die in a given year. If a large number of infants die at birth or during childhood, the life expectancy of that year's group will tend to be low.

Life expectancy throughout history has been low because of environmental hazards, wars, accidents, food and water scarcity, inadequate sanitation, and contagious diseases. During biblical times, the average life expectancy was approximately 20 years. Some people did live significantly longer, but 40 years was considered a good long life. By 1776 when the Declaration of Independence was signed, life expectancy had risen to 35 years. It was not uncommon for people to live into their sixties. By the 1860s, at the time of the American Civil War, life expectancy had increased to 40 years. The 1860 census revealed that 2.7% of the American population was over 65. By the beginning of the 20th century, life expectancy had increased to 47 years, and 4% of the American population was 65 years of age or older. In a span of more than 2000 years, life expectancy had increased by only 27 years.

Since the beginning of the 20th century, advances in technology and health care have changed the world dramatically, especially in industrialized nations where food production exceeds the needs of the population. Diseases such as cholera and typhoid have been eliminated or significantly reduced by improved sanitation and hygiene practices. Dreaded communicable diseases that at one time were often fatal (e.g., smallpox, measles, whooping cough, diphtheria) are now preventable through immunization. Even pneumonia and influenza are no longer the fatal diseases they once were. Today, vaccines can be given to those who are at higher risk, and treatment can

TABLE 1-1

The 25 Most Longevous Nations

Rank and country	Percentage of the population over age 65
1. Sweden	18
2. Norway	16
3. United Kingdom	15
4. Denmark	15
5. West Germany	15
6. Switzerland	15
7. Austria	15
8. Belgium	14
9. Italy	14
10. Greece	14
11. Luxembourg	14
12. France	13
13. East Germany	13
14. Finland	13
15. Hungary	13
16. Netherlands	12
17. Spain	12
18. United States	12
19. Ireland	12
20. Bulgaria	12
21. Portugal	12
22. Faroe Islands	12
23. Uruguay	11
24. Czechoslovakia	11
25. Canada	11

From the U.S. Bureau of the Census, International Data Base, 1987.

be given to those who become infected. Hopefully, changes in the geopolitical climate of the world will lessen the number of deaths due to war.

Life expectancy in the United States is among the highest in the world (Table 1-1). Many areas of the world have not yet benefited from advanced technology as have Europe, Canada, and the United States. During the 20th century, the life expectancy of Americans has increased approximately by 28 years. A child born in the United States in 1995 has an average life expectancy of nearly 75.8 years.

Age cohort is a term used by demographers to describe a group of people born within a specified period of time. The most significant cohort today is the "Baby Boomers." This cohort consists of people who were born after World War II between 1946 and 1964. Baby Boomers comprise approximately *one third* of all Americans today. Because of its size, this group has

had, and will continue to have, significant influence in all areas of society. The oldest Baby Boomers are now entering their fifties. By the year 2011, slightly more than a decade from now, the oldest will reach age 65. The implications of this for all areas of society, particularly health care, are unprecedented.

Approximately 12% of the U.S. population is now over 65 years of age, and those over 85 years of age comprise the fastest-growing segment of the population. By 2030 over 21% of the population will be over 65, and there will be as many people over age 85 as there currently are over age 65. We are becoming an increasingly elderly society (Fig. 1-2).

The Administration on Aging projects that minority populations will represent 25% of the elderly population by 2030, an increase from 13% in 1990. Whereas the percentage of the white, non-Hispanic population in the United States is expected to increase by 91%, the non-Hispanic, black population is expected to increase by 159%, the Hispanic population by 570%, and the Asian/Pacific Islander population by 643%.

The elderly population is not equally distributed throughout the United States. Climate, taxes, and other issues regarding quality-of-life influence where the elderly choose to live.

All regions of the country are affected by the increases in life expectancy but not to the same degree. About half of the over-65 population reside in only nine states. In order of elderly population, these states are California (over 3 million), Florida and New York (over 2 million each), Pennsylvania, Texas, Ohio, Illinois, Michigan and New Jersey (over 1 million each). Population distribution data show that Florida leads the nation, with more than 18% of its population over 65 years of age. Eleven states, including Nevada, Alaska, Hawaii, Arizona, Utah, Colorado, New Mexico, Wyoming, Delaware, North Carolina, and Texas have shown a rapid increase in the over-65 population.

Approximately 76% of the elderly population live in metropolitan areas, only slightly less than younger populations. About 30% reside in the central city and 46% in suburban areas. The remaining quarter of the elderly live in rural or semi-rural areas. Since the 1980s more elderly people have been leaving the cities to live in rural areas. Elders who live in rural areas have a higher incidence of chronic illness and disability than do those who live in urban areas. This may be due to attitudes held by rural elders or possibly to the increased distance that must be traveled to obtain health care. See Box 1-2 and the critical thinking box on p. 11 for details about U.S. demographic trends.

The populations of men and women are not equal. Women outnumber men in all but five states (Alaska, Hawaii, Nevada, North Dakota, and Nebraska). In the over-65 age group, this disproportion is very notice-

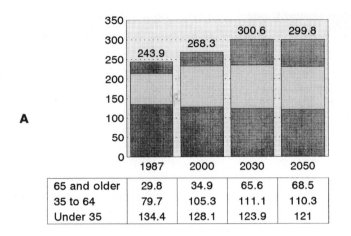

	1987	2000	2030	2050
65 and older	29.8	34.9	65.6	68.5
35 to 64	79.7	105.3	111.1	110.3
Under 35	134.4	128.1	123.9	121

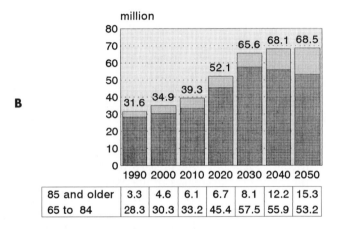
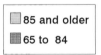

	1990	2000	2010	2020	2030	2040	2050
85 and older	3.3	4.6	6.1	6.7	8.1	12.2	15.3
65 to 84	28.3	30.3	33.2	45.4	57.5	55.9	53.2

FIG. 1-2   National population projections. **A,** All ages, 1987 to 2050. **B,** Older adults, 1990 to 2050. (Data published by the US Bureau of the Census, 1989.)

BOX 1-2

Summary of U.S. Demographic Trends

1. The life expectancy of Americans is increasing rapidly.
2. The percentage of individuals over 65 years of age is increasing.
3. The median age is increasing.
4. The Baby Boom generation will reach age 65 within the next 20 years. Because of its size, this cohort will have a major impact on all aspects of society.
5. The rural-farm population is older than the urban population.
6. Certain states and regions have larger elderly populations than others.
7. Women outlive men and comprise the largest group of the old-old population.

---

able. Women currently outlive men by about 7 years, but projections to the year 2000 increase this gap to 15 years. In 1994 almost half of all older women were widows, with the ratio of widow to widowers at 5:1.

THE ECONOMICS OF AGING

The stereotypical belief that the elderly are poor is not necessarily true. The economic status of elderly persons is as varied as that of other age groups. Some of the poorest people in the country are old, but so are some of the richest. As of 1995, 5% of elderly households had an income of under $10,000 whereas 10% had an income over $75,000. In 1995, the median income of households headed by a person 65 years of age or older was slightly over $28,000. The major sources of income for the elderly include Social Security (42%), pensions (19%), earnings (18%), asset income (18%), and miscellaneous sources (3%).

In 1995, the poverty rate for persons over 65 years of age was 10.5%. This is slightly lower than the 11.4%

---

1. What impact will the changing demographics have on you personally?
2. How is your community's age distribution changing?
3. Are you a member of the Baby Boom cohort? Is this an advantage or a disadvantage as you age?
4. Were you born after the Baby Boom? Before the Baby Boom? What difficulties do you expect to encounter as you age?

---

poverty rate for adults younger than 65 years of age. Elderly people who live alone are more likely to be poor than is the average older person; 39% of those who live alone have a median income of less than $10,000. Elderly women are the most severely affected group, with a median income of $9355.

Older adults who are racial minorities are more likely to be poor or near-poor than is the average older adult. Studies show that only 9% of the white elderly population have an income below the poverty line, but 24% of the Hispanic elderly population and 25% of the black elderly population have incomes below the poverty line. Poverty rates are highest in the South, where eight states—Mississippi, Louisiana, Alabama, Arkansas, Tennessee, Kentucky, South Carolina, and Georgia—have poverty rates in excess of 20%.

Economic well-being is usually measured in terms of income, which is the amount of money a household receives on a weekly, monthly, or yearly basis. This measurement is not always a reliable indicator of financial security in the elderly. People over 65 years of age generally have more discretionary income (i.e., money left after paying for necessities such as housing, food, medical care) available than do younger people. Younger individuals may have a higher income, but they also have higher nondiscretionary demands.

Although many elderly people receive less cash on a yearly basis from Social Security and pensions than some younger individuals earn, a substantial number have accumulated assets and savings from their working years. Frugal lifestyles and self-reports by the elderly of being "poor" must be viewed cautiously. Some individuals are in fact impoverished, whereas others have significant estates to leave to their children or to charities.

Approximately 78% of households headed by a person over 65 years of age own their home. Most of these homes, which have a median value of over $75,000, are owned outright. The home is usually an elderly person's biggest asset. Many elderly people choose not to sell their houses because they fear they will have nowhere to live. Many prefer to remain "house rich and cash poor," making do on a limited income, rather

BOX 1-3
Legislation That Has Helped Older Adults

1965	• Medicare and Medicaid established
	• Administration on Aging established
1967	• Age Discrimination Act passed
1972	• Supplemental Security Income Program instituted
	• Social Security indexed to reflect inflation, Cost of Living Adjustment
1972	• Nutrition Act, which allows for providing nutrition programs for older adults, passed.
1973	• Council on Aging established
1978	• Mandatory retirement age changed to 70 years
1986	• Mandatory retirement age eliminated for most employees
1988	• Catastrophic health insurance became part of Medicare

than selling their home. Additional considerations regarding home ownership and housing options are discussed in more detail later in this chapter.

The Federal Housing Authority and other lending agencies have proposed the use of reverse mortgages, which are plans that allow the elderly to remain in their homes and receive monthly payments based on their equity in the property. Monthly income realized from these plans could range from as little as $100 to as much as several thousand dollars, depending on the value of the property and the age of the residents. This money could be a much-needed income supplement for older adults. Plans such as this are likely to become more common in the future when more elderly people recognize their economic benefits.

Legislation (Box 1-3) and political activism among older people have helped improve the economic outlook for the elderly. Through activist organizations (Box 1-4), older adults have joined together to consolidate their political power and to use the power of the vote to initiate programs that benefit them. Over the

---

BOX 1-4

Politically Active Senior Citizen Groups

AARP—AMERICAN ASSOCIATION OF RETIRED PERSONS
- Consists of members who are at least 50 years of age and spouses regardless of age
- Currently has 30 million members
- In the future, could have 76 million members when Baby Boomers reach age 50
- Uses volunteers and employs lobbyists to advance the political and economic interests of older adults
- Provides a wide variety of membership benefits, including insurance programs and discounts

NCSC—NATIONAL COUNCIL OF SENIOR CITIZENS
- Has 4.5 million members
- Focuses on political and legislative issues

NASC—NATIONAL ALLIANCE OF SENIOR CITIZENS
- Has 2 million members
- Focuses on a variety of issues of concern to older adults

OWL—OLDER WOMEN'S LEAGUE
- Has 20,000 members
- Focuses on needs of aging women

GRAY PANTHERS
- Has 75,000 members
- Consists of local groups and a national organization
- Attempts to increase public awareness of the needs of older adults by means of demonstrations, door-to-door canvassing, and other attention-getting methods

---

BOX 1-5

Factors That Influence the Economic Conditions of Older Adults

1. Many elderly bought their homes when housing costs and inflation were low. If they paid off their mortgages before retirement, their housing costs are limited to taxes, maintenance, and utility bills.
2. The number of older adults who receive pensions is greater now than it will be in the future. The current changes in business conditions are resulting in the offering of smaller pensions to fewer employees.
3. Older adults qualify for several tax breaks that are unavailable to younger people.
   —Most older adults pay no social security taxes, whereas younger working adults pay increasingly higher rates.
   —Social security and government pensions are largely exempted from taxation.
   —Taxpayers over 65 years of age can take extra tax deductions.
   —A one-time capital gains tax exclusion applies when the house is sold.
4. Most older adults qualify for government income programs.
   —The income from Social Security exceeds the program contributions of most recipients.
   —Medicare covers 70% of medical costs.
   —Programs such as Social Security, SSI, Medicare, housing programs, and energy assistance provide an annual average of $9000 per every older adult.

THE ROLE OF THE NURSE IN FINANCIAL ISSUES

Sensitivity is needed when dealing with the financial issues of older adults. The critical thinking box on p. 13 should help you assess your attitudes, and thus your sensitivity, toward these kinds of situations. Many older adults who find it easy to talk about their intimate physical and medical problems are reluctant to discuss finances. Nurses may become suspicious of financial need if an elderly person lacks adequate shelter, clothing, heat, food, or medical attention. When an economic problem causes real or potential dangers, nurses must be prepared to respond appropriately.

Because regulations covering assistance programs change frequently, it is difficult for elderly clients and the nurses trying to help them to keep current and up to date. Nurse may be called on to help the elderly deal with the paperwork required when applying for

---

past 25 years, these groups have done much to improve the economic welfare of older adults.

Elderly people may choose not to seek help despite the availability of assistance programs designed to aid them. Many of the elderly are suspicious of "getting something for nothing" or are reluctant to disclose the details of their financial status, which is necessary in order to qualify for most assistance programs. Many elderly people feel that asking for help is humiliating. Some may fear they will lose what little they have if they seek assistance. Factors that can impact the financial well-being of older adults are described in Box 1-5.

assistance, to provide emotional support as they work through the frustration of bureaucratic processes, or to arrange transportation to the appropriate agencies. Nurses are not usually expected to be experts in this area, but they should know how to locate appropriate resources. Nurses working in community health should be aware of community agencies that provide assistance to the elderly so appropriate referrals can be made. Nurses working in hospitals and nursing homes can initiate referrals to social workers or other professionals who are knowledgeable about assistance programs.

HOUSING AND THE ELDERLY

When asked where the elderly live, most people will say that they live in senior citizen housing or nursing homes. They are wrong. More than two thirds of the elderly (68%) live independently in a family setting. Twenty-seven percent live in modified but not institutional settings, including senior citizen housing, group homes, and apartments, or with family members. About 5% are institutionalized, and this percentage increases with advancing age. Only 1% of 65- to 74-year-old individuals are institutionalized. This increases to 6% of individuals 75 to 84 years of age and reaches 24% of people over age 85.

Elderly individuals will often try to keep their homes despite the physical or economic difficulties in doing so. A house is more than just a physical shelter; it represents independence and security. The home holds many memories. Being in a familiar neighborhood close to friends and church is important. A sense of community is important to many aging people, to whom it is unpleasant to think of leaving security for the unknown. The physical exertion and emotional trauma involved in moving can be intimidating, even overwhelming, to the elderly. Moving to a different, often smaller residence is a difficult decision, particu-

larly when it involves giving up precious possessions due to lack of space.

For some elderly people, keeping the family home is not a sensible option for many reasons. Many of the houses owned by the elderly are in central cities with high crime rates. Expenses, including increasingly high property taxes and ongoing maintenance costs, often present excessive strain on elderly persons with limited financial resources. Home maintenance, including even simple tasks such as housecleaning, becomes increasingly difficult with advancing age or illness. Ownership may require more effort in terms of money and time than some elderly people possess, yet many will struggle to remain independent and keep their houses.

Some elderly individuals remain in their own houses and refuse to give them up long after it is safe for them to be alone. They may be able to cope as long as family, friends, and neighbors are willing to help. However, if there is a change in their support system, dangerous, life-threatening situations may arise. Some elderly people try to live in their houses despite broken plumbing, inadequate heat, and insufficient access to food. Families, health care professionals, and social service agencies may have to step in to protect the welfare of these aging individuals.

Some elderly people recognize the problems associated with living alone and decide to seek housing arrangements that are more in keeping with their needs and abilities. They may choose to move into an apartment, condominium, senior citizen complex, or some other type of housing. As the elderly population grows, a variety of new types of housing and living arrangements are evolving (Fig. 1-3). The critical thinking box on p. 14 should help you determine your attitudes toward housing for the elderly.

Independent or **assisted living centers** are becoming common. These centers combine privacy with easily available services. Most consist of private apartments that are either purchased or rented. For additional charges the residents can be served meals in restaurant-style dining rooms and receive laundry and housekeeping services. Different levels of medical, nursing, and personal care services are available. Health care services may include assistance with hygiene, routine medication administration, and even preventive health clinics. Many centers have communal activity rooms, art and craft hobby centers, swimming pools, lounges, beauty salons, minigrocery stores, greenhouses, and other amenities. Transportation to church, shopping, and other appointments is provided by some of these facilities.

Life-lease or **life-contract facilities** are another housing option. For a large initial investment and substantial monthly rental and service fees, elderly persons or couples are guaranteed a residence for life. Independent residents occupy apartment units, but extended-care units are either attached to this apart-

ment complex or are located nearby for residents who require skilled nursing services. If one spouse needs skilled care, the other may continue to live in the apartment and can easily visit the hospitalized loved one. When the occupants die, control of the apartment reverts to the owners of the facility. The costs for this type of housing are high and may be out of the range of the average older adult. Despite the costs, however, many find this option satisfactory because it meets their needs for independence, socialization, and services. Many find security in knowing that skilled care is easily available if needed.

Less well-to-do people are more limited in their housing options. Some older adults qualify for **government-subsidized housing** if they meet certain financial standards and limits. Government-subsidized housing units may be simple apartments without any special services or they may have limited services, such as access to nursing clinics and special

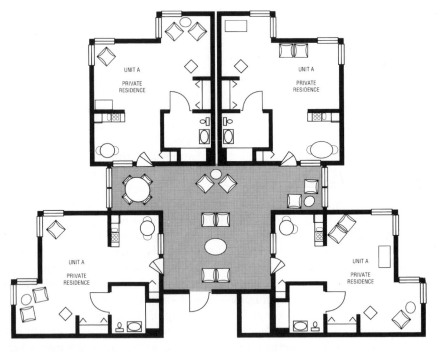

FIG. 1-3   The floor plan for one type of alternative housing. (Courtesy of Arvid Elness Architects, Minneapolis, Minn.)

CRITICAL THINKING
YOUR ATTITUDES TOWARD HOUSING FOR THE ELDERLY

1. Is it safe for the elderly to remain in their own houses indefinitely?
2. When should an elderly person sell his or her house?
3. Once a house is sold, what are the best type of living accommodations for the elderly?
4. What kinds of alternative housing for the elderly are available in your community?
5. Should the elderly live in housing that is separated from people in other age groups? Why? Why not?

transportation arrangements. Most communities are finding that the demand for these facilities exceeds the availability. Waiting lists and 1- to 2-year delays are common. Interpretation of government regulations is causing some concern with regard to senior citizen housing. Residences originally intended for the elderly may be required to accept a variety of medically handicapped people, regardless of age. Some of these younger residents suffer from psychiatric or drug-related problems, and the presence of these individuals may leave the elderly residents feeling threatened and fearful for their own safety and well-being.

Some older adults who are not related to each other are forming **group-housing plans.** In this type of arrangement, two or more unrelated people share a household where they have private bedrooms but share the common recreational and leisure areas as well as the tasks involved in home maintenance. Some communities offer services to help match people who are interested in this option. Roommates are selected so that the strengths of one individual compensate for the weaknesses of the other. In some cases, a large house may shelter 10 or more residents. Not all of these arrangements are limit to the elderly. In some situations, younger adults who need reasonable housing may be included. By providing services for the elderly residents, the younger residents are able to reduce their rental costs. Both younger and older individuals who have chosen this option report benefits from the extended-family atmosphere.

A more formal type of group home called a **community-based residential facility** (CBRF) is available in some communities. For a monthly fee, this type of facility provides services such as room and board, help with activities of daily living, assistance with medications, yearly medical examinations, information and referrals, leisure activities, and recreational or therapeutic programs. Fees for this type of housing may be paid by the individual or may be provided by county or state agencies.

The most dependent elderly require more extensive assistance, which is typically provided in **nursing homes** or **extended-care facilities.** Nursing homes provide room and board, personal care, and medical and nursing services. They are licensed by individual states and regulated by both federal and state laws. Three levels of care are provided by nursing homes. *Basic care facilities* provide the level of care and supervision necessary to maintain the residents' safety and well-being. They provide assistance with activities of daily living, including hygiene, ambulation, nutrition, elimination, and other basic needs. This level of care is typically provided by nursing assistants and licensed vocational or practical nurses. *Skilled care facilities* provide skilled nursing care on a regular ba-

sis. Interventions such as administration of medication and skilled treatments or procedures that require the expertise of registered and practical nurses are provided in this type of facility. Skilled care facilities also provide services performed by specially trained professionals such as speech, physical, occupational, and respiratory therapists. *Subacute care facilities* provide comprehensive inpatient care designed for individuals who have an acute illness, injury, or exacerbation of a disease process. Subacute care falls between the traditional care provided in an acute care facility and that provided in a skilled nursing home.

HEALTH CARE AND AGING

Health care has become a major issue in the United States. The costs of health care have increased dramatically in recent years. More money is spent on health care in the United States than in any other country in the world, yet health care is not provided for all U.S. citizens. Many other nations do a better job than the United States of meeting their citizens' health care needs.

Approximately $500 billion is spent annually on health care in the United States. This exceeds the amount spent on any other activity, including defense. Currently one third of this (more than $150 billion) is spent on the 12% of the population that is over 65 year of age. These numbers are staggering considering how quickly the number of older adults is increasing. Unless some type of reform is instituted we can expect to spend 20% of the Gross Domestic Product (GDP) on health care for the elderly by the year 2000.

The government program that provides health care funding for the elderly is called **Medicare.** Almost all Americans over 65 years of age qualify for Medicare. Medicare has two distinct programs, neither of which covers all of the health care costs. Medicare **Part A** covers inpatient hospital care; extended care in a skilled nursing facility; some home health services such as visiting nurses, occupational, speech, or physical therapists; and hospice services—but only after the patient pays an initial deductible, which often exceeds $500.

During the 1980s Medicare instituted the **diagnosis-related group** system in an attempt to contain hospital costs. Under this system, a hospital is paid a set amount based on the patient's admitting diagnosis. If the patient is discharged in fewer days than predicted, the hospital may keep the excess money. If the patient needs to stay longer than projected, the hospital must absorb the additional costs. Although diagnosis-related groups have resulted in some cost reduction, they have also resulted in the quicker discharge of sicker people than in the past. Many elderly people are released from the hospital before they have actually recovered from their illnesses, placing an increased health care burden on families and home health agencies.

Medicare **Part B** covers 80% of the "customary and usual" rates charged by physicians after deductibles are met. In addition to physicians' fees, services covered by Medicare Part B include medically necessary ambulance transport; physical, speech, and occupational therapy; home health services when medically necessary; medical supplies and equipment; and outpatient surgery or blood transfusions. The patient is responsible for the remaining 20% of the costs plus the difference between the actual fee and the government's "customary and usual" rate. The actual costs of medical care often exceed the amount the government pays.

Supplemental Medicaid (Title 19) assistance may be available for those elderly who meet certain financial need requirements. Many of those who have assets do not qualify; they are left with a "Medicare gap" that they must pay themselves. Many elderly people buy private medical insurance—often at unreasonable prices—to pay medical bills that are not covered by Medicare.

Not all elderly people use the available health care resources equally. A majority of the health care services are consumed by the very ill or terminally ill minority, many of whom happen to be elderly. Studies by the Health Care Financing Administration indicate that 2% of the over-65 population receiving Medicare accounts for 34% of the costs. Overall, 72% of the total resources are used by only 10% of the aging population. More than 25% of the Medicare budget is used for terminally ill patients. Serious questions are being raised about the appropriateness of using intensive, expensive interventions to extend the lives of terminally ill elderly people.

Financial concerns are forcing health care providers and society to face ethical dilemmas regarding the allocation of limited health care resources. This is a highly emotional issue with no easy answers. Many people are alive today because of advances in medical technology. Some of those who benefit are young, whereas others are old. Some go on to lead lives of high quality; others never lead normal lives again. By virtue of their training, physicians are inclined to try to cure everyone. Most doctors do not feel comfortable allowing a person to die, regardless of his or her age. Most doctors will use all available technology to save a life.

Reputable authorities, ethicists, and politicians have widely differing points of view on this issue. Some feel that health care restrictions on the elderly are the ultimate in age discrimination. Others argue that the benefits gained, which can usually be measured in months, do not outweigh the costs. Private citizens examining this dilemma are equally confused. Those who believe that health care costs are excessive still want everything possible done to save the lives of their own loved ones. This dilemma is moral, ethical, and legal with no simple right answer. The critical thinking box on this page is designed to increase your awareness and insight into these problems.

Advance Directives

All adults who are 18 years of age or older and "of sound mind" have the right to make decisions regarding the amount and type of health care they desire. Because the elderly are more likely to experience significant health problems, the question of what and how much medical care to administer must be addressed. Such important decisions are best made during a stress-free time when the individual person is alert and experiencing no acute health problems. A person's wishes can best be communicated using advance directives, which are legally recognized, written

---

CRITICAL THINKING
YOUR UNDERSTANDING OF THE HEALTH CARE DILEMMA

1. Should an 80-year-old person have coronary bypass surgery at a cost of approximately $100,000?
2. Should dialysis be provided to individuals over 65? over 75? over 85?
3. Should people over 65 be candidates for organ transplants?
4. Should a respirator be used on a terminally ill patient?
5. Are feeding tubes a part of basic physical care or are they extraordinary means?
6. Should the individual, the family, or the physician decide the type and amount of medical intervention necessary?
7. What should be the role of the government in health care?

How to Use a Living Will

The Living Will should clearly state your preferences about life-sustaining treatment. You may wish to add specific statements to the Living Will in the space provided for that purpose. Such statements might concern:

- Cardiopulmonary resuscitation
- Artificial or invasive measures for providing nutrition and hydration
- Kidney dialysis
- Mechanical or artificial respiration
- Blood transfusion
- Surgery (such as amputation)
- Antibiotics

You may also wish to indicate any preferences you have about such matters as dying at home.

THE DURABLE POWER OF ATTORNEY FOR HEALTH CARE

The durable power of attorney is an optional feature that permits you to name a surrogate decision maker (also known as a proxy, health agent, or attorney-in-fact) to make health care decisions on your behalf if you lose that ability. Because this person should act according to your preferences and in your best interests, you should select this person with care and make certain that he or she understands your wishes and your Living Will.

You should not name someone who is a witness to your Living Will. You may want to name an alternate agent in case the first person you select is unable or unwilling to serve. If you do name a surrogate decision maker, the form must be notarized. (It is a good idea to notarize the document in any case.)

From *A Living Will, Concern for the Dying,* New York, New York, with permission

documents that specify the types of care and treatment that the individual desires when that individual cannot speak for him- or herself.

Two formal types of advance directive are recognized: (1) the durable power of attorney for health care and (2) the living will (Box 1-6). Information about both power of attorney for health care and living wills is typically provided when a person enters the hospital. Each patient is expected to make a decision about the type and extent of care to be administered if his or her condition becomes terminal.

These written documents are designed to help guide the family and medical professionals in planning care. The family is often relieved to have this information when making difficult decisions during a stressful time. Advance directives are generally recognized and respected, but various agencies, individual physicians, or health care providers may have beliefs or policies that prohibit them from honoring certain advance directives. Individuals should discuss their wishes with their health care providers when these documents are written. Open communication reduces the risk of questions, conflict, or legal repercussions at a later time. If irreconcilable differences exist between an individual and the care provider, changes in either the document or the care provider must be considered.

Durable power of attorney for health care transfers the authority to make health care decisions to another person called the "health care agent." The agent may only act in situations in which the person is unable to make decisions for him- or herself. Because the health care agent must be trusted to follow through with the elderly person's wishes, the agent specified in the document is usually a family member or friend. These wishes are specified in writing and usually witnessed by unrelated individuals to reduce the risk of undue influence. Standardized legal forms are available to initiate a power of attorney for health care.

A living will informs the physician that the individual wishes to die naturally if he or she develops an illness or receives an injury that cannot be cured. Living wills prohibit the use of life-prolonging measures and equipment when the individual is near death or in a persistent vegetative state. Living wills go into effect only when two physicians agree in writing that the necessary criteria are met.

Usually either of these documents is adequate to communicate one's wishes; both are not needed. Those who choose to initiate both documents should ensure that there is no conflict between the directions provided. Either document can be revoked at any time. Directions to accomplish this are usually provided on the specific forms. An advance directive should be stored in a safe place where it can be located easily if the need arises. A safe deposit box is not recommended for this purpose. Ideally, family members and the family lawyer should know the substance of the document and its location. An advance directive should be provided to the physician so it becomes part of the patient's permanent medical record.

Nurses should be aware of the legal standing of such documents in the particular state where they practice and should understand any legal ramifications engendered by these documents.

> ### BOX 1-7
>
> #### Demographic Changes Affecting the Family
>
> 1. Extended life spans are leading to more older family members.
> 2. There are more people who are living with chronic conditions and who need some degree of care or assistance.
> 3. The number of people in the younger generations is decreasing in proportion to the number of older members.
> 4. There is an increasing number of widows who may be unprepared to provide for their own needs and who therefore need assistance.
> 5. The role of women is changing. As women increasingly must work outside the home, many are attempting to meet the demands of their parents, home, children, *and* workplace.

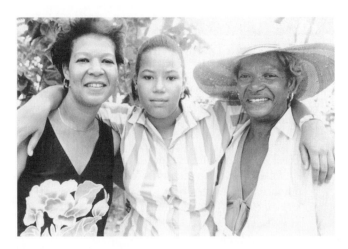

FIG. 1-4   Three generations of one family. (Courtesy of American Society on Aging.)

TABLE 1-2

The Family

80+ years of age	Parents
60+ years of age	Children
40+ years of age	Grandchildren
20+ years of age	Great-grandchildren
Less than 20 years of age	Great-great-grandchildren

THE AGING FAMILY

The family is undergoing significant change in our society. Many factors, including increasing divorce rates, single parenting, and a mobile population, are creating a less stable, less predictable family structure. Blended families, extended families, and separated families all present challenges. In addition to these societal changes, the demographic changes discussed earlier are having, and will continue to have, repercussions we can only begin to appreciate (Box 1-7).

Families today face historically unprecedented situations. Because of the lifespan extension, it is not uncommon for four or five generations of a family to be alive at one time (Fig. 1-4). Until recently this was an unheard-of occurrence.

Using 20 years as a typical generation, a family might resemble one such as that described in Table 1-2. If the generation time is less than 20 years, even more generations might potentially be alive at the same time.

PERSONAL REFLECTION

Some years ago, as death was approaching for a 91-year-old gentleman, his family gathered at the hospital. His wife of 69 years asked that "the children" come into the room. This sounded rather strange because "the children" were all in their sixties, the grandchildren were all mature adults, and the great-grandchildren were fast approaching adulthood. It sounded even stranger to me because this elderly man was my grandfather, and my father was "the baby" of the family.

It is estimated that 80% of older adults who need care will receive assistance from their families. The problems encountered in such situations can differ widely depending on the respective ages of the family members. In some families, the "children" who are attempting to provide care for the oldest members are likely to be over 65 themselves. They may have health problems of their own that make caregiving difficult or impractical.

Middle-aged family members often become the caregivers. The generation in their forties is often called the "sandwich generation" because its members are caught in the middle—trying to work, trying to raise their own dependent children, and often trying to provide assistance to one or two generations of aging family members. In some cases, they are also trying to help raise grandchildren by giving financial or physical assistance, or both.

Although the financial, psychologic, and physical demands of assisting aging relatives affect all family members, women are likely to be most affected. Regardless of whether it is fair, women still are the primary caregivers in the family. Typically, sons will contribute financially, but the brunt of the emotional and physical care burden falls to the daughters. It is estimated that as the population ages, women will spend more time caring for their parents than they did caring for their children.

Families try to help aging family members in a variety of ways. If the aging family member is able to live alone, families may demonstrate concern by visiting frequently and assisting with transportation to shopping and doctor appointments. Some prepare meals, do the heavy housecleaning, and make major home repairs. Running between two households and trying to maintain both can be mentally and physically exhausting to younger family members, but many are willing to help their loved ones in any way they can.

A family crisis may occur when the aging person is no longer able to live alone. Important decisions must be made. Most families who try to "do the right thing" find that there is no perfect solution.

The two most common options are bringing the aging parent into the home of one of the children or placing the parent in a long-term care facility. There are problems and concerns with both of these options. It is essential that the family making this difficult decision consider many factors. The amount of care needed by the parent; the availability of a willing and able family member; the amount of available space in the children's homes; the added financial burden of an additional household member; the wishes of the parent, the child, and his or her family; and the interpersonal dynamics within the family must be considered before a decision is made.

Children often take elderly parents into their homes when the older adults can no longer maintain their own houses or apartments. Although this arrangement works well in some families, in others it is problematic for everyone involved. The familiar roles and responsibilities often reverse when children step in and attempt to take care of their parents. This places the aging person into the role of the "child," which he or she usually resents strongly. "Don't tell your mother what to do!" or "I'm still your father!" is often heard in aging parent-child interactions.

Loss of independence is probably the most significant issue that aging parents and their children must face. The aging family members have spent 40, 50, 60, or even 70 years making their own decisions as adults. As independent adults they could make their own choices about where to live, what to do, and when to do it. They chose what to eat, obtained their food, and prepared it without interference. They went to bed when and where they chose. They went to places they wanted to go without asking anyone's permission. They had control of their lives. Independence is what being an adult is about. Most independent adults do not want to ask anyone for help.

As physical change or disease affects the older adult, some or all of his or her independent function may be lost. Aging persons find it difficult to accept the fact that they can no longer do the things that they

once did. It is also distressing for the family to watch their loved ones change. While the aging person tries to cope with these changes in him- or herself, the family tries to determine how to respond to these changes. If "the right thing to do" is not known, all family members begin to have many mixed feelings and confusion. Feelings of grief, anger, frustration, and loss are common in all individuals.

When an aging family member moves in with a child's family, the dynamics within the home are always changed. The ability of the family to adapt and cope with an additional member of the household varies greatly from situation to situation. If all parties are agreeable to the move and if the older adult can have enough privacy to maintain independence, the blending of the elderly person into the child's home may be successful. Some families feel that a resident grandparent is rewarding and enriching. However, if the presence of the elderly person intrudes excessively on the family unit, the situation may be unpleasant for both the family and the elderly person.

If the elderly family member requires a substantial amount of physical care, the demands on family members can be intense. Yet many children feel duty-bound to care for their aging parents. This sense of obligation may be based on cultural, religious, or personal beliefs. If the childern determine that they are unable to care for their parents and instead opt for nursing home placement, children often feel that they have failed in their responsibilities. This can lead to intense feelings of guilt, even if nursing home placement is the most realistic and reasonable option.

The Nurse and Family Interactions

When we as nurses care for the elderly, particularly in hospital or nursing home settings, we only see the person as he or she is now. We tend to forget that these people have not always been old. They lived, loved, worked, argued, and wept as each of us does. Frequently the elderly persons we care for are very ill or infirm, and as nurses we tend to focus on their *physical* needs, cares, and treatments. In our preoccupation with our duties, we can easily lose our perspective of the elderly patient as both a person and a member of a family.

In hospitals and nursing homes, family members come and go. Some families show a great deal of interest and concern for their aging members, visiting regularly and interacting with the patient and the staff. This allows us to increase our understanding and appreciation of our patients as people. Other elderly individuals never have family members visit them. They seem to be alone in the world, even though the charts list children and their telephone numbers for emergencies. Even in home settings, family attention and interaction vary greatly. In some households, a great deal of interest is given to each family member, whereas in others little or none is shown. Why do we see such a wide variation of family attention?

The answer often lies in family dynamics and processes that began long ago when the elderly person was a young spouse and parent. Some families are very stable and cohesive. They are together often and share close, loving bonds. They have developed healthy methods for interacting, responding, and meeting each other's needs. Because of the strong bonds that have developed over many years, these families remain interested in and supportive of aging members.

Other families never develop the closeness that is ideal in a family. The family unit may have been disrupted by divorce, mental illness, or other serious problems. There may have been problems with abuse, alcoholism, or drugs. In fact, many families today are troubled by these problems, which may have been caused by the behavior of younger family members or by the behavior of the elderly person. Long-term problems that have developed over time do not go away when a person gets old. When the family unit is weak, supportive behavior from family members is unlikely.

Most families we interact with fall somewhere between these extremes. Few families are perfect, and few are terrible. Families are made up of human beings who respond to stress in many different ways. Coping with the stresses related to aging is difficult both for the aging individual and for his or her family. The behavior we see at any given time is the best that the person is capable of *at that time*. That does not mean that it is the best that they will be capable of at some other time. We as nurses need to examine the stresses affecting the family so that we can best respond to the needs of all family members. The critical thinking box on this page should help us determine what our stress factors will be.

ELDER ABUSE

Self-Neglect

Abuse and neglect are usually something done *to* someone, but self-neglect is unfortunately too common a problem in the elderly population. Self-neglect is more likely to be seen when an elderly person has few or no close family or friends, but it can occur despite their presence. Because our society has laws to protect the rights of adults it may be difficult for concerned parties to intervene until a situation has reached critical, or even life-threatening proportions.

Self-neglect is defined as failure to provide for the self due to a lack of ability or lack of awareness. Indicators of self-neglect include (1) the inability to maintain activities of daily living such as personal care, shopping, meal preparation, or other household tasks; (2) the inability to obtain adequate food and fluid as indicated by malnutrition or dehydration; (3) poor hygiene practices indicated by body odor, sores, rashes, or inadequate or soiled clothing; (4) changes in mental function such as confusion, inappropriate responses, disorientation, or incoherence; (5) the inability to manage personal finances as indicated by the failure to pay bills or hoarding, squandering, or giving away money inappropriately; (6) failure to keep important business or medical appointments; and (7) life-threatening or suicidal acts such as wandering, isolation, or substance abuse.

Self-neglect in the community is most likely to be recognized by neighbors and reported to the police, public health nurses, or social workers. It may also be suspected by emergency room nurses who see these individuals after they are found injured on the street, after a fire, or in some other state of distress.

Self-neglect is frequently connected with some form of mental illness or dementia. Once the problem is recognized, legal action through the courts is needed to place the person in the custody of a family member or adult protective services.

Abuse or Neglect by the Family

It is estimated that 10% of the elderly will need some form of long-term care in the home. Attempts to meet these demands may be accompanied by high levels of stress for the caregivers. Increased demands on limited resources, physical exhaustion, or mental fatigue can result in deviant behaviors on the part of the caregiver. Inappropriate behavioral responses include **abuse** and **neglect** of the elderly family members. A Senate subcommittee that studied the problem of elder abuse estimated that as many as 1 million elderly Americans are being abused in some way by their families.

Intentional abuse occurs when any person deliberately plans to mistreat or harm another person. Abusive behavior cannot be justified at any time or in any way. Intentional abuse is most likely to occur in families with preexisting behavioral or social problems. High-risk families include those with members who have a history of violence or substance abuse and those with severe financial problems or unemployment.

Not all forms of abuse are intentional, but even unintentional abuse is devastating to the elderly. Unintentional abuse or neglect is most likely to occur when the caregiver lacks the necessary knowledge, stamina, or resources needed to care for an elderly loved one. Often the caregiver is an elderly spouse or an aging child who physically cannot meet the high-level care demands. Situations that trigger abuse are more likely when the elderly person requiring care is confused or needs continual care.

Continuous demands on caregivers can make them virtually prisoners within their own home. Stress builds, leaving the caregiver feeling trapped, frustrated, or angry. Unable to cope with the stress of these continual demands, caregivers may strike out at the elderly, lock them in a room, restrain them in a chair, or leave them unattended. When stress is high and coping ability is low, caregivers may not be able to identify any better options. They may not intend to hurt the elderly person or may rationalize that they are only doing it to "keep Dad from hurting himself," but the end result is still abuse.

Abuse can be physical, financial, and psychologic, or emotional. Neglect and abandonment also constitute forms of abuse.

Physical abuse

There are many types of physical abuse. Physical abuse is any action that causes physical pain or injury. Abuse may take the form of physical attacks in which elderly people who lack the strength to defend themselves are beaten by younger, stronger family members. Elderly people may be locked in bedrooms, clos-

ets, or basements. Elderly women may be sexually abused or even raped by family members. Some elderly people are starved by family members or given food that is unsuitable or unfit for human consumption. Failure to provide adequate food or fluids also constitutes physical abuse.

Neglect

Physical abuse involves one or more actions that cause harm. Neglect is a passive form of abuse in which caregivers fail to provide for the needs of the elderly person under their care. Neglect includes situations in which caregivers fails to meet the hygiene or safety needs of the elderly person. Examples include situations in which a bedridden person is left wet and soiled with body wastes for days at a time without care or when an elderly person suffers from exposure because he or she lacks adequate clothing for protection from the elements. Failure to provide necessary medical care may constitute neglect because with no means of going to the doctor or pharmacy the elderly person may suffer or even die. It is not considered neglect, however, if the elderly person refuses treatment. Neglect may be deliberate on the part of the caregiver, or it may result from lack of knowledge, inadequate financial resources, or an insufficient support system.

Emotional abuse

Even when physical abuse is absent and adequate physical care is provided, emotional abuse may be present. Emotional abuse is more subtle and difficult to recognize than is physical abuse or neglect. It often includes behaviors such as isolating, ignoring, or depersonalizing the elderly. Emotional abusers may forbid visitors and isolate the elderly person from more responsible and sympathetic friends or family members. They may prohibit use of the telephone or interfere with communication by mail.

Emotional abusers can use verbal or nonverbal means to inflict their damage. Verbal abuse includes shouting or voicing threats of punishment or confinement. Often emotional abusers threaten the elderly person with all manner of horrors if they tell anyone about their plight. Displeasure, disgust, frustration, or anger can be communicated nonverbally through sighing, head shaking, door slamming, or other negative body language. Repeatedly ignoring what the elderly person has to say or avoiding social interaction with the individual are subtle forms of abuse.

Negative communications are devastating because they can attack the elderly person's mind and emotions. These messages can be so subtle and so routine that people may not even recognize them as abusive.

Emotional abuse is insidious in that it can damage the elderly person's sense of self-esteem and can even destroy the will to live without leaving any obvious signs.

Financial abuse

Financial abuse exists when the resources of an elderly person are stolen or misused by a person whom the elder trusts. Such incidents are reported every day in the news. Children and grandchildren may take money from the elder, rationalizing that money is owed to them for providing care or that it will eventually be theirs anyway. People who expect to benefit from the elderly person's estate may be afraid that the needs of the elderly person will consume all the money and leave them nothing, so they better take it while they can. Regardless of the caregivers' rationalizations in these situations, it is financial abuse if the elderly person's money is taken and spent by others for their own purposes. It is not abusive to use the elderly person's resources to provide for his or her own personal needs.

Many elderly are overly trusting of family members, often refusing to believe that their children would steal from them. This state of denial often continues despite clear evidence to the contrary. Frequently, all of the savings have been spent, the house has been sold, and any objects of value have disappeared before they will accept the truth. Even then, some elderly make excuses to try to cope with the harsh reality. Abusive caregivers frequently abandon the elderly person once all of his or her assets are gone. The elderly are left homeless, penniless, and in despair.

Abandonment

Abandonment occurs when dependent elderly persons are deserted by the person or persons responsible for their custody or care under circumstances in which a reasonable person would continue to do so. Abandonment usually leaves the elderly person physically, emotionally, and financially defenseless. Elders who have been abandoned by their families usually become wards of the state.

Responses to abuse

It is natural to think that an elderly person suffering from one or more forms of abuse would complain, but this is rarely the case. Fear of being treated even worse or fear of being institutionalized or abandoned may prevent the victim from seeking help (see the following clinical situation box).

Elderly people who manifest signs of abuse must be assessed carefully (Box 1-8). They may try to protect and defend the abuser, deny that abuse is occurring, or seem resigned to the situation, believing that there is no better alternative.

All questioning and assessment must be done with great tact and sensitivity. The rights of elderly people to determine their own affairs to the full extent of their abilities must be respected. Information obtained must be kept confidential and shared only with agencies as authorized by the client or necessitated by law.

All observations, both objective and subjective, must be carefully documented in case legal action is required. Detailed records should be kept regardless of whether legal action is anticipated. Data may only become significant at a later date when they are im-

CLINICAL SITUATION

An 84-year-old woman was admitted to the hospital for dehydration and malnutrition. Six months earlier she had suffered a mild stroke. Since then, her 86-year-old husband had been caring for her at home. On admission, the woman weighed 91 lbs. Stage 2 pressure ulcers were present on both buttocks. Her clothing and undergarments were soiled, and she was in serious need of a bath. She reported episodes of incontinence of bladder and bowel. Her only reported activity consisted of sitting in a lounge chair watching TV. She was wearing a wig, which covered hair that was matted tightly on her scalp. After several days of carefully combing out the snarls, shoulder-length hair that had not been washed in months was revealed. Her husband explained, "I tried to do my best, but since she had always done all of the cooking, I didn't know what to do." He made sure she took her prescribed medicines, and he tried to see to it that she had enough to eat and drink, but he said that she was "picky." He also stated that he was unsure just how to take care of his wife's hygiene needs: "I tried to wash her up, but she said she wanted to be left alone." He explained that he stopped for groceries when she was asleep. He was afraid that if he called anyone for help, they would place his wife in an institution, and he couldn't cope with this idea. She had not complained to anyone for the same reason. Their children all lived out of state and had not visited since she had the stroke. The patient and her husband had assured their children by phone that everything was all right. It was only when she complained of chest pain that they sought medical attention.

possible to reconstruct if not appropriately recorded. Photographs may be necessary to provide proof of neglect or abuse. These may include pictures of wounds, injuries, or living conditions. It is wise to avoid using the term *abuse* when working with the elderly because they may become defensive and will probably deny it. Using words like "problems" or "concerns" is more likely to yield truthful information.

When there is any question of abuse, an experienced professional who is skilled in dealing with elder abuse should oversee the case. Physical and financial abuse are criminal offenses. Nurses have a moral, legal, and ethical responsibility to report any suspected cases

of abuse. See the clinical thinking box on this page for more information. Nurses who provide care to at-risk groups, particularly the young and the elderly, must be aware of their legal obligations with regard to suspected abuse. Nurses must know the state laws pertaining to abuse, the proper authorities to contact, and how to contact them. Once the responsible authorities are notified they are obligated by law to investigate and pursue any legal action necessary to protect the safety of the abused and protect them from further harm.

Abuse by Unrelated Caregivers

One would like to think that everyone seeking employment as caregivers to the elderly were responsible, caring individuals, but unfortunately this is not the case. People who are hired to provide for the safety and well-being of the elderly can sometimes become their greatest threat. Increased use of nonrelated caregivers exposes the elderly to additional risks.

As the number of older adults increases and as more frail elderly people remain in their homes, the demand for nursing assistants, home health aides, and housekeepers increases. Most people who work as nursing assistants or housekeepers are decent, caring individuals who provide difficult services for little reward. The salaries paid to nursing assistants and housekeepers are generally low, the hours are long, and the work is emotionally and physically demanding. Under these conditions, it is hard to find caring, responsible people who are willing to provide these types of service. When the demand for caregivers exceeds the supply of desirable workers, employers may be forced to hire some people who are willing to take these jobs only because they cannot find other employment.

Specific federal and state laws designed to prevent undesirable persons from contact with vulnerable people such as the young and elderly are in force today, but sometimes people with criminal records, inadequate training, or other serious shortcomings somehow manage to gain employment despite safe-

---

BOX 1-8

Signs That May Indicate Elder Abuse

1. The older person demonstrates *excessive* agreement or compliance with the caregiver.
2. The older person shows signs of poor hygiene such as body odor, uncleanliness, or soiled clothing or undergarments.
3. The older person has malnutrition or dehydration.
4. The older person has burns or pressure sores.
5. The older person has bruises, particularly clustered on trunk or upper arms.
6. The older person has bruises in various stages of healing that may indicate repeated injury.
7. The older person lacks adequate clothing or footwear.
8. The older person has had inadequate medical attention.
9. The older person verbalizes lack of food, medication, or care.
10. The older person verbalizes being left alone or isolated in some way.
11. The older person verbalizes fear of the caregiver.
12. The older person verbalizes his or her lack of control in personal activities or finances.

CRITICAL THINKING • YOUR KNOWLEDGE OF ELDER ABUSE

1. Is elder abuse increasing today? If so, why?
2. What would you do if you thought a close friend or relative was an elder abuser?
3. What do you think is the best way to reduce the incidence of elder abuse? Why?
4. What would you do if you suspected that a nursing assistant was abusing patients?
5. What can you as a student nurse do to prevent elder abuse?
6. What resources are available in your community to help prevent elder abuse?

guards such as state registries, employment histories, and reference checks. These untrustworthy individuals may unwittingly be hired by families and even health care institutions to provide care for the elderly.

In home settings, unscrupulous caregivers have been known to take money and personal belongings from defenseless elderly people under their care. They may physically abuse the elderly person and threaten him or her with physical harm if the abuse is reported. They may threaten to quit, leaving the elderly person in fear of being placed in an institution. Using threats enables these individuals to remain undetected until they have caused serious harm. When they are discovered, they often disappear only to reappear somewhere else and repeat their pattern of abuse.

Even health care institutions are not immune to problems of elder abuse. One assumes that because hospitals and nursing homes are licensed and regulated, this type of behavior does not occur. Unfortunately, this is wishful thinking. Many institutions have difficulty hiring enough people to meet the required staffing levels. Although most health care institutions and agencies screen applicants in an attempt to find the most qualified individuals and to avoid hiring anyone with a history of abusive or criminal behavior, some unscrupulous people manage to avoid detection and are employed as caregivers to the elderly.

These unsuitable caregivers may victimize the elderly before they can be detected. Nurses who supervise other caregivers must constantly be on the lookout for abusive behaviors (Box 1-9). Any indication of abuse in an institutional setting must be reported as soon as it is suspected so that appropriate action can be taken and the abusive person removed. The importance of this nursing responsibility cannot be stressed enough.

PREVENTION OF ELDER ABUSE

To reduce abuse and to meet the emotional and physical needs of the elderly and their caregivers, a wide variety of services have evolved. The types of services available vary from area to area, with some farsighted cities offering many services. Nurses who work with older adults should become knowledgeable about the services that are available in their communities. Resources may include education programs designed to improve awareness of the problem of elder abuse, support groups for caregivers of the elderly, respite care programs, and senior day care centers. Many hospitals and health care agencies (e.g., Red Cross) provide educational programs in nutrition, medication administration, bedside care, and other aspects of caring for the elderly. The need for these programs is growing as the elderly population increases.

BOX 1-9

Abusive Behaviors in Health Care Settings

1. Use of sedative or hypnotic drugs that are not medically necessary
2. Use of restraints when they are not medically indicated
3. Use of derogatory language, angry verbal interactions, or ethnic slurs
4. Withholding of privileges such as snacks or cigarettes
5. Excessive roughness in handling during care or during transfers
6. Delay in taking a resident to the bathroom or allowing a resident to lie in body waste
7. Consumption of a resident's food
8. Theft of money or personal belongings
9. Physical striking or any other assaultive behavior of or toward a resident
10. Violation of a resident's right to make decisions
11. Failure to provide privacy

Support Groups

Caregivers to the elderly are often isolated from other people. The demands of providing care prevent them from getting the rest, encouragement, and support they need. Caregivers who want or need to share their experiences and their frustrations have started forming support groups to help each other cope with stress. These support groups may be specialized (e.g., for caregivers of people with Alzheimer's disease) or more general in nature. Support groups allow the caregivers time to share their feelings and to learn strategies for improving their coping skills. Some groups schedule speakers to discuss topics of common interest or offer social activities to promote stress reduction.

Respite Care

Respite care allows the primary caregiver to have time away from the constant demands of caregiving, thereby decreasing caregiver stress and the risk of abuse. Many caregivers are unable to lead normal lives because they cannot leave their responsibilities for more than a few minutes without fear of some disaster occurring. Respite care gives the primary caregiver the opportunity to attend church, shop, conduct personal business, obtain medical care, and participate in other activities that most people take for granted.

Respite care may be provided by family members, volunteers, or one of the many services agencies that have proliferated within the past few years. Caregivers may be reluctant to use respite care out of guilt, fear, or other misguided emotions. Nurses should encourage caregivers to protect their own health and well-being by taking advantage of respite care on a regular basis.

SUMMARY

Aging is described in many ways. Chronologic age is not always the most reliable way to measure aging because the number of years a person has lived provides little information about his or her physiologic or functional ability. A large segment of today's aging population lives a more dynamic, positive lifestyle than ever before. Stereotyping and negative perceptions of aging and elderly persons appear to be on the decline, yet subtle forms of ageism still exist and need to be addressed. As the elderly become an increasingly larger segment of the population, they are having significant impact on politics, economics, and social family dynamics. Although many positive changes have occurred, the most frail elderly remain vulnerable to physical, emotional, and financial abuse.

READINGS AND REFERENCES

Adamchak D: Demographic aging in the industrial world: a rising burden? *Generations* 17:6, 1993.

American Association for Retired Persons: Understanding senior housing for the 1990s, Washington, DC, 1993, The Association.

American Association for Retired Persons: A profile of older Americans, Washington, DC, 1993, The Association.

American Association for Retired Persons: A matter of choice, Washington, DC, The Association.

Atchley RC: The myth of fixed income, *Aging Today* 13:10, 1992.

Bradley M: Elder abuse, *BMJ* 313:548, 1996.

Butler RN: Dispelling ageism: the cross-cultural intervention, *Generations* 17:75, 1993.

Cannon N: Older Americans Act reauthorization targets more services to minorities, *Aging* 365:58, 1993.

Crown WH: Projecting the costs of aging populations, *Generations* 17:32, 1993.

Crozier M: Respite care keeps elders at home longer, *Perspect Aging* 11: Sept/Oct, 1982.

Cutler S, Coward R: Availability of personal transportation in households of elders: age, gender, and residence differences, *Gerontologist* 32:77, 1992.

deLuce J: Ancient images of aging: did ageism exist in Greco-Roman antiquity? *Generations* 17:31, 1993.

Ebersole P, Hess P: *Toward healthy aging: human needs and nursing response,* ed 5, St Louis, 1998, Mosby.

Ferraro K, LaGrange R: Are older people most afraid of crime? Reconsidering age differences in fear of victimization, *J Gerontol* 47:S233, 1992.

Gailbraith M: Elder abuse: perspectives on an emerging crisis, Kansas City, Mo, 1986, Midwest Congress on Aging.

Gurland BJ, Breuer A, Cachkes E: *Columbia University College of Physicians and Surgeons complete home medical guide,* ed 3, New York, 1995, Crown Publishers.

Hamilton A: *Legal guide for senior citizens,* Topeka, Kan, 1991, Kansas Department on Aging.

Himes CL: Social demography of contemporary families and aging, *Generations* 23:13, 1992.

Jones PS: Where doctors are few and far between, *Aging* 365:12, 1993.

Kupetz BN: Bridging the gap between young and old, *Children Today* 22:10, 1993.

Longino CF: Myths of an aging America, *American Demographics,* August, 1994.

Lueckenotte A: *Gerontologic nursing,* St Louis, 1996, Mosby.

National Research Council: Research committee views aging population's effect on future policies, *Public Health Rep* 109:830, 1994.

Patrick G: Keep the focus on our patients: not the big picture, *Med Ec* 70:27, 1993.

Procino J: Designs for living, *Mod Matu* 36:24, 1993.

Senior living alternatives: Winter/Spring, Southfield, Mich, 1997.

Vladeck BC: End of life care, *JAMA* 274:449, 1995.

THEORIES OF AGING

LEARNING OBJECTIVES

1. Discuss how a theory is different from a fact.
2. Describe the most common biologic theories of aging.
3. Describe the most common psychosocial theories of aging.
4. Discuss the relevance of these theories to nursing practice.

Like other living organisms, humans age and then die. The maximum life expectancy for humans today appears to be 110 years, but why is this the case? Studies of families and identical twins show that there is a strong correlation in the life expectancies of genetically related people. If your grandparents and parents live to be 60, 70, 80, or 90 years of age, you are likely to have a similar lifespan. This is not always the case, however. Some individuals fail to meet genetic expectations, whereas others significantly exceed expectations. Biologic and environmental factors are being studied to explain these variations.

Although there is no question that aging is a biologic process, sociologic and psychologic components play a significant role. All of these areas—genetic, biological, environmental, and psychosocial—have produced theories that attempt to explain the changes seen with aging. Despite extensive interest in this topic, the specific causes and processes involved in aging are not yet completely understood. Because we do not have definitive and reproducible evidence indicating exactly why we age, all of the following remain theories.

BIOLOGIC THEORIES

Biologic theories of aging attempt to explain why the physical changes of aging occur. Researchers are trying to identify which biologic factors have the greatest influence on longevity. It is known that all members of a species suffer a gradual, progressive loss of function over time because of their biologic structure. Many of the biologic theories of aging overlap because most assume that the changes that cause aging occur at a cellular level. Each theory attempts to describe the processes of aging by examining various changes in cell structures or function.

Some **biologic theories** look at aging from a genetic perspective. The *programmed theory* proposes that every person has a "biologic clock" that starts ticking at the time of conception. In this theory each individual has a genetic "program" specifying an unknown but predetermined number of cell divisions. As the program plays out the person experiences predictable changes such as atrophy of the thymus, menopause, skin changes, and graying of the hair. A closely related theory is the *run-out-of-program theory,* which proposes that every person has a limited amount of genetic material that will run out over time. The *gene theory* proposes the existence of one or more harmful genes that activate over time, resulting in the typical changes seen with aging and limiting the lifespan of the individual.

The **molecular theories** propose that aging is controlled by genetic materials that are encoded to predetermine both growth and decline. The *error theory* proposes that errors in RNA protein synthesis cause errors to occur in cells in the body, resulting in a progressive decline in biologic function. The *somatic mutation theory* is similar but proposes that aging is due to DNA damage caused by exposure to chemicals or radiation and that this damage causes chromosomal abnormalities that lead to disease or loss of function later in life.

Cellular theories propose that aging is a process that occurs because of cell damage. When enough cells are damaged, overall functioning of the body is decreased. The *free radical theory* provides one explanation for cell damage. Free radicals are unstable molecules produced by the body during the normal processes of respiration and metabolism or following exposure to radiation and pollution. These free radicals are suspected to cause damage to the cells, DNA, and immune system. Excessive accumulation of free radicals in the body is purported to cause or contribute to the physiologic changes of aging and a wide variety of diseases such as arthritis, circulatory diseases, diabetes, and atherosclerosis. One free radical named *lipofuscin* has been identified to cause a buildup of fatty pigment granules that cause "age spots" in the elderly. Individuals who support this theory propose that the number of free radicals can be reduced by the use of antioxidants such as vitamins, carotenoids, selenium, and phytochemicals.

One variation of this theory is the *crosslink* or *connective tissue theory,* which proposes that cell molecules from DNA and connective tissue interact with free radicals to cause bonds that decrease the ability of tissue to replace itself. This results in the skin changes typically attributed to aging such as dryness, wrinkles, and loss of elasticity. Another variation, the *Clinker theory,* combines the somatic mutation, free radical, and crosslink theories to suggest that chemicals produced by metabolism accumulate in normal cells and cause damage to body organs such as the muscles, heart, nerves, and brain.

Wear-and-tear theory presumes that the body is similar to a machine, which loses function when its parts wear out. As people age, their cells, tissues, and organs are damaged by internal or external stressors. When enough damage occurs to the body's parts, overall functioning decreases. This theory also proposes that good health maintenance practices will reduce

---

BOX 2-1

Common Theories of Aging

BIOLOGIC THEORIES

Programmed theory: Proposes a biologic "time clock" or genetic program that starts at conception and is set with an unknown but predetermined number of cell devisions.

Run-out-of-program theory: Proposes a limited amount of genetic material that is used up over time.

Gene theory: Proposes the existence of one or more harmful genes that cause the physiologic changes of aging and limit the lifespan.

Error theory: Proposes that errors in protein synthesis result in errors in the body's cells, causing a progressive decline in biologic function.

Somatic mutation theory: Proposes that DNA is damaged by exposure to chemicals or radiation, causing chromosomal damage that leads to loss of function in later life.

Free radical theory: Proposes that substances called free radicals, which are produced during normal metabolism, are not eliminated from the body; these free radicals interfere with normal body function and result in cell damage.

Crosslink/connective tissue theory: Proposes that cellular DNA and connective tissues interact with free radicals, decreasing the body's ability to replace itself.

Wear-and-tear theory: Proposes that cells wear out through exposure to internal and external stressors, including trauma, chemicals, and buildup of naturally occurring wastes.

Immunologic theory: Proposes that the aging immune system is less capable of distinguishing between self and non-self; consequently autoimmune disease and allergies become more common.

PSYCHOSOCIAL THEORIES

Disengagement theory: Proposes that society withdraws from elderly people and elderly people withdraw from society.

Activity theory: Proposes that aging results from decreased activity, interest, and involvement.

LIFE-COURSE OR DEVELOPMENTAL THEORIES

Erickson's theory: Proposes that aging is a normal stage in the course of life wherein the elderly person either gains acceptance of his or her life and maintains integrity or fails to gain this acceptance and experiences anger or despair.

Havighurst's theory: Proposes specific tasks for aging, including adjusting to loss, adapting to change, and maintaining social relationships

Newman's theory: Proposes specific tasks for aging, including coping with physical changes and role changes, accepting life experiences, and preparing for death.

---

the rate of wear and tear, resulting in longer and better body function.

Immunologic theory proposes that aging is a function of changes in the immune system. According to this theory, the immune system—an important defense mechanism of the body—weakens over time to make an aging person more susceptible to disease. Immunologic theory also proposes that the increase in autoimmune diseases and allergies seen with aging is caused by changes in the immune system.

PSYCHOSOCIAL THEORIES

Psychosocial theories of aging do not explain why the physical changes of aging occur, but rather they attempt to explain why older adults have different responses to the aging process.

Some of the most prominent psychosocial theories of aging are the disengagement theory, activity theory, life-course or developmental theories, and a variety of other personality theories.

The highly controversial *Disengagement theory* was developed to explain why aging persons separate from the mainstream of society. This theory proposes that older people are systematically separated, excluded, or disengaged from society because they are not perceived to be of benefit to the society as a whole. This theory further proposes that the elderly desire to withdraw from society as they age, so that the disengagement is mutually beneficial. Critics of this theory believe that it attempts to justify ageism, oversimplifies the psychosocial adjustment to aging, and fails to address the diversity and complexity of older adults.

Activity theory proposes that activity is necessary for successful aging. Active participation in physical and mental activities helps maintain functioning well into old age. Purposeful activities and interactions that promote self-esteem improve overall satisfaction with life, even at an older age. "Busywork" activities and casual interaction with others were not shown to improve the self-esteem of older adults.

Life-course theories are perhaps those best known

to nursing. These theories trace personality and personal adjustment throughout a person's life. Many of these theories are very specific in identifying life-oriented tasks for the aging person. Three of the most common theories—Erickson's, Havighurst's, and Newman's—are worth exploring.

Erickson's theory identifies eight stages of developmental tasks that an individual must confront throughout the lifespan: (1) trust versus mistrust, (2) autonomy versus shame and doubt, (3) initiative versus guilt, (4) industry versus inferiority, (5) identity versus identify confusion, (6) intimacy versus isolation (7) generativity versus stagnation, and (8) integrity versus despair. The last of these stages is the domain of late adulthood, but failure to achieve earlier in life tasks can cause problems later in life. Late adulthood is the time when people normally review their lives and determine whether they have been negative or positive overall. The most positive outcomes of this life review are wisdom, understanding, and acceptance; the most negative outcomes are doubt, gloom, and despair.

Havighurst's theory details the process of aging and defines specific tasks for late life, including (1) adjusting to decreased physical strength and health, (2) adjusting to retirement and decreased income, (3) adjusting to the loss of a spouse, (4) establishing a relationship with one's age group, (5) adapting to social roles in a flexible way, and (6) establishing satisfactory living arrangements.

Newman's theory identifies the tasks of aging as (1) coping with the physical changes of aging; (2) redirecting energy to new activities and roles, including retirement, grandparenting, and widowhood; (3) accepting one's own life; and (4) developing a point of view about death.

IMPLICATIONS FOR NURSING

Physical theories of aging indicate that although biology places some limitations on life and life expectancy, other factors are subject to behavior and life choices. Nursing can help individuals achieve the longest, healthiest lives possible by promoting good health maintenance practices and a healthy environment.

Psychosocial theories help explain the variety of behaviors seen in the aging population. Understanding all of these theories can help nurses recognize problems and provide nursing interventions that will help aging individuals successfully meet the developmental tasks of aging.

SUMMARY

Many biologic, environmental, and psychosocial theories have been proposed to explain why we age (Box 2-1). These remain theories because the exact processes that cause the changes seen with aging are not completely understood. Further research and study will be needed to determine which theory or combination of theories is most accurate. Once this is determined we will be able to institute measures to slow aging and prolong the human lifespan.

READINGS AND REFERENCES

Charlesworth B: Evolutional mechanisms of senescence, *Genetica* 91:11, 1993.

Cookson C: In search of eternal youth, *Financial Times*, p 14, August, 1996.

Curtsinger JW, et al: Genetic variation and aging, *Ann Rev Genet* 29:553, 1995.

Dixon B: Why on earth do we grow old? *BMJ* 308:861, 1994.

Evans JG: Metabolic switches in ageing, *Age Ageing* 22:19, 1993.

Found a clue to why people age, *US News & World Report*, p 20, April 22, 1996.

Levine SA, Kidd PM: *Antioxidant adaptation: its role in free radical pathology.* San Leandro, Calif, 1986, Allergy Research Group.

Martensen RL: The emergence of old age as a scientific struggle, *JAMA* 274:1907, 1995.

Raloff J: Oxygen's radical role in cancer and aging, *Science News* 146:407, 1994.

Reiter RJ: A review of the evidence supporting melatonin's role as an antioxidant, *J Pineal Res* 18:1, 1995.

Reiter RJ: Oxidative processes and antioxidative defense mechanisms in the aging brain, *FASEB J* 9:536, 1995.

PHYSIOLOGIC CHANGES

LEARNING OBJECTIVES

1. Describe the most common structural changes observed in the normal aging process.
2. Discuss the impact of normal structural changes on the older adult's self-image and lifestyle.
3. Describe the most commonly observed functional changes that are part of the normal aging process.
4. Discuss the impact of normal functional changes on the older adult's self-image and lifestyle.
5. Identify the most common diseases related to aging in each of the body systems.
6. Differentiate between normal changes of aging and disease processes.
7. Discuss the impact of age-related changes on nursing care.

The changes in body function that occur with aging are not random and do not develop suddenly or without warning. Rather, they are part of a continuum that begins at the moment life begins. From the moment of conception, tissues and organs develop in an orderly manner. When fully developed, these organs and tissues perform specific functions and interact together in a predictable way. Throughout life, human growth and development occur methodically.

Early in life, the physical changes are dramatic. In only 9 months of gestation, the human organism develops from two almost invisible cells into a unique, functioning individual measuring about 20 inches in height and weighing usually between 6 and 9 pounds. For the next 13 to 15 years, rapid physical growth continues. By approximately age 18, the human body reaches full anatomic and physiologic maturity.

The peak years of physiologic function last from the late teens through the thirties—the so-called prime of life. Physiologic changes are still occurring during this time, but they are subtle and not easily recognized. Because these changes do not happen as rapidly or as dramatically as do those that occur early in life, they are more likely to be ignored.

As a person moves into his or her fifth and sixth decades of life, these physiologic changes become more apparent. In the seventh and eighth decades and beyond, they are significant and no longer deniable.

It is important to recognize that although age-related changes are predictable, the *exact* time at which they occur is not. Just as no two individuals grow and develop at exactly the same rate, no two individuals show the signs of aging at the same time. There is wide person-to-person variation in when—and to what degree—these changes will occur. Heredity, environment, and health maintenance significantly affect the timing and magnitude of age-related changes. Some people are chronologically quite young but appear old. The most severe cases of this occur in a rare condition called **progeria.** When they are only 8 or 9 years of age, children with progeria have the physiology and appearance of 70-year-olds. At the other extreme, there are persons in their sixties, seventies, and even older who are vigorous and appear much younger than their chronologic age. Most people show the signs of aging at a rate somewhere between these two extremes.

We can observe many normal changes in the body's physical structure and function during the aging process. There are also changes that indicate the onset of disease or illness. Nurses are expected to be able to tell the difference between normal changes and abnormal changes that signify a need for medical or nursing intervention. To identify these differences, nurses must have a good understanding of the normal structures and functions of the body. This knowledge should help nurses understand how normal and abnormal changes affect the day-to-day functional abilities of older adults.

It is essential that nurses learn that each aging person, just like each younger person, is unique. The type and extent of changes seen with aging are specific and unique to each person. Nurses must avoid falling into the trap of stereotyping elderly individuals. Stereotyping is very dangerous because it leads us to accept as inevitable some changes that are *not* inevitable. It can also cause us to mistake early signs of disease as a part of aging.

As nurses, we must be aware of the physical changes that are likely to occur, assess each individual to determine the extent to which these changes have occurred, and then make our care plans in response to that specific person's needs.

THE INTEGUMENTARY SYSTEM

The integumentary system, which includes the skin, hair, and nails, undergoes significant changes with aging. Because many of these structures are visible, changes in this system are probably the most obvious and are evident to both the aging individual and others.

NORMAL BODY STRUCTURE AND FUNCTION

The **epidermis,** the outermost layer of the skin, is an important structure that provides protection for internal structures, keeps out dangerous chemicals and microorganisms, functions as part of the body's fluid regulation system, and helps regulate body temperature and eliminate waste products. It also contains melanocytes that produce the pigment **melanin,** which provides protection from ultraviolet radiation.

The **dermis** contains **collagen** and elastin fibers, which give strength and elasticity to the tissues. The **sebaceous** (oil-producing) and eccrine (sweat-producing) glands are located in the subcutaneous tissue, as are the hair and nail follicles and the **sensory**

nerve receptors. Hair and nails are composed of dead **keratinized** cells. Hair pigment, or color, is related to the amount of melanin produced by the follicle and, like skin pigmentation, is hereditary. Nails are rigid structures that protect the sensitive, nerve-rich tissue at the tips of the fingers and toes. Nails also aid dexterity in fine finger manipulation.

Subcutaneous tissue consists of **areolar connective tissue,** which connects the skin to the muscles, and **adipose tissue,** which provides a cushion over tissue and bone. Subcutaneous tissue provides insulation to regulate body temperature. It is here that **white blood cells** (WBCs) are available to protect the body from microbial invasion through the skin. Blood vessels in the subcutaneous tissue supply the tissue with nourishment and assist in the process of heat exchange. These superficial blood vessels dilate or constrict as needed to release heat or to conserve heat lost through convection.

NORMAL AGE-RELATED CHANGES

With aging, the epidermis becomes more fragile, increasing the risk of skin damage such as tears, maceration, and infection. Rashes due to contact with chemicals such as detergents or cosmetics are increasingly common in older individuals. Skin repairs more slowly in older than in younger individuals, also increasing the risk for infection.

Melanocyte activity declines with age, and in whites the skin may become very pale, making older individuals more susceptible to the effects of the sun. Clusters of melanocytes can form areas of deepened pigmentation, a condition called **senile lentigo;** these areas are often referred to as "age spots" or "liver spots" and

are most often seen on areas of the body that are most exposed to sunlight. In a condition called **seborrheic keratosis,** slightly raised, wartlike macules with distinct edges appear (Fig. 3-1). These lesions, which can range in color from light tan to black, are most often observed on the upper half of the body and may cause discomfort and itching. Skin tags, or **cutaneous papilloma,** are small brown or flesh-colored projections of skin that are most often observed on the necks of older adults.

Aging results in decreased elastin fibers and a thinner dermal layer (Table 3-1). With loss of elasticity, the skin starts to become less supple. "Crow's feet," or

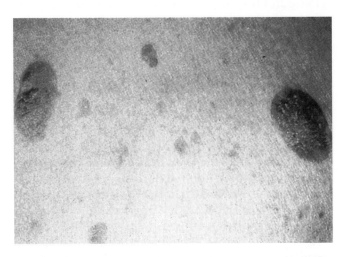

FIG. 3-1 Seborrheic keratoses usually appears at about the fifth decade of life and gradually increase in number with age. These superficial, benign growths can enlarge to 20 mm in diameter and have a convoluted surface. (From Eaglstein WH, McKay M, Pariser DM: *Patient Care* 28[7]:104, 1994.)

TABLE 3-1

Integumentary Changes Associated with Aging

Physiologic change	Results
Decreased vascularity of dermis	Increased pallor in white skin
Decreased amount of melanin	Decreased hair color (graying)
Decreased sebaceous and sweat gland function	Increased dry skin; decreased perspiration
Decreased subcutaneous fat	Increased wrinkling
Decreased thickness of epidermis	Increased susceptibility to trauma
Increased localized pigmentation	Increased incidence of brown spots (senile lentigo)
Increased capillary fragility	Increased purple patches (senile purpura)
Decreased density of hair growth	Decreased amount and thickness of hair on head and body
Decreased rate of nail growth	Increased brittleness of nails
Decreased peripheral circulation	Increased longitudinal ridges of nails; increased thickening and yellowing of nails
Increased androgen: estrogen ratio	Increased facial hair in women

wrinkles, develop. Very dry skin or skin that has had excessive exposure to sunlight or harsh chemicals is more likely to wrinkle at a younger age. Hair color tends to fade or "gray" because of pigment loss, and hair distribution patterns change. Color changes and hair loss patterns tend to be hereditary. The hair on the scalp, pubis, and axilla tends to thin in both men and women. Hairs in the nose and ears often become thicker and more noticeable. Some women experience the growth of facial hair, particularly after menopause. Fingernails grow more slowly, may become thick and more brittle, and ridges or lines are commonly observed. Toenails may become so thick that they require special equipment for trimming. Sweat gland function decreases, and thus the amount of perspiration decreases. This results in heat intolerance because of the body's less efficient cooling system through the process of evaporation.

A decrease in the function of sebaceous and sweat gland secretion increases the likelihood of dry skin, or **xerosis** (Fig. 3-2). Dry skin is probably the most common skin-related complaint among the elderly, particularly when it is accompanied by itching, or **pruritus.** This problem is often more severe on the lower extremities due to diminished circulation.

The walls of the capillaries become increasingly fragile with age and may hemorrhage, leading to **senile purpura,** the red, purple, or brown areas commonly seen on the legs and arms.

By 70 years of age, the body has approximately 30% fewer cells than at age 40. The remaining cells enlarge so that body mass appears approximately the same. Total body fluid decreases with age. Plasma and extracellular volume remain somewhat constant, but intracellular fluid decreases. This loss of intracellular fluid increases the risk of dehydration. Tissue changes include a decrease in subcutaneous tissue that is visible in the eye orbits, hollows in the supraclavicular space, and sagging of breasts and neck tissue.

ABNORMAL CONDITIONS COMMON WITH AGING

Basal Cell Carcinoma

It is important to distinguish normally occurring changes in the skin from the lesions that may be precancerous or cancerous. Cases of basal cell carcinoma are frequently observed in elderly people who have spent significant amounts of time in the sun. Any pigmented area that is enlarging, elevated from the skin, bleeds when touched, or is in any other way suspicious should be documented and reported so that it can be examined promptly by a physician.

Pressure Ulcers

Shrinkage in the cushion provided by subcutaneous tissue places the elderly person at increased risk for pressure ulcers—breakdown of the skin and tissues located over bony prominences (Fig. 3-3). This is a significant problem for immobilized people such as those who are bedridden or confined to wheelchairs. Special precautions to prevent this type of problem will be discussed in Chapter 11.

Inflammation and infection

Changes in the integumentary system increase the elderly person's risk for skin inflammation and infection. Skin inflammation and infection frequently occur on visible surfaces of the body such as the face, scalp, and arms, making the conditions very distressing to the elderly person.

Common types of inflammation include rosacea and various forms of dermatitis. **Rosacea** appears as redness, dilated superficial blood vessels, and small "pimples" on the nose and center of the face (Fig. 3-4). It may spread to cover the cheeks and chin. Left untreated, it can lead to swelling and enlargement of the nose or conjunctivitis. There is no known cause for this disorder, but it is most common in postmenopausal women, people who flush easily, and those taking vasodilating medication. Treatment includes avoidance of actions that trigger vasodilation such as stressful situations, extreme heat, sun exposure, spicy foods, and alcoholic beverages.

Several forms of dermatitis are common in the elderly, including contact, allergic, and seborrheic dermatitis. **Contact** and **allergic dermatitis** appear as

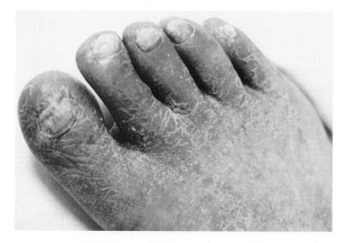

FIG. 3-2   Xerosis. (From Ebersole P, Hess P: *Toward healthy aging: human needs and nursing response,* ed 5, St Louis, 1998, Mosby.)

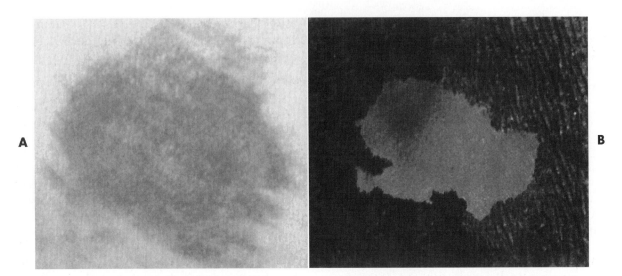

FIG. 3-3 **A,** Early-stage pressure ulcers, or stage 1 lesions, are frequently dismissed as minor abrasions because their primary attribute is nonblanchable erythema. **B,** On dark skin, even a stage 2 ulcer, which is characterized by some skin loss, may be difficult to identify accurately because of its resemblance to a blister or abrasion. (From Eaglestein WH, McKay M, Pariser DM: *Patient Care* 28[7]:103, 1994.)

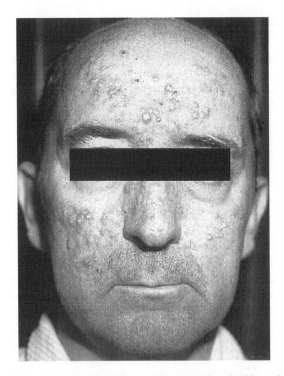

FIG. 3-4 Fairly longstanding rosacea is evident in this patient. The acneiform eruptions have spread over the entire face, and the bulbous red nose of rhinophyma is present. (From Eaglstein WH, McKay M, Pariser DM: *Patient Care* 28[7]:110, 1994.)

rashes or inflammation that is either localized to certain areas of the body or generalized (Fig. 3-5). Clues to the causative substance are gained from the unique pattern presented on each individual. Identification of the particular irritant may be difficult because of the number of chemicals, drugs and other substances to which an individual is exposed. Treatment consists of avoiding the offending substance.

Seborrheic dermatitis is an unsightly skin condition characterized by yellow, waxy crusts that can be either dry or moist (Fig. 3-6). Caused by excessive sebum production, seborrheic dermatitis can occur on the scalp, eyebrows, eyelids, ears, axilla, breasts, groin, and gluteal folds. There is no known cure, but treatment with special shampoos and lotions will help control the problem.

Infectious diseases of the skin and nails commonly seen in the elderly include herpes zoster (also called shingles); fungal, yeast, and bacterial infections; and infestation with the scabies mite. Each of these diseases has a unique cause, characteristic appearance, and specific treatment that are beyond the scope of this text.

Hypothermia

The decrease in the amount of subcutaneous tissue reduces the older adult's ability to regulate body temperature. Very thin elderly people lose the insulation provided by subcutaneous and adipose tissue. This loss of insulation is most likely to result in hypothermia if

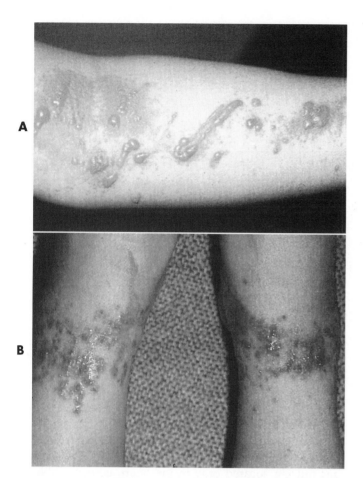

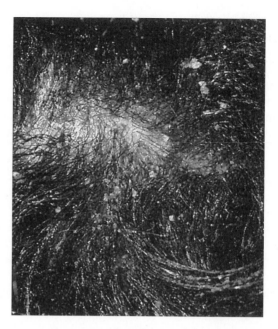

FIG. 3-6 Seborrheic dermatitis is characterized by itching and patches of scales that exfoliate. The most common sites are on the scalp, behind the ears, and on the midface, including the eyebrows and lashes. (From Eaglstein WH, McKay M, Pariser DM: *Patient Care* 28:114, 1994.)

FIG. 3-5 The incidence of contact dermatitis may increase with age, possibly due to increased exposure to outdoor agents associated with leisure activities. **A,** Erythema and vesiculation are common in the acute stage of irritant contact dermatitis, as shown on this patient's forearm. **B,** Extremely localized reactions, such as these behind a patient's knees, indicate a possible fiber allergy (e.g., to wool socks or trousers). The linear tracks from scratching may spread the allergen to adjacent areas. (From Eaglestein WH, McKay M, Pariser DM: *Patient Care* 28[7]:113, 1994.)

the person is exposed to an environment that is too cold.

THE MUSCULOSKELETAL SYSTEM

The musculoskeletal system performs many functions. The bones of the skeleton provide a rigid structure that gives the body its shape. The red bone marrow in the cavities of spongy bones produces red blood cells (RBCs), platelets, and WBCs. Structures such as the ribs and pelvis protect easily damaged internal or-

gans. The muscles provide a power source to move the bones. The combined functions of bones and muscles allow free movement and participation in the activities necessary to maintain a normal life.

NORMAL STRUCTURE AND FUNCTION

Bones

Bone consists of protein and the minerals calcium and phosphorus. Calcium is necessary for bone strength, muscle contraction, myocardial contraction, blood clotting, and neuronal activity. It is normally obtained by eating dairy products and dark green leafy vegetables. Vitamin D is needed for absorption of calcium and phosphate through the small intestine; vitamins A and C are needed for **ossification,** or bone matrix formation.

For the long bones to remain strong, adequate dietary intake of these nutrients is important. Dietary intake of minerals alone will not maintain bone strength, however. It is also necessary to apply stress to the long bones in order to keep the minerals in the bones. This needed stress is best provided by weight-bearing activities such as standing and walking. The calcium that is needed for clotting and nerve and muscle functions is constantly being withdrawn from the bone and moved into the bloodstream to maintain consistent blood levels. Calcium is normally redeposited in the bone at an equal rate, replacing the calcium that is lost. As long as this movement of calcium is in balance, bone remains strong.

Hormones also play an important role in bone maintenance. **Calcitonin,** which is produced by the thyroid gland, slows the movement of calcium from the bones to the blood and lowers the blood calcium level. Parathyroid hormone increases the movement of calcium from the bones to the blood and increases the blood calcium level. Parathyroid hormone also increases the absorption of calcium from the small intestine and kidneys, thus further increasing the blood calcium level. Insulin and thyroxine aid in the protein synthesis and energy production needed for bone maintenance. Estrogen and testosterone, produced by the ovaries and testes, respectively, help retain calcium in the bone matrix.

Vertebrae

The spinal column consists of a series of small bones, called **vertebrae,** that stack up to form a strong, flexible structure. The spinal column supports the head and allows for flexible movement of the back. The segments of the spinal column consist of cervical, thoracic, lumbar, and sacral vertebrae. The muscles that move the back connect at bony processes that protrude

from each vertebra. The **spinal cord,** the nerve tissue that extends downward from the brain, passes through the **vertebral canal,** which runs through an opening in each vertebra. The bones of the spinal column protect this nerve tissue from injury.

Fibrous pads called **intervertebral disks** are located between the vertebrae and cushion the impact of walking and other activities.

Joints

Joints are the places where bones meet. The freely moving synovial joints are lined with **cartilage,** which allows free movement of the joint surfaces. Many of these joints contain a **bursa,** which is a fluid sac that provides lubrication to enhance joint mobility (Fig. 3-7).

Tendons and Ligaments

Tendons are structures that connect the muscles to the bone, and **ligaments** are structures that connect bones to other bones.

Muscles

There are three types of muscle tissue in the body: cardiac muscle, smooth muscle, and skeletal muscle. **Cardiac muscle,** located only in the heart, is responsible

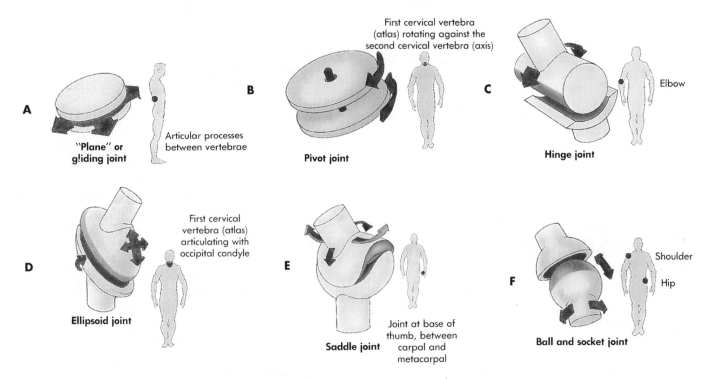

FIG. 3-7   Types of synovial joints. **A,** Plane, or gliding joint. **B,** Pivot joint. **C,** Hinge joint. **D,** Ellipsoid joint. **E,** Saddle joint. **F,** Ball-and-socket joint. (From Tate P, Seeley RR, Stephens TD: *Understanding the human body,* St Louis, 1994, Mosby.)

for the pumping action of the heart that maintains the blood circulation. **Smooth muscle** is found in the walls of hollow organs such as the blood vessels, stomach, intestines, and urinary bladder. Because cardiac and smooth muscle cannot normally be stimulated by conscious effort, they are called **involuntary** muscle.

Skeletal muscle comprises the largest amount of muscle tissue in the body. The major function of skeletal muscle is to move the bones of the skeleton. Because their actions can be controlled by conscious effort, skeletal muscles are considered **voluntary** muscles. Muscles are connected to bones by tendons. Contraction or relaxation of muscles causes the bones to move. Controlled and coordinated movement of bones and muscles allows us to perform the wide variety of movements required for activities of daily living. Special effort and practice allow us to perform special activities such as dancing, playing sports, and playing the piano.

The amount of muscle mass and the type of muscle development differ greatly among individuals. Men normally have larger muscles, or more muscle mass, than do women, particularly in the muscles of the upper body. The male hormone testosterone stimulates muscle development. In both men and women, the largest and strongest skeletal muscles are found in the legs and upper arms; the smallest and weakest are located in the lower back.

Muscle tissue is normally in a state of slight contraction. This muscle tone is necessary to support the head, to keep the spine erect, and to perform any controlled movement. Muscle mass is built and muscle tone maintained by means of exercise. There are two general types of exercise: **isometric exercise,** which involves muscle contraction without body movement; and **isotonic exercise,** which involves muscle contraction with body movement. Isometric exercise helps maintain muscle tone and strength but does little to increase muscle size. Isotonic exercise maintains muscle tone and strength and also increases muscle mass if it is done repetitively. **Aerobic** exercise is isotonic exercise that occurs for 30 minutes or longer. Aerobic exercise strengthens the skeletal, cardiac, and respiratory muscles. People who lead inactive or sedentary lifestyles suffer from the lack of isotonic exercise. Regardless of age, unless people undertake an exercise program, they will manifest poor muscle development and strength.

Muscle movement is controlled by impulses from the parietal lobes of the cerebrum and is coordinated by impulses from the cerebellum. **Muscle sense** is a term used to describe the brain's ability to recognize the position and action of the muscles without conscious effort. Receptor cells in the muscles called **proprioceptors** send information to the brain that enables it to integrate all body movements. This coordinative function of the brain allows us to walk, bend, or eat without consciously thinking about all of the separate movements and feeling all of the different positions.

Muscles need energy to function. The most abundant source of muscular energy is glycogen. **Adenosine triphosphate** (ATP), the direct energy source for muscular contraction, is a product of glycogen metabolism. Glycogen is first broken down into glucose. During cell metabolism, glucose interacts with oxygen transported in the bloodstream by hemoglobin or oxygen stored in the muscle fibers as myoglobin. This reaction involves the production of ATP, heat, water, and carbon dioxide. If muscle fibers do not receive enough oxygen, glucose may not be oxidized completely and a chemical intermediate, **lactic acid,** is produced. Elevated levels of lactic acid may result in muscle fatigue and soreness.

NORMAL AGE-RELATED CHANGES

The major bone-associated change related to aging is loss of calcium (Table 3-2). This change begins between 30 and 40 years of age. With each successive decade the skeletal bones become thinner and relatively weaker. Women lose approximately 8% of skeletal mass each decade, whereas men lose about 3%. Some parts of the skeleton, including the epiphyses, vertebrae, and jaw bones, contribute more to increased risk of fracture, loss of height, and loss of teeth.

The intervertebral disks shrink as the thoracic verte-

TABLE 3-2

Musculoskeletal Changes Associated with Aging

Physiologic change	Results
Decreased bone calcium	Increased osteoporosis; increased curvature of the spine (kyphosis)
Decreased fluid in intervertebral disks	Decreased height
Decreased blood supply to muscles	Decreased muscle strength
Decreased tissue elasticity	Decreased mobility and flexibility
Decreased muscle mass	Decreased strength; increased risk of falls

brae slowly change with aging. This results in a condition called **kyphosis,** which gives the elderly person a stooped or hunchback appearance, with the head dropping forward toward the chest. The combination of disk shrinkage and kyphosis results in loss of overall height. A person can lose as many as 2 inches by age 70. People who are concerned about their appearance find these changes disturbing. When clothing no longer fits properly, and it becomes increasingly difficult to find flattering styles.

Connective tissues tend to lose elasticity, and this restricts joint mobility. Loss of flexibility and joint mobility begins as early as the teens and is common with aging. Regular stretching exercises can help slow or even reverse flexibility problems.

Muscle tone and mass typically decrease with aging, and this is directly related to decreased physical activity and exercise. People of all ages who exercise regularly have better muscle mass and tone. Hormonal changes, particularly the decrease in testosterone level, tend to reduce muscle mass in aging men. Reduction in blood supply to the muscles as a result of aging or disease can lead to changes in muscle function. Less glycogen is stored in aging muscles, thereby decreasing the fuel available for muscle contraction. Any condition that restricts oxygen availability (e.g., anemia or respiratory problems) can lead to excessive production of waste products such as lactic acid and carbon dioxide. This can increase the incidence of muscle spasms and muscle fatigue with minimal exertion. Decreased endurance and agility may result from a combination of these factors. Neuronal changes in the areas of the brain responsible for muscle control can result in alterations of muscle sense, which may be observed in the elderly as an unsteady gait and impairment of other activities that require muscular coordination.

As a person ages, muscle mass decreases and the proportion of body weight due to fatty, or **adipose,** tissue increases. This is significant in the administration of medications. Intramuscular injection sites may not be as well muscled, and fatty tissue tends to retain medication differently than does lean tissue. Absorption and metabolism of drugs can be significantly different from that in younger persons.

CONDITIONS COMMON WITH AGING

Osteoporosis

Excessive loss of calcium from bone combined with insufficient replacement results in **osteoporosis.** People with inadequate dietary calcium intake, post-

menopausal women, and immobilized or physically inactive individuals are most at risk for developing this condition. Osteoporosis is characterized by porous, brittle, fragile bones that are susceptible to breakage. Spontaneous fracture of the vertebrae or other bones can occur in the absence of obvious trauma. In fact, spontaneous hip fractures may lead to a fall, rather than the fall leading to the hip fracture. Simple falls or other traumas are more likely to result in fractures in people who have osteoporosis. Common fracture sites include the hip (usually the neck of the femur), ribs, clavicle, and arm (when trying to break a fall).

Degenerative Joint Disease

The incidence of **osteoarthritis,** the most common form of arthritis, increases with age. It affects men and women equally. The cause of osteoarthritis is unknown; however, chemical, genetic, hormonal, and mechanical factors are involved. People employed in jobs that involve placing a high amount of physical stress on certain joints are likely to experience changes in those joints later in life. As most people age, they experience some symptoms of osteoarthritis because of this wear and tear on the joints. After years of normal joint use, the cartilage on the bones' articulating surfaces thins and begins to wear out. Calcium and cartilage fragments may form within the joint, and the synovial membrane of the bursa may become inflamed. This is particularly true in the weight-bearing joints of the spine, hips, knees, and ankles. **Heberden's nodes,** which are caused by abnormal cartilage or bony enlargement, may be seen in the distal joints of the fingers. Pain may occur with activity or exercise of the affected joints and may worsen with emotional stress. Osteoarthritis is treated by administering nonsteroidal antiinflammatory drugs (NSAIDs) by injecting corticosteroids into the joints, and by rest and heat. In severe cases, surgical joint replacements may be necessary.

Rheumatoid arthritis is a collagen disease that results from an autoimmune process. Its onset is typically earlier in life than that of osteoarthritis, and it is seen more commonly in women. Rheumatoid arthritis is characterized by periods of exacerbation during which the symptoms are severe and cause further damage, and **remission,** during which the progress of the disease halts. Rheumatoid arthritis can also result in muscle atrophy, soft tissue changes, and bone and cartilage changes.

The most serious deformities and problems are typically observed when an individual has suffered from this disease for an extended period of time. Rheumatoid arthritis is treated with heat, splinting, NSAIDs, gold salts, systemic corticosteroids, and a wide range of other modalities. Affected individuals are best treated by a **rheumatologist,** a physician who specializes in the disorder.

Bursitis, inflammation of the bursa and the surrounding fibrous tissue, can result from excessive stress on a joint or from a localized infection. Bursitis commonly results in joint stiffness and pain in the shoulder, knee, and elbow, ultimately leading to restricted or reduced mobility. While this problem can occur at any age, age-related changes in the musculoskeletal system make it a more common problem in older individuals. Treatment includes resting the joint and administering salicylates or NSAIDs. Corticosteroid preparations are occasionally injected into the painful areas to reduce inflammation. Mild range-of-motion exercise is encouraged to prevent permanent reduction or loss of joint function.

Gouty arthritis

Gouty arthritis is due to an inborn error of metabolism that results in elevated levels of uric acid in the body. Crystals of these acids deposit within the joints and other tissues, causing episodes of severe, painful joint swelling. Some joints, such as that of the great toe, are more commonly affected. Chills and fever may accompany a severe attack. Attacks of gout become more frequent as a person ages. If left untreated, this disease can result in destruction of the joints. It is observed more frequently in men but is also common in women after menopause.

THE RESPIRATORY SYSTEM

The respiratory system provides the body with the oxygen needed for life. Without oxygen, cells quickly die. The brain cells are the most sensitive cells in the body, and they will die if deprived of oxygen for as little as 4 minutes. Breathing, the process of inhaling to take in oxygen and exhaling to release carbon dioxide, occurs at a rate of 12 to 20 times per minute for our entire lives.

NORMAL STRUCTURE AND FUNCTION

The respiratory system is typically divided into two parts: the upper respiratory tract and the lower respiratory tract. The entire respiratory tract is lined with mucous membranes.

Upper Respiratory Tract

On its way to the lungs, air passes through the **upper respiratory tract,** which includes the air passages of the nose, mouth, and throat, all of which are located above the chest cavity. Mucous membranes line the nasal passages and warm and humidify the air that passes through the nose. Cilia and mucus in the nasal passages trap particulate matter (bacteria and debris) and sweep it toward the pharynx where it is routinely swallowed and destroyed by gastric acid. The cough and sneeze reflexes also help prevent debris and foreign objects from entering the respiratory tract. The **pharynx,** which is located at the back of the oral cavity, has three segments: the oropharynx, nasopharynx, and **laryngopharynx.**

The nasopharynx is connected to the middle ear by the **Eustachian tubes,** which help maintain proper air pressure in the middle ear. The **larynx,** or voicebox, is composed of cartilage rings and folds of tissue called **vocal folds.** The **epiglottis,** which is the uppermost cartilage ring, prevents food from entering the airway. During inhalation, the vocal folds move to the sides of the larynx to allow air to pass freely. During exhalation, we can speak and sing by controlling the distance between these folds, which vibrate when air is forced through them and produce sound.

Lower Respiratory Tract

The **lower respiratory tract** includes the lower trachea, bronchial passages, and alveoli, all of which lie within the chest cavity. The **trachea** is a cartilaginous passageway that connects the larynx to the bronchial passages of the lungs. The trachea branches into two major **bronchi,** which further divide like the branches of a tree into smaller and smaller **bronchioles.** At the ends of the bronchioles are the **alveoli,** or air sacs, which are the functional units of respiration. A thin layer of fluid lines each tiny air sac, which is surrounded by pulmonary capillaries to allow efficient exchange of gases by diffusion. It is here that oxygen enters the bloodstream for transport to body tissue; and it is here that carbon dioxide from the body leaves the bloodstream. This gaseous exchange is essential for normal cell function and for maintenance of the blood's acid-base balance.

Because the alveoli have a moist lining, their surfaces could adhere if they touched when the alveoli were empty. This is prevented by a special protein substance called **surfactant.**

Air Exchange (Respiration)

The movement of air into and out of the alveoli is called **ventilation.** Ventilation requires the action of muscles, primarily the **diaphragm** and the **intercostal muscles.** During inhalation, the diaphragm contracts and moves downward while the intercostal muscles pull the ribs upward and outward. These combined activities increase the size of the chest cavity until the air pressure inside the lungs is lower than the atmospheric pressure, and air is drawn into the lungs. This process is known as **inhalation** or **inspiration.** When the air pressure inside the lungs equals or exceeds atmospheric pressure, air ceases to enter the lungs. When the diaphragm and intercostal muscles relax, the diaphragm moves upward and the ribs move inward, making the chest cavity smaller. As the chest cavity becomes smaller, the pressure in the lungs becomes greater than the atmospheric pressure. Air is forced out of the lungs until the pressure in the lungs equals the atmospheric pressure. This action is known as **exhalation** or **expiration.** Regulation of respiration is both neurologic and chemical. The respiratory centers in the medulla and pons of the brainstem continuously monitor and control the rate and depth of involuntary respiration. Most breathing is unconscious and involuntary. If we had to think about inhaling and exhaling every breath, we would have little time to do anything else. However, breathing *can* be conscious and voluntary. When swimming, singing, or engaging in other activities that require breath control, we can temporarily alter our breathing patterns.

NORMAL AGE-RELATED CHANGES

With aging, changes are seen throughout the respiratory tract (Table 3-3). Years of exposure to air pollution, cigarette smoke, and other hazardous chemicals may take their toll on the air passageways and lung tissue. Mucous membranes in the nose become drier as the fluid content of body tissue decreases; thus the incoming air is not humidified as effectively. The number of cilia decreases, diminishing the ability of the cilia to trap and remove debris. Decreased vocal cord elasticity leads to changes in voice pitch and quality, and the voice develops a more tremulous character.

Musculoskeletal system changes that occur with aging alter the size and shape of the chest cavity. Kyphosis contributes to a barrel-chested appearance. Costal cartilage located at the ends of the ribs calcifies and becomes more rigid, thus reducing the mobility of the rib cage. Intercostal muscles atrophy, and the diaphragm flattens and becomes less elastic. All of these changes reduce lung capacity and interfere with respiratory function.

Structural changes involving decreases in ciliary movement, in airway and alveoli elasticity, and in the number of capillaries surrounding the alveoli can interfere with gas exchange. In addition, decreased physical mobility and elasticity in the lung tissue itself can lead to increased pooling of secretions, particularly in the lower lung lobes. Taken together, these factors increase the possibility of inadequate oxygenation and the risk of respiratory tract infections in the elderly.

CONDITIONS COMMON WITH AGING

Chronic Obstructive Pulmonary Disease

Chronic obstructive pulmonary disease is not a single disease but a group of three commonly occurring respiratory disorders: asthma, emphysema, and chronic bronchitis. Although they may appear independently, these disorders usually occur in combination. Chronic obstructive pulmonary disease is common in people who have a history of smoking or who have had a high level of exposure to environmental pollutants. In **asthma,** the trachea and bronchioles are extremely sensitive to a variety of physical stimuli and emotional stress that then cause constriction of

---

TABLE 3-3

Respiratory Changes Associated with Aging

Physiologic change	Results
Decreased body fluids	Decreased ability to humidify air
Decreased number of cilia	Decreased ability to trap debris
Decreased tissue elasticity	Decreased gas exchange; increased pooling of secretions in the lower lung lobes
Decreased number of capillaries	Decreased gas exchange
Increased calcification of cartilage	Increased rigidity of rib cage; decreased lung capacity

the bronchial passages and increase mucus production within the airways. This narrows the airways and restricts air flow. **Emphysema** is characterized by changes in the structure of the alveoli. The air sacs lose elasticity, become overinflated, and are ineffective in gas exchange. **Chronic bronchitis** involves inflammation of the trachea and bronchioles. Chronic irritation leads to excessive mucus secretion and a productive cough.

Individuals with chronic obstructive pulmonary disease manifest such symptoms as productive cough, wheezing, cyanosis, and dyspnea on exertion. They are at higher risk of developing respiratory tract infections; in severe cases, respiratory failure can occur.

Influenza

Influenza, often referred to as the "flu," is a highly contagious respiratory infection caused by a wide variety of influenza viruses. Many different strains of influenza have been identified, and new forms are being identified continually. The various forms of influenza, such as the Hong Kong or Beijing flu, are often named for the area where they are first recognized. Epidemics occur at regular intervals and are seen most often in the winter months. The virus is usually spread through airborne droplets and moves quickly through groups of people who live or work in close contact with each other. The incubation period is brief, often only 1 to 3 days from the time of exposure. The onset of symptoms is sudden; symptoms include chills, fever, cough, sore throat, and general malaise and may be dramatic and leave the victim feeling severely ill.

Elderly people are at higher risk for serious complications of influenza than are younger people. More than 90% of deaths due to influenza occur in the over-65 population. Influenza presents a special danger for elderly people with a history of respiratory disease or other debilitating conditions. Yearly "flu shots" are recommended for all persons over 65 years of age to reduce the chance of contracting the most common forms of influenza. Immunizations should be given in the fall so that the level of immunity is high before the risk of exposure occurs.

Some people refuse or are hesitant to take the vaccine because of the mild symptoms that may be experienced after inoculation. It is important to explain to the elderly that these symptoms are mild and will protect them from more severe problems later. Anyone who is allergic to eggs should not receive the vaccine. Influenza vaccine is cultured in egg protein and can cause a serious allergic reaction in allergic individuals. Given properly, these vaccines are 70% to 80% effective in preventing illness.

Pneumonia

Pneumonia is acute inflammation of the lungs caused by bacterial, viral, fungal, chemical, or mechanical agents. In response to the agent, the alveoli and bronchioles become clogged with a thick, fibrous substance that decreases the ability of the lung to exchange gases. Pneumonia can progress to a state in which the exudate fills the lung lobes and they become consolidated or firm. Pneumonia can be detected by radiologic examination. Breath sounds exhibit characteristic changes.

The symptoms of pneumonia differ with the causative organism. Viral pneumonia, sometimes called walking pneumonia, is most commonly seen following influenza or another viral disease. Symptoms include headache, fever, aching muscles, and cough with mucopurulent sputum. Treatment for viral pneumonia varies according to the symptoms.

Bacterial pneumonia can be caused by a number of organisms, most commonly *Staphylococcus, Streptococcus, Klebsiella,* and *Legionella.* The symptoms of bacterial pneumonia are abrupt and dramatic. Chills, fever up to 105° F, tachycardia, and tachypnea are common, as is pain with respiration, or dyspnea. The associated cough may be dry and unproductive or purulent and productive. The color of the sputum is significant and should be observed carefully. The type of microorganism involved can be determined by Gram's stains and sputum culture. Bacterial pneumonia is treated with bacteria-specific antibiotics and supportive medical and nursing care.

Aspiration pneumonia is an inflammatory process of the bronchi and lungs caused by inhalation of foreign substances such as food or acidic gastric contents. The risk of aspiration is highest in elderly people with a poor gag reflex and in those who must remain supine because these individuals can easily inhale or regurgitate food during oral or tube feeding. Aspiration of highly acidic gastric secretions can lead to cell membrane damage with exudation and ultimately to respiratory distress. Aspiration of large amounts of feeding solution is likely to trigger coughing or choking episodes and dyspnea. If these fluids are not removed immediately by suction, respiratory distress and death may result. Aspiration of small amounts of liquid can result in continued and progressive inflammation of the lungs. The person suffering from aspiration pneumonia typically has a fast pulse and respiratory rate. Sputum is frothy but free of bacteria; however, a superimposed bacterial infection may develop.

Tuberculosis

Tuberculosis is an infectious disease caused by the bacillus *Mycobacterium tuberculosis,* which spreads by means of airborne droplets. When an infected person coughs or sneezes, contaminated droplets are released into the air. These droplets are inhaled by other people, the bacillus lodges in their lungs, and the disease spreads. Malnutrition, weakening of the immune system, crowded living conditions, poor sanitation, and the presence of systemic diseases such as diabetes and cancer increase the elderly person's risk of contracting tuberculosis.

The symptoms of tuberculosis include cough, night sweats, fever, dyspnea, chest pain, anorexia, and weight loss. The cough may be nonproductive or productive. Sputum may be green or yellow; with hemoptysis, the presence of blood may impart a rusty color.

Because skin tests for tuberculosis are not reliable in the elderly, diagnosis is based on chest radiography or sputum cultures of acid-fast bacillus. Early detection is important to prevent further spread of the disease.

Treatment today consists of drug therapy using a variety of antimicrobial agents such as isoniazid, rifampin, ethambutol, and streptomycin. A combination of these drugs is usually administered and continued for many months. Many of these drugs are associated with numerous adverse effects, particularly in the elderly. Nursing care of the elderly person with tuberculosis focuses on maintaining good nutrition, monitoring compliance with the medication administration schedule, and detecting side effects.

Lung Cancer

Lung cancer, or bronchogenic cancer, is one of the most deadly forms of cancer in the United States. The age range at which diagnosis of lung cancer peaks is 55 to 65 years. Although lung cancer is more common in men, it has become increasingly common in women and has recently passed breast cancer as a leading cause of death. The survival rate after diagnosis of lung cancer is poor, rarely exceeding 5 years.

Lung cancer results from exposure to **carcinogenic,** or cancer-causing, agents, particularly tobacco smoke, air pollution, asbestos, and other hazardous industrial substances. Cough, chest pain, and blood-tinged sputum are typical symptoms, which can easily be missed because they resemble those of pneumonia and other common respiratory conditions of the elderly.

The treatment of choice is surgical resection of the lungs. This procedure is associated with a high mortality rate in the elderly. Radiation and chemotherapy are used in some patients, with varying amounts of success.

THE CARDIOVASCULAR SYSTEM

The cardiovascular system moves blood throughout the body. This continuous, closed system is responsible for the transportation of blood with oxygen and nutrients to all body tissue. It also transports waste products to the organs that remove them from the body. Through its action, the cardiovascular system helps maintain homeostasis within the body. The heart pumps the blood, and the blood vessels dilate or constrict to aid in the maintenance of blood pressure and exchange of materials between the blood and body tissue.

NORMAL STRUCTURE AND FUNCTION

Heart

The heart is a muscular organ located centrally in the thoracic cavity between the lungs. The **sternum,** or breastbone, protects its anterior surface. The heart's tip, or **apex,** projects toward the left side of the body and extends directly above the diaphragm muscle.

There are three **pericardial membranes** that form a sac around the heart. The innermost membrane is on the surface of the heart and is called the **epicardium,** or **visceral pericardium.** The middle membrane is the **parietal pericardium,** and the outermost membrane is the **fibrous pericardium.** The space between the epicardium and the parietal pericardium is the **pericardial cavity;** it contains a small amount of **serous fluid** that prevents the membrane surfaces from rubbing together during cardiac activity.

The heart, which is composed of cardiac muscle (called **myocardium),** is a hollow organ with four distinct chambers. The right side of the heart consists of the **right atrium** and **right ventricle,** which are separated by the **tricuspid valve.** The right side of the heart is a low-pressure pump that moves deoxygenated blood through the pulmonary valve and pulmonary artery and out to the lungs. After the blood is oxygenated, it returns to the left side of the heart via the **pulmonary vein.** Because less effort is required to move blood the short distance through the lungs of a healthy individual, the muscle wall of the right side of the heart is relatively thin. The left side of the heart also has two chambers, the **left atrium** and **left ventricle,** which are separated by the **mitral valve.** The pressure within the left side of the heart is higher than that in the right side because the left side is responsible for blood distribution to the entire body. Therefore, to provide the necessary force, the left ventricle has a thicker muscle wall than does the right ventricle. When blood leaves the left ventricle, it proceeds through the aortic valve into the **aorta** and its branches and out to the rest of the body.

The heart chambers and valves are lined with **endocardial** tissue. **Endothelial** tissue continues out from the heart and lines all of the blood vessels. This smooth layer allows the blood to flow freely and reduces the risk of clot formation.

Blood Vessels

The **arteries** are blood vessels that carry blood *away* from the heart. With the exception of the pulmonary artery, arteries carry oxygenated blood. The aorta, the largest artery in the body, leaves the heart and branches into a series of progressively smaller arteries and capillaries. These vessels run through the entire body and reach all organs and tissues.

Arterial walls are composed of three layers of tissue. The innermost layer is the **endothelium,** or **tunica intima.** This layer is a continuation of the endocardial tissue that lines the inside of the heart. The middle layer, or **tunica media,** is composed of smooth muscle and connective tissue. This smooth muscle is controlled by the autonomic nervous system and dilates or constricts the artery to maintain the blood pressure. The outermost layer, or **tunica externa,** is composed of strong fibrous tissue that protects the vessels from bursting or rupturing under high pressure. The relative thickness of the tunicae media and externa enables the arteries to perform properly.

The **veins** are vessels that carry blood *toward* the heart. With the exception of the **pulmonary vein,** veins carry deoxygenated blood. **Venules,** the smallest veins, are connected to the smallest capillaries. Veins and venules are composed of the same three layers of tissue seen in arteries. The veins use a system of **valves,** which are created by endothelial tissue folds, to aid in the return of blood to the heart. The valves prevent backflow of blood, which could be a problem when the blood is moving toward the heart against the force of gravity.

The smooth muscle layer of the veins is much thinner than that of the arteries because the veins are not as important in the regulation of blood pressure. The outer fibrous layer is also thinner because blood pressure in the veins is much lower than that in the arteries.

A special set of blood vessels, the **coronary arteries** and **veins,** supplies the heart with blood enriched with oxygen and nutrients. These arteries are the first branches of the ascending aorta. Because the heart

muscle works continuously, it has high oxygen demands. Any condition that obstructs the normal supply of blood to the heart can damage the myocardium. If it is severely deprived of oxygen and nutrients, heart muscle will die. Too much damaged or destroyed tissue will result in cardiovascular system failure and death.

Conduction System

To function effectively, the cardiovascular system must work in a controlled, organized, and rhythmic manner. The heart's rhythm is established by specialized cells within the heart muscle that make up the electric system of the heart. The body's natural pacemaker, the **sinoatrial node,** is a group of specialized cells in the right atrium. Impulses generated in the sinoatrial node travel across the atria to the **atrioventricular node** in the lower interatrial septum. From there they are conducted through the bundle of His, through the right and left bundle branches, through the Purkinje fibers, and finally to the ventricular myocardium. When the cells of the heart's electric system **depolarize,** the myocardium depolarizes and the heart contracts (systole), following which the special cells and the myocardium repolarize as the heart relaxes (diastole). This process alternately empties and fills the chambers, which pump blood through the circulatory system.

NORMAL AGE-RELATED CHANGES

The heart does not atrophy with aging as other muscles do. In fact, the heart muscle mass increases slightly with age and the thickness of the wall of the left ventricle also increases slightly. The increase in muscle mass may occur to offset some loss of tone. The aging heart may function less effectively even when there are no pathologic changes present (Table 3-4). Loss of tone typically leads to the decrease in maximum cardiac output seen in the elderly.

The heart valves show some degree of thickening and increased calcification with aging, resulting in mild degrees of mitral valve regurgitation.

As in other body tissues, the endocardium and endothelium lose elasticity with aging. When these tissues become increasingly fibrous and sclerotic, venous return from the peripheral areas of the body decreases. **Orthostatic hypotension** occurs because the circulation does not respond quickly to postural changes. Less effective pumping of the heart muscle combined with sclerotic changes in the veins can lead to **dependent edema** and to the appearance of **varicosities** in the lower extremities. Weakness of the valves in the rectal veins can lead to hemorrhoids.

TABLE 3-4

Cardiovascular Changes Associated with Aging

Physiologic change	Results
Decreased cardiac muscle tone	Decreased tissue oxygenation
Decreased cardiac output	Increased chance of heart failure; decreased peripheral circulation
Decreased elasticity of heart muscle and blood vessels	Decreased venous return; increased dependent edema; increased incidence of orthostatic hypotension; increased varicosities and hemorrhoids
Increased atherosclerosis	Increased blood pressure

CONDITIONS COMMON WITH AGING

Cardiovascular disease is the leading cause of morbidity and mortality in the United States, accounting for over 75% of all deaths in men and women over 65 years of age.

Coronary Artery Disease

Some degree of coronary artery disease is present in almost all persons over age 70. The coronary arteries supply blood to the heart. If these vessels become narrowed or obstructed because of atherosclerosis, the heart may not receive adequate oxygen and nutrients. Many elderly people have seriously obstructed coronary arteries, yet they remain essentially asymptomatic.

Once circulation to the heart muscle decreases significantly, the amount of oxygen delivered to the heart decreases and ischemia occurs. The pain that may be experienced with ischemia is referred to as **angina pectoris** (literally, chest pain). The symptoms of ischemia do include chest pain or pain radiating down the left arm, but such pain is not always present or recognized in the elderly. Vague gastrointestinal (GI) discomfort or shortness of breath may be reported, or there may be no symptoms at all. People experiencing an angina attack are advised to decrease their activity and rest until the episode passes. Physicians usually prescribe coronary vasodilators such as nitroglycerin, or β-adrenergic–blocking agents for people with ischemic heart disease.

When one or more coronary arteries become totally obstructed by atherosclerosis or embolus, the person is said to have a **myocardial infarction,** or heart attack. The mortality rate from myocardial infarction is four times higher in those over 70 years of age than in younger individuals. Symptoms of a heart attack in the elderly are more variable than in younger people.

Most elderly people are likely to present with symptoms including sudden-onset dyspnea or chest discomfort, confusion, and syncope; diaphoresis is uncommon. Many elderly individuals who have heart attacks die suddenly.

If severe atherosclerotic occlusion of the coronary arteries is detected prior to infarction, angioplasty, stent placement, or coronary bypass surgery may be performed. The age and overall health of the individual are considered before any of these surgical procedures is attempted. Myocardial infarction caused by an embolus that is detected quickly can be treated using thrombolytic agents such as tissue plasminogen activator, but the use of these drugs may increase the risk of stroke.

Total oxygen deprivation results in myocardial tissue necrosis. Cardiac tissue necrosis is irreversible. The types of problems experienced after a myocardial infarction depend on the location and extent of the damage to the heart muscle. Mild damage may not be associated with symptoms and may only be detectable on the electrocardiogram. This type of infarction is often referred to as a "silent heart attack." Moderate damage may limit a person's physical activity. Extensive damage or damage to a critical area of the heart may result in death.

Coronary Valve Disease

The valves of the heart become less pliant over time. In addition, calcium deposits may develop on the valves, preventing them from sealing completely. This can result in mitral valve prolapse, mitral regurgitation, ultimately congestive heart failure. Symptoms of mitral valve prolapse include chest pain, palpitations, fatigue, and dyspnea. Calcium deposits on the valves roughen the lining and increase the risk of clot formation in the chambers of the heart and in the blood vessels.

Cardiac Arrhythmias

Cardiac arrhythmias, including ventricular arrhythmias, atrial fibrillation, and conduction disturbances, are increasingly common with aging.

Heart block is a common conduction disturbance caused by disruption of the electric conduction system of the heart. This disruption can be caused by fibrotic tissue infiltration or myocardial infarction. Sinus node dysfunction, sometimes called "sick sinus syndrome," is the primary conduction disorder seen in the elderly. This condition causes a disturbance in the rate and rhythm of heart contraction, resulting in symptoms such as lightheadedness, fatigue, palpitations, and syncope. When the disturbance is severe, an artificial pacemaker may be used to regulate cardiac activity.

Congestive Heart Failure

Congestive heart failure (CHF) is primarily a problem of the aging population. It is estimated that over 2 million people suffer from this disorder, resulting in almost 1 million hospitalizations each year. The term *congestive heart failure* is descriptive of the disease process: the patient's lungs are often congested, and edema appears because the heart's pumping action is ineffective.

Congestive heart failure is not a single disease but a syndrome that accompanies and results from many other disorders. A variety of cardiovascular diseases can contribute to the development of CHF. Coronary artery disease, myocardial infarction, hypertension, valve disease, and cardiac infection or inflammation increase the risk of CHF. Diseases of other body systems, including bronchitis, emphysema, asthma, hyperthyroidism, liver disease, kidney disease, and anemia, can also lead to CHF. Metabolic changes and fluid and electrolyte imbalances seen with malnutrition can lead to CHF. Excessive sodium intake with fluid retention increases the risk of CHF. The effects of alcohol, digoxin, hormones, some antineoplastics, corticosteroids, and NSAIDs can directly or indirectly lead to CHF.

Congestive heart failure is associated with a wide range of symptoms, depending on the type and severity of the underlying disease. Mild **chronic CHF** tends to have a slow, insidious onset. Older adults who experience mild symptoms such as dyspnea, orthopnea, or paroxysmal nocturnal dyspnea often decrease their activity spontaneously. They may not recognize these symptoms as serious and may attribute them to "slowing down" with aging. Many elderly will not seek medical attention until they have serious problems and are unable to perform even minimal activities (Box 3-1). **Acute CHF** can result in severe pulmonary congestion or cardiogenic shock and is often fatal in the elderly. Chronic CHF can become acute CHF with

---

> **BOX 3-1**
>
> ### Signs and Symptoms of Congestive Heart Failure
>
> 1. Dyspnea (shortness of breath) with exertion
> 2. Orthopnea (dyspnea at rest when recumbant)
> 3. Coughing or wheezing with exertion or at rest
> 4. Fatigue, weakness, or generalized muscle weakness with minimal exertion
> 5. Peripheral edema
> 6. Weight gain without an increase in food intake (as a result of fluid retention)
> 7. Nausea, vomiting, or anorexia
> 8. Paroxysmal nocturnal dyspnea (extreme orthopnea during sleep)

---

increased physical or emotional stress. People with CHF are more susceptible to fluid and electrolyte imbalances, infections, and renal or liver failure.

Medical management of CHF includes dietary restriction of sodium to decrease fluid retention, administration of diuretics (e.g., furosemide) to reduce fluid overload, administration of cardiotonic medications (e.g., digoxin) to increase the pumping efficiency of the heart, and activity restriction to reduce cardiac workload.

Cardiomegaly

Although aging does not routinely affect the size of the heart, many elderly persons do develop **cardiomegaly,** or enlargement of the heart, which is frequently related to CHF. As we age, the muscular wall of the left ventricle thickens. Because arteries and veins lose elasticity with age, the heart must pump harder to move blood through the vessels. The muscles of the left ventricle hypertrophy in an attempt to improve the output of blood from the heart to meet the body's tissue demands for oxygenated blood.

The right side of the heart may also hypertrophy. Right-sided enlargement is a result of increased resistance in the pulmonary circulation. When one side of the heart is weakened, the other side is soon affected.

Peripheral Vascular Disease

Vessel changes with aging can lead to mild or severe problems. In arteriosclerosis, the walls of the arteries become less elastic and plaque forms in the lumen, further restricting blood flow. Excessive plaque is often related to lifestyle factors or to other disease conditions, most commonly obesity, high cholesterol intake, cigarette smoking, and diabetes mellitus (DM). If the lumen becomes too narrow, blood flow to peripheral sites, particularly the lower extremities, may be restricted. This decreased blood flow deprives the tissue of oxygen and nutrients and causes ischemia. If the lumen is completely obstructed, tissue death may result.

An early symptom of arterial occlusive disease is pain. **Intermittent claudication,** which manifests as a cramping pain in the legs during or after walking, is common with diminished peripheral circulation. Severe circulatory impairment can result in tissue necrosis that requires amputation.

Acute occlusion may occur if a thrombus or embolus obstructs the blood vessel. Sudden pain, pallor, pulselessness, loss of sensation, or a change in body temperature should be assessed and reported promptly.

Occlusive Peripheral Vascular Problems

Thrombus formation (clotting) in the lumen of a vein is a common problem, particularly in the immobile elderly. These clots can form quickly because of sluggish blood flow within the vessels. Increasing the patient's activity and using antiembolism stockings will help prevent problems related to venous stasis or pooling.

Thrombi form most frequently in the veins of the lower extremities, where they irritate and inflame the vessel and cause thrombophlebitis. Signs of thrombophlebitis include edema, swelling, warmth over the affected area, aching, cyanosis or pallor, and a positive Homan's sign (pain induced by dorsiflexing the foot of the affected leg).

Medical management of thrombophlebitis typically includes rest, elevation of the affected leg, application of elastic stockings or wraps, analgesics, anticoagulant therapy, and sometimes, application of heat.

If a thrombus breaks loose from the vein and travels in the circulatory system, it is referred to as an **embolus.** Emboli can be life-threatening. They are particularly dangerous if they reach small blood vessels in the lungs or brain, where they can occlude the blood supply to vital tissues.

Varicose Veins

Varicose veins are seen when blood pools in the veins and dilates or stretches them. The decrease in vascular muscle tone that occurs with aging increases the risk of this. Varicosities are most often seen as a twisting discoloration in the superficial veins of the lower extremities. Elderly persons who are obese, inactive, or spend a great deal of time standing are more likely to have varicosities.

Varicosities can result in leg cramps or a dull aching pain in the legs. Related problems can be reduced or prevented by avoiding constricting garments such as garters or rolled stockings, by refraining from sitting with crossed legs, by increasing activity, by resting with the legs elevated, and by wearing elastic stockings that promote venous return.

Aneurysm

Aneurysm, the pouching or ballooning of arteries, is common in elderly persons who suffer from arteriosclerotic blood vessel changes. Elderly people with a history of angina, myocardial infarction, or CHF are at increased risk of developing aneurysms. As parts of the muscular walls of the arteries develop plaque and become rigid, other areas of the vessels stretch, dilate, and weaken. The walls of the dilated areas become thin and prone to rupture.

Aneurysms of the abdominal aorta are most common in the elderly. These are sometimes observed as a pulsating mass near the umbilicus, or navel. Patients may have abdominal pain and GI complaints. Aneurysms can also develop in peripheral and cerebral blood vessels. Thrombi can form in aneurysms and block the flow of blood. Rupture of an aneurysm results in massive, life-threatening hemorrhage. Early detection and surgical repair of the damaged area provide the best chance for survival.

Hypertensive Disease

Hypertension is prevalent in the elderly population. It is estimated that more than 50% of the population over 65 years of age has some form of hypertensive disorder.

Hypertension is categorized as **essential** (primary) or **secondary.** Essential hypertension, the more common form, has no known cause. Many factors, including heredity, diet, obesity, stress, smoking, increased serum cholesterol levels, and abnormal sodium transport, are known to contribute to essential hypertension. Secondary hypertension occurs as a result of a coexisting disease process or other known cause. Renal, vascular, and endocrine pathologies are among the most common causes of secondary hypertension.

Essential hypertension tends to have a gradual onset and is often asymptomatic until complications arise. Most often, hypertension is discovered during a routine physical examination. It is diagnosed on the basis of two elevated blood pressure determinations on 3 separate days. A reading of 140/90 is considered the upper limit of normal in adults, but some physicians consider slightly higher readings normal in adults over 60 years of age.

Essential hypertension cannot be cured, but it can

be treated. Treatment includes nonpharmacologic approaches such as rest, smoking cessation, use of stress reduction techniques, weight loss, and dietary sodium restriction. Pharmacologic approaches typically include administration of oral diuretics and β blockers. The person experiencing hypertension must be monitored continuously to determine the effectiveness of therapy. Treatment of secondary hypertension is directed at the underlying pathology.

THE HEMATOPOIETIC AND LYMPH SYSTEMS

Body fluids distribute essential protective factors, nutrients, oxygen, and electrolytes throughout the body. The two major fluids of the body are lymph and blood. These fluids flow through the body within two parallel circulatory systems.

NORMAL STRUCTURE AND FUNCTION

Blood

Blood flows within the heart and vessels of the cardiovascular system. The general functions of blood include **transportation** of nutrients, waste products, blood gases, and hormones; regulation of fluid-electrolyte balance, acid-base balance, and body temperature; and **protection** against pathogenic attack by the WBCs, and against excessive blood loss through clotting mechanisms.

Blood is 91% to 92% liquid; the remaining 8% to 9% is solid. The liquid of the blood is called **plasma.** As a liquid, plasma is a substance in which many other substances can dissolve and be transported, including nutrients (e.g., glucose, amino acids, lipids), electrolytes (e.g., sodium, potassium, calcium, chloride), hormones, vitamins, antibodies, and waste products. Carbon dioxide is carried in the plasma as bicarbonate ion. Plasma contains a variety of proteins. **Albumin,** the most abundant plasma protein, is important in the maintenance of **osmotic pressure** needed to regulate blood pressure and volume. In the **fibrinogen** component are prothrombin, fibrinogen itself, and other clotting factors that circulate until they are required by the body. **Globulins** function as transport agents for lipids and fat-soluble vitamins; the γ-globulin fraction is composed of antibodies that provide immunity from pathogens.

The solid portion of the blood is composed of three types of blood cells: RBCs, WBCs, and platelets.

Erythrocytes

Erythrocytes, or RBCs, live for about 120 days; therefore, the body produces new RBCs throughout life. They are formed in the red bone marrow by **stem cells,** which undergo mitosis. For mitosis to occur, and thus for RBCs to form, vitamin B_{12} and folic acid are necessary for DNA synthesis. For maturation, the RBCs need adequate amounts of protein and iron.

When RBCs become old and fragile, they are removed from the circulation by the **reticuloendothelial cells** of the spleen, liver, and red bone marrow. Their iron is reused in new RBCs formed by the red marrow. Excess iron is stored in the liver for later use. The **heme** portion of the RBC is converted to bilirubin in the reticuloendothelial system and is then processed by the liver. The liver secretes the bilirubin, or **bile pigment,** with the other components of bile into the duodenum for use in digestion. This bile pigment helps give stool its characteristic brown color. If excessive numbers of RBCs are destroyed or if the liver does not function adequately, excessive amounts of bilirubin remain in the circulation. High bilirubin levels result in jaundice, a yellow discoloration of the sclera of the eyes and of the skin of light-skinned individuals.

Leukocytes

Leukocytes, or WBCs, have protective functions: they destroy dead or damaged tissue, detoxify foreign proteins, protect from infectious disease, and function in the immune response. WBCs are produced in the lymphatic tissue of the spleen, lymph nodes, thymus, and red bone marrow. The five types of WBCs are **neutrophils, eosinophils, basophils, lymphocytes,** and **monocytes.**

Platelets

Platelets, more properly called **thrombocytes,** are not whole cells but pieces of cells. They are produced when large cells called **megakaryocytes** fragment and enter the circulation. Platelets, which remain in circulation for approximately 10 days, play an important role in the blood's clotting mechanism.

The Lymph System

The lymph and circulatory systems are parallel and interdependent. In fact, the lymph system is sometimes considered part of the circulatory system because it is responsible for returning fluids from the tissues to the circulation. The major components of the immune system—lymphocytes and antibodies—are formed by the lymph system to protect the body from pathogenic microorganisms, malignant cells, and foreign proteins. The lymph system consists of the lymph vessels, fluid, nodes, and nodules; the spleen; and the thymus gland.

Lymph Fluid, Vessels, and Nodes

Lymph vessels are located in most tissue spaces. These very permeable vessels absorb fluid and proteins from the tissues. Muscular compression on the vessels moves this fluid through a series of lymph nodes and nodules that trap and phagocytize foreign materials before the fluid enters the circulatory system at the subclavian veins. Lymph nodes and nodules also produce lymphocytes and monocytes and phagocytize pathogens.

Spleen and Thymus

The spleen is responsible for producing lymphocytes and monocytes, which enter the bloodstream. It also contains fixed **plasma cells,** which produce antibodies to foreign antigens, and fixed macrophages, which phagocytize pathogens and other foreign substances in the blood. Although people can survive without a spleen, they may be more susceptible to certain bacterial infections, including pneumonia.

The thymus, which is located behind the thyroid gland, is large in fetuses and infants. The embryonic bone marrow and the spleen produce the initial **T lymphocytes,** or T cells, which are responsible for recognition of foreign antigens and for cell-mediated immunity. The thymus shrinks with age, but once the T cells are established in the spleen and lymph nodes they are self-perpetuating.

Lymphocytes and Immunity

B lymphocytes, or B cells, are also produced in embryonic bone marrow. These cells are responsible for the recognition of antigens located on a foreign cell and for humoral immunity. In humoral immunity, T cells and B cells often cooperate: Sensitive **helper T cells** detect antigens and induce the B cells to produce antibodies, which are then found in the globulin portion of plasma. When the antigen has been destroyed, **suppressor T cells** reduce helper T-cell activity and stop the immune process. Conversely, in cell-mediated immunity, antibodies are not produced. Instead, activated T cells divide into memory T cells (which recognize the pathogen) and killer T cells (which destroy bacteria by disrupting their cell membranes).

NORMAL AGE-RELATED CHANGES

The characteristics of blood change somewhat as a person ages (Table 3-5). Plasma viscosity increases

---

TABLE 3-5

Hematopoietic and Lymph Changes Associated with Aging

Physiologic change	Results
Increased plasma viscosity	Increased risk of vascular occlusion
Decreased red blood cell production	Increased incidence of anemia
Increased immature T cells	Decreased immune response

---

slightly and is most often related to a general decrease in total body fluid. Blood cell production in the bone marrow decreases slightly, resulting in a small decrease in total RBCs and WBCs. Unless extreme physiologic stress or disease is present, blood levels of RBCs, WBCs, and platelets remain within normal limits.

The number of T cells in the body does not appear to decrease with aging, but more of the cells are immature. The ratio of helper cells to suppressor cells is increased. These T-cell changes lead to a diminished immune response. Consequently, older adults are at greater risk for developing infections, particularly respiratory and urinary tract infections. Elderly individuals are also at increased risk of acquiring nosocomial infections. Studies have shown that women over 55 years of age have limited antibody titers to tetanus toxoid, raising questions about changes in humoral immunity with aging. If the ability to produce antibodies is affected by aging, changes in immunization practices for the aging population may be necessary.

Changes in the immune response may modify the usual signs and symptoms of infection. Such changes may be difficult to recognize in older adults: Body temperature may not become significantly elevated until the infection is severe, and pain may not be present to indicate infection. Some examples include the following: (1) older adults with pneumonia may not have a fever or chills; (2) dysuria is often absent in elderly people with urinary tract infections; (3) pain may be absent with peritonitis or appendicitis, even though the individual is obviously ill; (4) the physiologic response of the elderly to tuberculosis skin testing may be delayed or less intense than that of younger individuals.

CONDITIONS COMMON WITH AGING

Anemia

Anemia is defined as inadequate levels of RBCs or insufficient hemoglobin. The most commonly observed anemias in older adults are iron deficiency anemia, pernicious anemia, and folic acid deficiency anemia.

Iron deficiency anemia result from inadequate nutritional intake, blood loss, malabsorption, or increased physiologic demand. Pernicious anemia is associated with decreased intake or absorption of vitamin B_{12}. Folic acid deficiency anemia is usually caused by poor nutrition, chronic alcohol abuse, or malabsorption syndromes such as Crohn's disease. Anemia is common in the elderly population, and these problems are explored further in other chapters.

Leukemia

Leukemia is the result of excessive production of immature WBCs. There are both acute and chronic varieties, and leukemia is also classified by the type of abnormal cells present. Other blood disorders (e.g., anemia) and hemorrhage (related to a decrease in the number or function of platelets) are commonly seen with leukemia. **Chronic lymphocytic leukemia** is the form most often seen in older persons. About 75% of those diagnosed with chronic lymphocytic leukemia are over age 60. Depending on the stage of the disease and the patient's overall health, life expectancy may vary from a few to as many as 20 years after diagnosis.

THE GASTROINTESTINAL SYSTEM

Food and fluids containing the nutrients needed for survival normally enter the body through the GI tract. Although it is possible to live without food for several days, the cells require a regular supply of nutrients to support their normal physiologic activities.

As appealing as a banana split, turkey dinner, or bowl of strawberries may be to us, these foods are useless to our cells until they are broken down into simple, usable forms by the GI system. The GI tract prepares food for digestion. It then digests, processes, and absorbs the nutrients, which are used by the cells of the body. The GI system also stores and discards wastes and plays a major role in maintaining fluid balance by absorbing water. After we chew and swallow food, we do not need to think about its further processing because the GI system takes care of removing the nutrients and discarding the waste. In unusual situations, however, the GI tract can be bypassed by administering specially prepared nutrients directly into the bloodstream (parenteral nutrition, or hyperalimentation).

NORMAL STRUCTURE AND FUNCTION

The GI tract begins at the mouth and ends at the anus. Each part of the GI tract performs its own distinct functions.

Oral Cavity

Food normally enters the body through the **mouth** and is prepared for digestion in the **oral cavity.** The teeth mechanically process food by biting, tearing, grinding, and chewing it, a process called **mastication.** The normal adult has 28 to 32 permanent teeth with shapes and sizes that vary depending on their function. The **incisors** are used to bite, the **canines** to tear, and the **premolars** and **molars** to chew and grind. Each tooth is composed of a crown, which is the part visible above the gingiva (gum), and a **root,** which is imbedded in a socket in either the mandible or maxilla of the jaw. The periodontal membrane lines the tooth socket and holds the teeth in place. The crown of the tooth is protected by an extremely hard casing called **enamel.** The **pulp cavity** of the tooth contains blood vessels and nerve endings.

Tongue

The tongue is a highly flexible structure controlled by and composed primarily of skeletal muscle. **Papillae,** which contain the taste buds, are located on the upper surface of the tongue. Cranial nerves control the movement of the tongue and carry the impulses for the perception of taste. The tongue aids in mechanical digestion by positioning food between the teeth and by mixing it with saliva in the oral cavity.

Salivary Glands

Three pairs of **salivary glands** excrete **saliva** into the oral cavity. Saliva is composed primarily of water but also contains the enzyme **amylase,** which begins the digestion of starch. Saliva production normally increases in response to the sight or smell of food. Inadequate amounts of saliva result in a dry mouth and in difficult swallowing. When adequately mixed with saliva, food reaches a consistency that makes it more suitable for chemical digestion.

The tongue lifts against the hard palate, pushing the bolus of food to the pharynx at the back of the oral cavity. From here the bolus of food enters the esophagus.

Esophagus

Once in the **esophagus,** food is moved by a process called peristalsis, a wavelike motion of the smooth musculature that propels material through the entire GI tract. The esophagus is a hollow muscular tube that passes from the pharynx through the flat layer of diaphragm muscle and to the stomach. The esophagus is located above the diaphragm, and the stomach is located immediately below the diaphragm. The lower esophageal sphincter, also called the cardiac sphincter, is at approximately the same level as the diaphragm where the esophagus meets the stomach. It allows food to enter the stomach but prevents the stomach contents from moving backward (refluxing) into the esophagus.

Stomach

The **stomach** is a muscular sac in which both mechanical and chemical digestion take place. The stomach is lined with mucous membrane, which helps prevent damage to the muscle walls. Special stomach glands secrete mucus; others secrete enzymes, intrinsic factor, and hydrochloric acid. This mixture of enzymes and acids is called **gastric juice,** or **digestive juice.** The pyloric sphincter at the distal end of the stomach retains the bolus of food and the digestive juices within the stomach, where they can be churned, mixed, and further broken down for later digestion and absorption. Once the food has been processed in the stomach, it is referred to as **chyme.** After adequate mixing, small amounts of chyme are released through the pyloric sphincter into the small intestine.

Small Intestine

The **small intestine** is more than 20 feet long and is divided into three segments called the **duodenum,** the **jejunum,** and the **ileum** (in order of progression away from the stomach).

Additional substances are added to chyme in the small intestine to complete digestion. Intestinal digestive glands secrete intestinal juice, which is alkaline and contains many enzymes. The common bile duct and pancreatic duct converge and enter the duodenum at the sphincter of Oddi. **Bile,** which is produced in the liver and stored in the gall bladder, breaks down fat by **emulsifying** it. **Pancreatic juice** contains enzymes that break down proteins. The pancreas also

produces sodium bicarbonate; when released into the duodenum, it neutralizes the hydrochloric acid from the stomach. After all of these chemicals have acted on the material in the GI tract, the process of digestion is completed, and the nutrients are in elementary forms (e.g., glucose and amino acids) that can be used by the cells of the body.

Absorption of nutrients occurs primarily in the small intestine. Special **villi,** projections of the lining of the small intestine that are rich in capillaries and lymphatic vessels, increase the surface area of the lining. As the digested nutrients pass over these villi, they are absorbed into the blood and lymph by the capillary network and lymphatics.

Once the nutrients have been absorbed, undigested material and water are propelled into the large intestine by peristalsis. A structure called the **ileocecal valve** is located between the ileum of the small intestine and the cecum of the large intestine. This structure prevents waste products from moving backward into the small intestine.

Large Intestine

The **large intestine** is approximately 5 feet long and is divided into segments called the **ascending, transverse, descending,** and **sigmoid colon** and the rectum. The major functions of the large intestine are absorption of water, minerals, and vitamins, and storage and elimination of indigestible wastes.

As the **effluent,** or waste products, moves through the large intestine, water is absorbed and the mass becomes increasingly solid in consistency. It is stored in the sigmoid and descending colon. When peristalsis causes the effluent to enter the rectum, its presence there triggers the defecation reflex, in which strong peristaltic movements propel the mass from the rectum and through the anus. Another reflexlike action occurs when the stomach is distended with food, stimulating vigorous peristalsis of the rectum and a desire to defecate. The internal anal sphincter is an involuntary muscle that relaxes when the rectum is full. The external anal sphincter, which is usually under voluntary control after 2 to 3 years of age, may be contracted to prevent defecation. When the external sphincter relaxes, wastes are eliminated from the large intestine.

NORMAL AGE-RELATED CHANGES

Over time, changes in the GI tract can interfere with normal digestion (Table 3-6). In the oral cavity, gingival tissue may recede and the periodontal bonds that hold the teeth in place may loosen. If the teeth are not structurally sound, the ability to bite and chew can be impaired. Good oral hygiene can slow these changes.

TABLE 3-6

Gastrointestinal Changes Associated with Aging

Physiologic change	Results
Increased dental caries and tooth loss	Decreased ability to chew normally; decreased nutritional status
Decreased gag reflex	Increased incidence of choking and aspiration
Decreased muscle tone at the sphincters	Increased incidence of heartburn (esophageal reflux)
Decreased gastric secretions	Decreased digestion
Decreased peristalsis	Increased constipation and bowel impaction

---

It is no longer considered normal for elderly people to lose some or all of their teeth, which was common in the past.

Dental caries (cavities) can soften the enamel and expose nerves in the tooth pulp. The resulting pain can decrease the ability and the desire to eat.

Esophageal dilation and problems related to swallowing may be observed with aging. Commonly, the **gag reflex** is depressed in older adults, even in those without neurologic problems. This can lead to episodes of choking and to aspiration. The tone of sphincter muscles, particularly the cardiac sphincter, may decrease, possibly resulting in frequent esophageal reflux or heartburn.

In the stomach, atrophy of the gastric glands may result in decreased production of intrinsic factor and hydrochloric acid; this in turn can interfere with normal digestion and can also contribute to anemia. Peristalsis of the intestine slows with aging, increasing the likelihood of constipation and incomplete elimination of feces during a single bowel movement.

CONDITIONS COMMON WITH AGING

Hiatal Hernia

A **hiatal hernia** is the protrusion of the stomach into the thoracic cavity through the esophageal opening in the diaphragm (Fig. 3-8). Men over 50 years of age are most likely to experience problems with hiatal hernias, and as many as 40% to 60% of those 60 years of age or older may be affected. Some demonstrate no symptoms; others complain of severe distress that may be intermittent or continuous. Reflux episodes usually occur after meals, especially when the person lies down to rest immediately after eating. Complaints may include sour stomach, heartburn, or generalized epigastric distress. Sometimes the symptoms can resemble an angina attack. As mentioned, hiatal problems are most likely to occur after meals or when the

person is at rest; in contrast, angina attacks are most likely to occur with physical exertion. Vital signs do not normally change in response to problems with hiatal hernias.

Gastroesophageal reflux disease is a major problem that can occur with hiatal hernias. With gastroesophageal reflux disease the gastric contents move backward into the esophagus where they increase the risk of aspiration. This can present serious concerns in elderly persons who have diminished gag or cough reflexes. Occasionally the hernia through the diaphragm is reduced surgically, but typical treatment involves the use of antacids and dietary modifications. Fatty foods, carbonated beverages, alcohol, and foods that contain caffeine or caffeine-like substances (e.g., coffee, cola, chocolate) should be avoided to reduce problems with reflux. Smaller, more frequent meals are often beneficial because overeating is likely to enlarge the stomach and cause it to bulge into the diaphragm. It is recommended that food and fluids be restricted after the normal evening meal, and affected persons should avoid lying down too soon after eating. In severe cases, the head of the bed may need to be elevated during sleep to reduce the risk of aspiration.

Gastritis and Ulcers

Chronic atrophic gastritis is an inflammatory change in the mucous membranes of the stomach in which the mucosa becomes thin and abnormally smooth and may develop hemorrhagic patches. All or parts of the stomach may be involved.

Both **gastric** and **duodenal ulcers** can occur with aging, but gastric ulcers are more common. Many factors contribute to the development of gastric ulcers. Behavior such as smoking or alcohol ingestion, physical trauma such as surgery or fractures, disease processes such as pneumonia, and psychologic stress due to hospitalization or nursing home placement can increase the risk of ulcers. A bacteria, *Heliobactor pylori*, has been implicated as the cause of some gastric ulcers. Drug-induced ulcers related to the use of iron

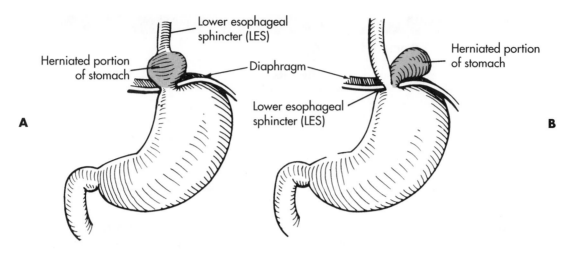

Fig. 3-8   Hiatal hernia. **A,** Sliding hernia. **B,** Paraesophageal hernia. (From Phipps WJ, et al: *Medical-surgical nursing: concepts and clinical practice,* ed 5, St Louis, 1995, Mosby.)

supplements, aspirin, and NSAIDs, are particularly common in the elderly.

Peptic ulcers in the elderly do not cause the classic epigastric pain that is seen in younger people. Elderly persons suffering from ulcers are more likely to complain of generalized pain and to exhibit a decreased activity level, decreased appetite, and weight loss. Vomiting, melena, and generalized signs of anemia may result from gastric bleeding. If a gastric ulcer progresses to the point of perforation, severe hemorrhage can result. If the person has already been weakened by occult bleeding, hemorrhage may be serious enough to result in death.

Early recognition and reporting of symptoms by the nurse is important so that treatment can be started before serious problems occur. Medical treatment of ulcers in the elderly is generally preferred to surgical correction (Box 3-2).

Diverticulosis/Diverticulitis

Diverticula are small pouches or sacs that develop because of weaknesses in the intestinal mucosa. Thirty percent to forty percent of persons over age 50 have some diverticula, and the incidence of diverticulosis increases with each decade of life. Most people with diverticula experience no symptoms, and there is no specific treatment unless symptoms occur. The patient should continue to eat a normal diet with adequate fluids and roughage. If rectal bleeding occurs, medical intervention is necessary to determine the source.

Diverticulitis involves inflammation of one or more diverticula. This inflammation may result in bowel obstruction, perforation, or abscess formation. In cases of severe diverticulitis, the patient may need to be hos-

---

BOX 3-2

Medical Treatment of Ulcers

- Dietary modifications, including avoidance of alcohol, caffeine, and other suspect foods that tend to irritate the problem or increase hydrochloric acid production
- Avoidance of tobacco, which stimulates acid release
- Administration of antacids to reduce acidity
- Administration of histamine (H_2)-blocking agents, such as cimetidine and ranitidine, to prevent ulcer formation or to promote ulcer healing
- Stress reduction programs

---

pitalized. Oral intake of food is restricted and intravenous fluids are administered to give the diseased area an opportunity to "rest." Surgical correction, including bowel resection or colostomy, may be required if conservative medical treatment is unsuccessful.

Cancer

The incidence of **colon cancer** begins to increase at 40 years of age and peaks between the ages of 60 and 75. Carcinoma of the colon is more common in women, whereas carcinoma of the rectum is more common in men. Any changes in bowel elimination should be viewed with suspicion, especially signs of obstruction or bleeding. Routine screening for rectal cancer is recommended for those older than 40 years of age.

Hemorrhoids

Hemorrhoids, sometimes called **piles** by the elderly, are common at all ages, but may be particularly troublesome to the elderly patient. People with chronic constipation and obese people are most likely to have problems with hemorrhoids. Pain and small amounts of bright red blood at the rectum are common complaints. Most patients with hemorrhoids do not require surgery. Diet changes, stool softeners, or bulk laxatives are usually effective in reducing problems related to constipation and hemorrhoids.

Rectal Prolapse

Bulging of the rectum through the anus is most likely to occur in women over age 60, especially those who have given birth to many children. Some form of medical intervention may be needed if this condition causes distress. Surgery may be performed to strengthen the musculature. Insertion of a wire loop at the anal sphincter may be attempted in very old people.

THE URINARY SYSTEM

The urinary system consists of two kidneys, two ureters, the urinary bladder, and the urethra. The urinary system supports homeostasis by eliminating wastes and excessive fluid from the body. The kidneys continuously filter the blood and selectively save or eliminate water, electrolytes, and wastes. Those substances not reabsorbed by the kidneys are eliminated from the body as urine.

NORMAL STRUCTURE AND FUNCTION

Kidneys

The kidneys are two bean-shaped organs located on each side of the spine behind the peritoneal lining of the abdomen and at the lower edge of the ribcage. The left kidney is usually located slightly higher than the right kidney. Each kidney is surrounded by an adipose tissue pad and is further protected from trauma by the muscles of the back. Within each kidney is a maze of nearly a million **nephrons,** the functional portion of the kidney. Blood is filtered in the glomerulus of the nephron, and this filtrate is destined to become urine. This highly vascular organ receives blood from the renal artery, which branches off of the abdominal aorta.

Blood returns to the circulation through the renal vein, which connects to the inferior vena cava. Adequate blood flow to the kidneys is very important; any condition that decreases renal blood flow will interfere with normal kidney function.

The kidneys play an important role in fluid and electrolyte balance and acid-base balance in the body. They remove nitrogenous wastes, excess glucose, and the drug metabolites from the bloodstream. They also help to regulate blood pressure. The kidneys typically produce between 1 and 2 L of urine every 24 hours. If excessive fluid is lost elsewhere (e.g., in perspiration or diarrhea), urine output normally decreases. Excessive fluid or alcohol intake tends to increase urine production. A single kidney can meet the needs of the entire body.

Ureters and Bladder

The **ureters** are tubes of smooth muscle that allow urine to drain from each kidney into the bladder. When the body is upright, urine drains by means of gravity. Pressure of the enlarging bladder against the lower portion of the ureter keeps the ureter closed and prevents urine from flowing back toward the kidneys.

The **bladder** is a hollow muscular sac located below the peritoneum and normally entirely within the pelvic cavity. The bones of the pelvis protect the bladder from trauma. In women, the bladder is located anterior to the uterus; in men it is superior to the prostate gland.

The muscular walls of the bladder are lined with mucous membrane and are capable of stretching to hold large volumes of urine (up to 1000 ml or more). Urine is retained in the bladder by means of the sphincter muscles. The **internal sphincter** is located at the outlet from the bladder into the urethra. Control of the internal sphincter is involuntary. The **external urethral sphincter** comes under voluntary control at about 2 to 3 years of age. Voluntary contraction of the external sphincter prevents urine from leaving the body. Relaxation of the external sphincter allows urine to drain from the body. Voluntary control of urination may be overcome if the bladder becomes overly enlarged with urine. In adults the urge to urinate typically occurs when urine volume in the bladder reaches approximately 200 to 400 ml.

The urethra is a tubelike passage that leads from the bladder to the outside of the body. At the point of exit, it is referred to as the urinary meatus. The female urethra is 1 to 1.5 inches long; the male urethra is 7 to 8 inches long. The urethra is part of the reproductive system in men and is used to transport semen as well as urine; however, ejaculation and urination cannot take place at the same time. The prostate gland surrounds the urethra. Although this normally causes no problems, an enlarged prostate can interfere with urination.

Characteristics of Urine

Urine is approximately 95% water, with the remainder composed of waste products and salts. The specific gravity (which measures the amount of solids dissolved in water) of urine is normally maintained within very close limits. A specific gravity of 1.010 to 1.025 is considered normal. Dilute urine will have a low specific gravity, concentrated urine will have a high specific gravity. Urine is normally clear, and its color ranges from pale yellow to dark amber. It may be alkaline or acidic, depending on the diet of the individual. High-protein diets tend to make the urine more acidic; vegetarian diets tend to lead to alkaline urine, which is more susceptible to infection.

NORMAL AGE-RELATED CHANGES

The kidneys lose approximately one third of their efficiency by age 70 but usually are able to remove wastes adequately to maintain normal blood levels. As a person ages (Table 3-7), the number of functional units or nephrons decreases. In addition, the kidneys lose mass and decrease in size. Vascular changes, such as those which occur with atherosclerosis or arteriosclerosis, lead to decreased blood supply to the kidneys. Decreased blood flow results in an altered **glomerular filtration rate.** At 90 years of age the glomerular filtration rate can be as little as half of what it was at age 20. The **blood urea nitrogen** remaining in the blood increases markedly with age, from a normal of 10 to 15 mg/dl in young adulthood to 21 mg/dl by age 70.

The nephrons and collecting system of the aging body are less sensitive to the effects of antidiuretic hormone. Less sodium and water are reabsorbed and more potassium is lost, resulting in the production of less concentrated urine with aging.

Aging results in reduced urinary bladder size, which leads to decreased **bladder capacity,** the volume of urine the bladder can hold before a person experiences the urge to void. Many elderly people need to void when only 100 ml of urine is present. In addition, overactivity of the detrusor muscle can result in contraction of the bladder before the bladder is full. Either or both of these factors can lead to the urinary urgency and frequency that is common in older adults. To further aggravate the situation, loss of muscle tone can impair voluntary control of the external sphincter muscle. Atonic muscular changes may also occur in the wall of the bladder. Loss of tone may result in reduced urinary stream, incomplete or unsuccessful voiding, continuous dribbling of urine, or urinary retention with overflow voiding (a condition in which the person voids frequently but never completely empties the bladder).

Urinary retention contributes to the risk for urinary tract infections, especially in the elderly, because retained urine is a good medium for bacterial growth.

The prostate gland enlarges with age. Most men over 60 years of age experience some degree of prostate gland enlargement due to **benign prostatic hyperplasia** or cancer. Because it surrounds the urethra, an enlarged prostate gland can compress and narrow the passageway, which in turn causes problems with voiding. Hesitancy, frequency, the inability to maintain a steady stream of urine, and urinary retention are common indicators of prostatic hypertrophy.

CONDITIONS COMMON WITH AGING

Urinary Incontinence

Urinary incontinence, the involuntary loss of urine, is not a routine or normal occurrence with aging. Incontinence may occur as a result of physiologic changes, other medical problems such as a urinary tract infections, neurologic problems, or changes in the ability

---

TABLE 3-7

Urinary Changes Associated with Aging

Physiologic change	Results
Decreased number of functional nephrons	Decreased filtration rate
Decreased blood supply	Decreased removal of body wastes; increased concentration of urine
Decreased muscle tone	Increased volume of residual urine
Decreased tissue elasticity	Decreased bladder capacity
Increased size of prostate	Increased risk of infection; decreased stream of urine; increased hesitancy and frequency of urination

to function. Several classifications of medication can contribute to incontinence. Urinary incontinence will be discussed in greater detail in Chapter 12.

Urinary Tract Infection

The incidence of urinary tract infections increases significantly with age. Only 3% of women in their forties experience urinary tract infections, whereas close to 15% experience them by age 60. Men also develop urinary tract infections, but they are less common in men and develop at older ages.

Both the normal changes of aging and the increased incidence of health problems contribute to this increased incidence of urinary tract infections (Box 3-3).

Chronic Renal Failure

An increasing number of people over 70 years of age are being treated with dialysis for chronic renal failure. This was an age-restricted treatment in the past; today, however, many older adults receive life-prolonging hemodialysis or peritoneal dialysis depending on their needs and their physicians' judgment.

Chronic renal failure may be a result of other chronic health conditions such as hypertension, diabetes mellitus, chronic urinary tract infections, or urinary tract obstructions. It may also result from acute renal failure caused by hypovolemia, hypotension, or antibiotic toxicity.

The symptoms of chronic renal failure are extensive and often mimic those of other conditions. These symptoms include changes in urine output; muscle weakness; edema; nausea and vomiting; itchy and dry skin; and numerous neurologic symptoms. Blood tests reveal significant changes, particularly elevated levels of blood urea nitrogen and creatinine.

BOX 3-3

Risk Factors for Urinary Tract Infections

- Inadequate or improper hygiene related to difficulty in cleansing after toileting
- Urinary stasis and incomplete emptying of bladder due to physiologic changes and decreased mobility
- Coexisting diseases such as diabetes, hypertension, stroke, and dementia
- Medical interventions, including catheterization and repeated use of antibiotics (which can lead to resistant strains of bacteria)
- Increased exposure to microorganisms in hospitals or extended-care facilities

---

THE NERVOUS SYSTEM

The nervous system processes and controls body functions and links us with the outside world. Through our nervous systems we perceive sensations and detect changes in our environment. We store information about the world within our nervous systems and use this information to respond to the world. A functioning nervous system is necessary for survival. Internally, the nervous system and the endocrine system maintain homeostasis.

Many of the functions of the nervous system (e.g., regulation of heart beat or body temperature) occur at an unconscious level. Other activities, such as writing, working with tools, or singing, can be done only with conscious thought and effort. Some activities, such as breathing, occur unconsciously but can also be consciously controlled. The nervous system functions at an unconscious or reflex level at birth; neurologic control is gained with maturation. With advanced age the nervous system becomes prone to deterioration and is susceptible to many types of injury and illness. Because of the serious consequences of age-related neurologic problems, it is important to examine this system in greater detail.

The nervous system is composed of highly specialized cells called **neurons.** Each neuron consists of a **cell body,** which contains the cell nucleus; multiple **dendrites,** which are fibers that transmit impulses (messages) to the cell body; and one **axon,** which carries impulses away from the cell body.

Nerve impulses are electrochemical in nature. An impulse travels through the neuron by fast-moving ion shifts across progressive segments of the cell membrane until it reaches the end of the axon. Axons and dendrites do not touch each other. A small gap called a **synapse** separates these structures. Special chemicals called **neurotransmitters** are released by the axon to stimulate a **receptor site** on another nerve cell. This allows the nerve impulse to move from one nerve cell to another. When the receptor has been stimulated, the neurotransmitter activity is halted by an inactivating chemical that stops prolonged transmission of impulses. In the peripheral nervous system, the most common neurotransmitters are **acetylcholine** and norepinephrine. In the central nervous system, dopamine, serotonin, and **norepinephrine** are important. Each neurotransmitter has a specific inactivator.

The nervous system consists of two major divisions: the central nervous system and the peripheral nervous system.

NORMAL STRUCTURE AND FUNCTION

Central Nervous System

The **central nervous system** is composed of the **brain** and the spinal cord. The brain is the master integrator of the nervous system. Thought, decision making, behavior, and all life processes are controlled by the various segments of the brain.

Medulla

The **medulla oblongata** extends from the spinal column to the pons of the brain. This area controls many vital functions, including heart rate, constriction of blood vessels (which affects blood pressure), and respiration. Reflex centers for coughing, vomiting, swallowing, and sneezing are also located in this area. Severe trauma to this area of the brain is life-threatening.

Pons and Midbrain

The **pons** also exerts control over respiratory patterns and works with the medulla to regulate breathing rhythm. The **midbrain** integrates visual and auditory reflexes and helps maintain balance and equilibrium.

Cerebellum

The **cerebellum** works to coordinate body movement at an unconscious level. It allows excitation of muscles by neurons higher in the brain while it inhibits unnecessary impulses; thus it enables smooth movements without jerkiness. Picking up a cup of coffee and bringing it to your mouth in a coordinated way is an example of the activity of the cerebellum. If you had to think consciously of all of the individual movements to accomplish this activity, the coffee would be cold before you could drink it.

Hypothalamus

The **hypothalamus,** a small area of the brain above the pituitary gland, is the coordinating center for the autonomic nervous system. It also secretes releasing and inhibiting hormones that affect the secretions of the pituitary gland (such as growth hormone–releasing factor) and thus results in various effects on the endocrine system. Other hormones are produced in the hypothalamus, move to the pituitary, and are released by that gland, including antidiuretic hormone and oxytocin. The hypothalamus regulates body temperature, controls food intake, and is involved with visceral responses such as the increased heart rate that occurs with anger.

Cerebrum

The cerebrum is the largest part of the human brain. It is divided into lobes, which are named according to the cranial bones they lie under. Because of the manner in which nerve impulses are routed in the central nervous system, the left lobes control the right side of the body and the right lobes control the left side of the body—they function **contralaterally.** The **frontal lobes** control voluntary motor activity; **Broca's area,** which controls the movements related to speech, is found on the left frontal lobe in right-handed individuals. The **parietal lobes** interpret impulses and sensations from the skin and muscles. Taste sensation overlaps both the parietal and temporal lobes of the brain. The **temporal lobes** receive auditory (hearing) and olfactory (smelling) impulses. The **occipital lobes** deal with vision, depth perception, and three-dimensional perception.

Peripheral Nervous System

The **peripheral nervous system** consists of the cranial and the spinal nerves and includes the **somatic nervous system,** as well as the **autonomic nervous system.** The peripheral nervous system is a relay system that detects changes in both the internal and external environments and relays this information to the central nervous system. It also transmits impulses from the brain and spinal cord to the appropriate end organs. To prevent messages from short-circuiting each other in the peripheral nervous system and to speed impulse conduction, the axons of many types of nerves are surrounded by **Schwann cells,** which form the protective **myelin sheath.** Probably because of the myelin sheath, injured peripheral nerves can be surgically repaired or they may even regenerate spontaneously if the damage is not too severe. Neurons in the central nervous system lack this guiding sheath; if damaged they will usually die.

NORMAL AGE-RELATED CHANGES

Many cellular changes have been observed in the aging brain, including a reduction in its size and weight due to a decrease in the volume of the cerebral cortex. Brain shrinkage has been linked to a decrease in the number of functional cortical neurons (Table 3-8). Mental function is often changed as these cells are lost or undergo functional changes. Cerebral blood flow decreases with aging due to the gradual accumulation of fatty deposits called **arteriosclerosis.** Decreased blood flow also results in a slower rate of cerebral metabolism. A progressive decrease in the number of branches and the connections between dendrites occurs over time. Studies of neurotransmitters

TABLE 3-8

Neurologic Changes Associated with Aging

Physiologic change	Results
Decreased number of brain cells	Decreased reflexes
Decreased number of nerve fibers	Decreased coordination
Decreased amounts of neuroreceptors	Decreased perception of stimuli; decreased motor responses

show that levels of serotonin increase with aging, and norepinephrine levels decrease. Levels of monoamine oxidase, which metabolizes catecholamines, increase. In the peripheral nervous system, the velocity of nerve conduction decreases as much as 30% between 20 and 90 years of age.

Because of these physiologic changes, motor responses take longer in older individuals. Simple actions such as walking and talking often become slower with age. Reflex movements become sluggish, and reactions are slowed. Some loss of coordination is common. Tasks that require quick perception of stimuli and highly coordinated responses (e.g., driving in rush-hour traffic) may pose a risk to those with significant neurologic loss. Many aging people recognize these changes and modify their lifestyles to avoid potentially dangerous situations.

CONDITIONS COMMON WITH AGING

Parkinson's Disease

Parkinson's disease, also called **paralysis agitans,** is a progressive, degenerative disorder of the central nervous system. The cause of Parkinson's disease is unknown. Specific neurons in the brain that produce the neurotransmitter dopamine are lost. Symptoms usually begin after age 40 and appear gradually. The incidence of Parkinson's disease increases in older age groups.

People suffering from Parkinson's disease may manifest a wide variety of symptoms. The initial signs of the disease tend to be unilateral and include slight tremors on one side in addition to a more general weakness and slowing down. As the disease progresses, these tremors become typical and obvious when the person is at rest, decrease with conscious movement, and are totally absent during sleep. Emotional stress or fatigue often worsens the tremors. Later in the course of the disease, both sides of the body become affected. Tremor increases, the body becomes more rigid, and movements become slower.

The face takes on a flat, open-mouthed, masklike expression, and eye blinking decreases in frequency. Speech slows and may be unclear. Swallowing may be affected. Many have trouble either starting to walk or stopping once they have begun. Gait changes, and the affected individual appears to lean forward and walk with short, shuffling steps that occur faster and faster until the person almost runs in an attempt to avoid falling. It is common for people with Parkinson's disease to fall both forward and backward because with increasing rigidity they lose the ability to compensate for shifts in their center of gravity. In severe cases, the affected person may become extremely rigid and unable to move.

Changes in mental processes may accompany physical changes. Although intelligence is not consistently affected by the disease, as many as 50% of persons suffering from parkinsonism experience some form of dementia late in the disease. Personality changes, frustration, and depression are common.

Medical treatment aimed at decreasing the symptoms of Parkinson's disease includes medications such as levodopa (combined with carbodopa), amantadine, bromocriptine, and anticholinergic drugs. These medications may allow less severely affected individuals to function almost normally. Unfortunately, the effects of these drugs lessen over time or the symptoms worsen. Various combinations of medications are often ordered to maximize benefit. Because stress worsens the symptoms, it is particularly important to minimize frustration and emotional upset in these individuals.

Dementia

Dementia is a general term for a permanent or progressive organic mental disorder. Dementia is characterized by personality changes; confusion; disorientation; deterioration of intellectual functioning; and impaired control of memory, judgment, and impulses. Dementia can be a result of drug intoxication, trauma, or other disease processes. Some forms are treatable, whereas others do not respond to any known form of treatment.

Multi-infarct dementia, or vascular dementia, results from hemorrhage or ischemic brain lesions, is more common in men than in women, and is most common after age 70. Persons with hypertension or other types of cerebrovascular disease are most likely to develop this form of dementia. Signs of depression are common, and sufferers may be suicidal.

Alzheimer's Disease

Alzheimer's disease or **senile dementia, Alzheimer's type,** is the most common form of dementia and is typically seen in individuals over 60 years of age. From ages 65 to age 85 the incidence of Alzheimer's disease doubles approximately every 5 years. It is estimated that as many as 2 million people in the United States suffer from this disorder. The cause is unknown, but the apoliprotein E gene has been implicated as a risk factor. Children of people with Alzheimer's disease have four times the risk of developing the disease. Traumatic head injuries, immunologic changes, and environmental causes are suspected. Some researchers believe that Alzheimer's is not a single disease, but that it may have more than one form.

Alzheimer's is a chronic, progressive, degenerative disease in which large numbers of brain cells and tissues are affected by atrophy, senile plaques, and neurofibrillary tangles. The brain level of the neurotransmitter acetylcholine decreases, leading to a disturbed ability to reason and to retain new information. Levels of norepinephrine and dopamine are also decreased in Alzheimer's disease.

Transient Ischemic Attack

Transient ischemic attacks (TIAs) are brief episodes of cerebrovascular insufficiency that are usually caused by obstruction of the cerebral blood vessels. Such obstruction is usually caused by an embolus or atherosclerotic plaque. TIAs occur most frequently in middle-aged and elderly people.

Transient ischemic attacks occur without warning. Most episodes last only a few minutes, but some may last as long as 24 hours. A person may have several attacks within a day or may go for months without experiencing another attack.

A wide variety of symptoms may indicate a TIA. Blurred, tunnel, or double vision; blindness; vertigo, transient numbness and weakness; aphasia or slurred speech; and gait disturbances are common. The person generally remains conscious throughout the attack. The symptoms of TIAs disappear spontaneously and do not cause permanent neurologic damage.

Transient ischemic attacks may be warnings of an impending stroke, but this is not necessarily the case. Some individuals who suffer from TIAs never have a stroke.

BOX 3-4

Right Brain Hemisphere Damage

- Left hemiparesis (weakness of the left arm and/or leg)
- Impaired sense of humor
- Disorientation to time, place, and person
- Difficulty recognizing people
- Visual/spatial problems, including loss of depth perception
- Neglect of the left visual field (may not see objects or hazards on the left side of body)
- Loss of impulse control (may strike out, cry, or shout if upset)
- Unawareness of neurologic function loss (may try to stand or walk despite hemiparesis)
- Poor judgment (may deny illness or problems or tend to overestimate the ability to perform activities)
- Inappropriate responses (may smile continually or demonstrate euphoric behavior even in serious or tragic situations)
- Confabulation (may make up detailed but inaccurate explanations to compensate for memory losses, which can be very believable to persons who are not aware of the facts)

Cerebrovascular Accident

A cerebrovascular accident (CVA), commonly called a stroke, is a disturbance of the blood supply to the brain. Most CVAs are related to atherosclerosis, hypertension, diabetes, or a combination of these. They can occur at any age, but they most commonly affect individuals over age 65. CVAs are frequently fatal and are a leading natural cause of death in the United States. The likelihood of CVA fatality increases with advanced age. CVAs occur slightly more often in men than in women. Blacks are affected more often than other groups, possibly because there is a higher incidence of hypertension in the black population. Even if they are not fatal, CVAs are a leading cause of disability.

There are several specific types of CVAs that are categorized by the process that disturbs the blood flow: (1) cerebral infarction caused by either an embolus or a thrombus, (2) cerebral insufficiency due to atherosclerotic changes that restrict blood flow, or (3) cerebral hemorrhage caused by weakened vessels or aneurysms that rupture spontaneously or as a result of hypertension.

If a CVA is suspected, care is directed at supporting essential life functions: maintaining an open airway, providing adequate oxygenation, and preventing

BOX 3-5

Left Brain Hemisphere Damage

- Right hemiparesis (weakness of the right arm and/ or leg)
- Language disturbances:
  Aphasia—defective or absent language skills that may be expressive (motor), in which words cannot be formed; receptive (sensory), in which language is not understood; or mixed, in which both processes are affected
  Agraphia—loss of the ability to write
  Alexia—inability to comprehend written words; reading problems
- Neglect of the right visual field (may not see objects or hazards on the right side of body)
- Behavior changes (slow, cautious, and anxious when attempting new activities)
- Mood changes (tendency toward worry or depression; verbalization of feelings of worthlessness or guilt; anger and frustration)

trauma. Hospitalization is necessary during the acute post-CVA phase. The need for rehabilitation or extended care is determined by the physician and is based on the individual's particular situation. The onset of a CVA may be sudden, or symptoms may progress gradually. The nature of the symptoms varies with the type of CVA, the area of the brain that is affected, and the extent of the damage (Boxes 3-4 and 3-5). Some individuals manifest mild symptoms, whereas in others the symptoms are more severe. A few victims of CVA recover completely, but most have some lingering deficits. Most improvement occurs within the first 6 months after a CVA. Any deficit lasting longer than 6 months is likely to be permanent. Because recurrence of CVAs is common, each occurrence is likely to cause additional problems.

Because the two sides of the brain serve very different functions, the symptoms depend on which side is affected. Effects of CVAs are contralateral: Damage to the right hemisphere will affect the left side of the body; damage to the left hemisphere will affect the right side of the body.

THE SPECIAL SENSES

The special senses, including sight, hearing, balance, smell, and taste, are integrally connected to the central nervous system by the cranial nerves. The other senses include touch, pressure, and proprioception, which is the awareness of body movement and position in space. These senses are the means by which we gather information from the world around us and our relationship to this world. The special senses provide our first line of protection against hazards in the environment. Unless all of these senses provide us with good information and all function properly, we are at risk of suffering from these hazards.

It is important to understand the visual and auditory changes that occur with aging because these changes may have serious implications for safety. A great deal of the information we receive and respond to in the world comes to us through our senses of sight and hearing. We may think elderly people are confused or senile when merely their sensory perceptions are impaired because of the changes associated with aging.

NORMAL STRUCTURE AND FUNCTION

The Eyes

The **eyes** are two globe-shaped structures located in the orbits of the skull on each side of the nose. Because the eyes are so important, they have surrounding structures designed to protect them from both physical and biologic hazards.

The **eyelids** are controlled by skeletal muscle and are lined with a smooth mucous membrane called the **conjunctiva.** The eyelids can close; thus they and the eyelashes located on their margins provide protection from dust and flying debris. Tears are produced by the **lacrimal glands** located at the upper and outer corner of the eye. These glands lubricate the eye, prevent particles of debris from scraping the surface, and inhibit the growth of bacteria by means of the enzyme **lysozyme.** Tears leave the eye at the medial corner through the **lacrimal sac** and the nasolacrimal duct that drains into the nose.

The eye itself is composed of three layers. The outermost layer, the sclera (commonly called the white of the eye), is composed of fibrous connective tissue and supports the inner structures of the eye. The anterior part of the sclera is the **cornea,** a transparent structure that **refracts,** or bends, light rays. The sclera contains small capillaries that are sometimes visible on its surface. The cornea does not contain any capillaries or nerves.

The middle layer of the eye, the **choroid,** contains pigments that absorb light and keep the interior of the eye dark. The choroid is highly vascular and supplies nourishment to the surrounding tissue. Located in the anterior portion of the choroid are the **iris** (the colored portion), the **pupil** (an opening in the iris through which light enters the eye), the **lens** (a transparent oval disk), and the **ciliary body** (muscles that change the shape of the lens to refract light waves). The lens does not contain any capillaries or nerves.

The innermost layer of the eye is the **retina.** This structure covers the posterior two thirds of the eye and contains the visual receptors, highly specialized structures called **rods** and **cones.** These receptors use chemical changes in their pigments to detect light. Cones are most abundant near the center of the retina. They detect color and discriminate among different colors based on the wavelength of the incoming light. Rods are more abundant near the periphery of the retina and detect the presence or absence of light. Vitamin A is essential to the formation of the pigment in the rods that enables their response. Rods are important for vision when there is limited light. Nerves in the retina transmit messages from the rods and cones to the optic nerve, which sends the information to the vision centers of the brain. The macula lutea (yellow spot) is a small area, less than 2 mm in size, located near the center of the retina that provides us with sharp central vision.

The greatest part of the eye mass is made up of two fluid-filled cavities. The small **anterior cavity** is located between the cornea and the lens, and it contains **aqueous humor,** a fluid formed by capillaries in the choroid. This fluid passes from the **posterior chamber** through the pupil to the **anterior chamber,** and it supplies the nourishment for the lens and cornea, which do not have a blood supply. Because aqueous humor is produced continuously, some must be absorbed or else the amount of fluid would becomes excessive. Normally, absorption takes place through small veins located at the juncture of the iris and cornea. The presence of excess fluid increases the pressure within the anterior chamber.

The posterior cavity of the eye, the **vitreous,** is much larger and contains a gelatinous substance called the **vitreous humor.** Vitreous humor holds the retina in contact with the choroid of the eye.

Refraction

The eye functions much like a camera. Light waves enter the eye through the cornea and then pass through the aqueous humor, lens, and vitreous humor to the retina. When light waves strike the retina, they stimulate the receptors in the cones and rods. The rods react chemically to the amount of light and regulate nerve impulses to the brain based on this information. Different cones respond to different wavelengths of light rays (different colors) and thus determine the perceived color of objects. Based on information gathered from the rods and cones, the image projected on

the retina is translated into nerve impulses by the retina, which then sends the information via the optic nerves to the visual centers of the cerebral cortex in the **occipital region.** The optic nerves from both eyes meet at the **optic chiasm** just under the pituitary gland. At the optic chiasm, the medial fibers (from the image on the part of the retina closest to the nose) cross to the opposite side of the brain and the lateral fibers (from the outside part of the retina) do not cross. This allows visual centers on both sides of the brain to process messages from both eyes and is important for binocular vision. Because of position, each eye "sees" things somewhat differently than the other and sends slightly different messages to the brain. The brain receives messages from both eyes, correlates the information, and makes sense of it. Binocular vision is also important for **depth perception,** the sense of how far you are from another person or object.

For information to be received accurately, all of the eyes' structures must function together to focus the light rays. The shape of the lens is controlled by the ciliary body, whose muscles relax or contract to change the shape of the lens so it can bend the light waves correctly and bring an object into clear focus. This change in lens shape is called **accommodation. Refractive errors,** or errors in focusing ability, occur when the cornea is misshapen or when the lens cannot appropriately change shape to focus images.

NORMAL AGE-RELATED CHANGES IN THE EYE

With aging, many structural and functional changes may occur in the eye (Table 3-9). The eyelids become less elastic and sag. Eyelashes tend to be shorter, thinner, and in some cases absent. A grayish haze of the peripheral cornea, **arcus senilis,** develops with aging and is more common in darkly pigmented races (Fig. 3-9).

A decrease in tear production is common in the elderly because the volume of body fluids and secretions decreases with age. An 80-year-old person produces only 25% of the tears he or she produced during the teenage years. Many elderly people complain of dry, burning, or itching eyes caused by friction from the lids or from small particles of debris. The decline in tear production reduces the antibacterial protection provided by enzymes and can lead to decreased resistance to bacterial eye infections.

Almost all people over 50 years of age experience some degree of farsightedness, or presbyopia, which means "elderly eye." Refractive errors are increasingly common as the ciliary muscles lose their ability to contract easily and progressive rigidity of the lens restricts accommodation. A combination of these

TABLE 3-9

Vision Changes Associated with Aging

Physiologic change	Results
Decreased number of eyelashes	Increased risk of eye injury
Decreased tear production	Increased risk of eye irritation
Increased discoloration of lens	Decreased color perception
Decreased tissue elasticity	Increased blurring
Decreased muscle tone	Decreased diameter of pupil; increased refractive errors; decreased night vision; increased sensitivity to glare

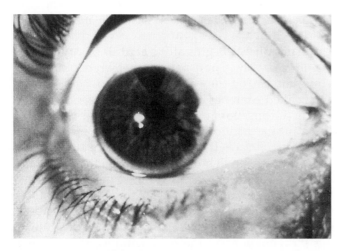

FIG. 3-9 Arcus senilis in a patient with a peripheral iridectomy. (From Stein HS, Slatt BJ, Stein RM: *The ophthalmic assistant: fundamentals and clinical practice*, ed 6, St Louis, 1994, Mosby.)

changes makes focusing on close objects, performing detailed close work, or reading increasingly difficult. Presbyopia is usually corrected by use of contact lenses or glasses which help the aging person focus on close objects.

Astigmatism, a malformation of the cornea, causes blurring of images at all distances. People of all ages can have astigmatism, but younger people compensate for it by quickly refocusing the blurred and unblurred images. When this ability decreases with aging, astigmatism appears to worsen. Corrective lenses help with this.

Older adults may have poor **dark adaptation** responses and may experience a decrease in the ability to adjust from light to darkness and darkness to light. **Night blindness,** the inability to see well at night or in dim light, grows increasingly common with aging.

The lens of the eye tends to yellow with age, possibly leading to misperception of colors. All dark colors may be perceived as black, and subtle differences in shades may not be detectable. Younger people who

find blue-haired women amusing should look at them through a lens that is slightly tinted yellow. Amazingly, the hair looks clean and "white."

Peripheral vision and depth perception often decrease with aging. It is important to recognize these changes because they significantly increase the risk of accidents and injuries.

Another common occurrence with aging is "**floaters.**" Many elderly people report seeing flecks, spots, cobwebs, or brilliant crystals within their eyes. These are harmless but can be very frustrating because they interfere with many visual activities such as reading, sewing, or other detailed crafts.

EYE CONDITIONS COMMON WITH AGING

Diplopia

Diplopia, or double vision, is not normal and indicates some disturbance of the nervous system that requires further investigation by a physician.

Cataracts

Cataracts, a clouding of the lens of the eye, are increasingly common with aging. Studies done in the United States show that 5% of people between 52 and 62 years of age develop cataracts. By age 75 to 85, the incidence of cataracts increases to 46%.

Cataracts develop over time and result in progressive, painless loss of vision. The amount of vision loss will depend on the degree of lens opacity and the area of the lens that is affected. Vision in bright light or glare may be particularly difficult with certain types of cataracts. Individuals with cataracts will require frequent changes in eyeglass prescriptions while the cataract matures. When vision is severely affected, surgical removal of the cataract or the lens is the medical treatment of choice. Today this surgery is common and in most cases can be performed on an outpatient basis. Once the cataract is removed, vision is corrected by means of surgically implanted lenses, contact lenses, or cataract glasses.

Glaucoma

Glaucoma is a disease characterized by increased fluid pressure (intraocular pressure) within the eye that may result in damage to the retina. Initially, peripheral vision is affected. Tunnel vision and eventually permanent blindness may result. Persons with glaucoma seldom experience obvious symptoms, so serious damage usually occurs before the disease is even recognized. However, a test for increased intraocular pressure can be performed easily. The test for glaucoma is simple, painless, and takes only minutes. It is normally part of a routine ophthalmic examination, and everyone over 40 should be tested routinely for glaucoma.

Macular Degeneration and Retinal Detachment

The **macula,** the small area in the center of the retina where visual acuity is best, is susceptible to damage and destruction. **Macular degeneration** occurs most often in aging people and is the leading cause of legal blindness in Americans over age 55. The exact cause of macular degeneration remains unknown, but two types of the disorder have been identified. The atrophic form is a result of inadequate nutrient supply or waste removal due to vascular changes. When cells atrophy or die, the macula is damaged and central vision is significantly diminished. Vision is restricted but not totally lost because noncentral vision remains.

The neovascular form of macular degeneration results from abnormal growth of tiny blood vessels under the retina. These vessels ruin vision by leaking fluid and blood, which cause the retina to become swollen and distorted. This form is more likely to cause severe vision loss. Laser surgery or microsurgery may be attempted to seal leaking vessels, slow their growth, and prevent further vision loss.

Circulatory changes in the blood vessels of the eyes are common with DM, resulting in a condition called **diabetic retinopathy.** This condition is characterized by hemorrhaging of small blood vessels into the vitreous humor and has effects similar to neovascular macular degeneration, (i.e., loss of vision). Diabetics are two to three times more likely to develop blindness as a result of retinopathy.

Normal shrinkage of the eye and changes in the consistency of the vitreous humor are common with aging and may result in **retinal detachment,** which is

separation of the retina from the choroid. Any or all of these changes can result in loss of central vision.

NORMAL STRUCTURE AND FUNCTION OF THE EAR

The ear is composed of three distinct portions, the **outer ear, middle ear,** and **inner ear.** The two main functions of the ear are the detection of sound and the maintenance of balance.

The outer ear consists of the visible curved structure, called the **pinna,** or **auricle,** and the **external ear canal.** The pliable auricle is made of cartilage. The size or shape of the external ear has little influence on hearing.

The middle ear begins at the **eardrum,** or **tympanic membrane.** This transparent membrane stretches across the end of the ear canal and separates it from an air-filled chamber called the **middle ear.** Air pressure in the middle ear is controlled through the **Eustachian tube,** which connects the middle ear to the nasopharynx. Attached to the tympanic membrane is a series of three small bones, the **malleus** (hammer), **incus** (anvil), and **stapes** (stirrup). Sound waves enter the ear through the external ear canal and cause the tympanic membrane to vibrate. This in turn causes movement of the three small bones, which then transmit the vibrations to the **oval window,** the opening into the inner ear.

The inner ear is a complex, fluid-filled structure that has several functions. A portion called the **cochlea** contains the hearing receptors, which consist of hair cells with fine movable projections that are set in motion when sound waves reach their fluid surroundings. When these hairs move, impulses are carried via the auditory nerve (a cranial nerve) to the midbrain and then to the temporal lobe of the brain where the sound is "heard."

Other specialized hair cells are found elsewhere in the inner ear: the vestibule and the **semicircular canals.** Hair cells from these structures transmit information in response to gravity, change of position, and motion via the cranial nerves. The central nervous system processes this information and maintains equilibrium.

NORMAL AGE-RELATED CHANGES IN THE EAR

Just as other body tissues become thinner with age, so does the tympanic membrane (Table 3-10). The small muscles that support the membrane show signs of atrophy with advanced age. Arthritic changes affect the

---

TABLE 3-10

Auditory Changes Associated with Aging

Physiologic change	Results
Decreased tissue elasticity	Decreased ability to distinguish high-frequency sounds
Decreased joint mobility	Decreased hearing ability
Decreased number of hair cells in the inner ear	Increased problems with balance

---

joints between the small bones of the middle ear, and hair cells in the inner ear often deteriorate.

Presbycusis, defined as an alteration in hearing capacity related to aging, affects an estimated 13% of people over 65 years of age. Men appear to be more affected by this problem than are women. The aging person with presbycusis loses the ability to perceive tones of higher frequencies. Speech sounds such as *s, sh, ch,* and soft *t* may not be audible, so the aging person may only hear parts of spoken words. Simple words like *cat, hat, sat,* and *that* may all sound the same. If other noises are present in the environment, sounds become even less distinct. The aging individual may have difficulty sorting out words and making sense of what is being said.

EAR CONDITIONS COMMON WITH AGING

Otosclerosis

Otosclerosis, a hardening or fixing of the stapes to the oval window, interferes with sound wave transmission into the inner ear. This condition occurs slightly more often in women than in men. Surgical correction is possible.

Tinnitus

Tinnitus, or ringing in the ears, is frequently reported by aging people. Tinnitus may be a result of trauma to the ear, pressure from cerumen against the eardrum, otosclerosis, presbycusis, or Meniere's disease. Tinnitus can also be caused by certain medications.

Deafness

Deafness, the inability to hear sounds fully, may be temporary or permanent, depending on the cause. Deafness can be unilateral, affecting one ear only, or bilateral, affecting both ears.

Conductive hearing loss occurs when something interferes with transmission of the sound waves. A plug of **cerumen** (earwax) in the external canal, rupture or scarring of the eardrum, the presence of fluid or an infection in the middle ear, or any condition that interferes with movement of the small bones of the middle ear may result in conductive hearing loss or deafness.

Nerve deafness occurs when either the receptors in the inner ear or the cranial nerves are damaged or destroyed. Some antibiotics and viral infections can cause nerve deafness. Chronic exposure to loud noise can speed up the degeneration of the hair cells. Many young people today are experiencing significant hearing loss from excessive exposure to extremely loud music, and this will have serious implications as they age. Work-related noise has also been shown to have negative effects on hearing. Many elderly men who worked in foundries or other noisy places may have suffered employment-related hearing loss. The Occupational Safety and Health Administration now requires employers to protect employees from excessive exposure to loud noise on the job.

Central deafness is caused by trauma or disease in the temporal lobes of the brain. This may be due to tumors, CVA, or injury. Central deafness is not common.

Ménière's disease

Ménière's disease is a fairly common chronic disorder of the inner ear observed in people over 40 or 50 years of age. Persons suffering from this disorder experience severe vertigo (not simple dizziness) to the point that they may be unable to stand or walk. They may also report nausea, tinnitus, hearing loss, and a sensation of pressure in the ear. Diaphoresis, vomiting, and **nystagmus** (rapid, involuntary eye movement) may also be observed. Episodes generally appear suddenly and may last for minutes or hours. The frequency of attacks is unpredictable. Meniere's disease tends to affect one ear, and it can result in nerve deafness that sometimes persists even if treatment relieves the other symptoms.

NORMAL FUNCTION OF TASTE AND SMELL SENSES

The receptors for our sense of taste are located in the papillae, or taste buds, on the superior surface of the tongue. In these papillae are chemical receptor cells that are sensitive to salty, sweet, sour, or bitter chemicals. When mixed with moisture like saliva or water, food releases chemicals that are detected by these receptors. Foods get their subtle flavors by their unique interaction with various receptors. The detection of odors occurs when the olfactory receptors in the upper nasal cavities respond to airborne chemicals. When vapors escape from food or other volatile substances, they enter the nose and stimulate the receptors.

Information from both taste and smell receptors is then transported to the nervous system via the cranial nerves. When these senses are intact and functioning well, many people salivate and can "taste" a meal while it is being prepared. Without a sense of smell, food has little flavor. Most of us have had severe nasal congestion from colds or allergies, and have found that without smell, food has either a strange taste or no taste at all. Some individuals with chronic nasal congestion report ongoing problems with appetite because food has little flavor or appeal. People with permanent damage to the olfactory senses report permanent changes in taste that often result in loss of appetite.

NORMAL AGE-RELATED CHANGES

With aging there is a decrease in the number of functional receptors in both the nasal cavities and papillae on the tongue (Table 3-11). The changes in taste particularly affect the receptors for sweet and salty tastes. Because salt enhances the flavor of food, elderly persons frequently add salt in an attempt to add flavor. Complaints of flavorless food are common even if the food seems well prepared and tasty to younger individuals. In addition, alterations in taste sensation are a side effect of many medications.

TABLE 3-11	
Olfactory Changes Associated with Aging	
Physiologic change	**Results**
Decreased number of papilla on tongue	Decreased ability to taste
Decreased number of nasal sensory receptors	Decreased ability to detect smells

THE ENDOCRINE SYSTEM

The endocrine system and the nervous system perform the major integrating and regulating functions of the body. The endocrine glands secrete chemical substances called **hormones** to regulate body processes. Hormones are secreted directly into the capillaries of the bloodstream, where they circulate until they reach their target organs and cause specific effects. Some endocrine glands produce a single hormone; others produce several different hormones. Some hormones have only one target organ; others target multiple organs. The production of hormones is regulated by a negative feedback process in which the endocrine glands constantly monitor the effects of hormones circulating in the system. If the effect is adequate, the gland decreases production. If it is inadequate, the gland increases production. The process of regulation is similar to a system consisting of a thermostat and a furnace in a home. When the temperature reaches that for which the thermostat is set, the thermostat signals the furnace to stop producing heat. If the temperature drops below the preset level, the thermostat signals the furnace to produce more heat. In a highly complex manner, the endocrine glands constantly monitor the effects and the levels of the many hormones circulating in the body and increase or decrease production as needed to meet body demands.

NORMAL STRUCTURE AND FUNCTION

Pituitary Gland

The pituitary gland is often referred to as the master gland of the body because of the many functions it regulates. It is located within the skull cavity and is connected directly to the hypothalamus. There are two major segments of the pituitary gland: the **anterior pituitary** and the **posterior pituitary.** The posterior pituitary is the site of connection between the nervous system and the endocrine system. The posterior pituitary hormones are actually produced in the hypothalamus of the brain and are stored in the posterior pituitary until needed. The major secretion of the posterior pituitary gland is **antidiuretic hormone.** This hormone maintains fluid balance in the body by causing the kidneys to reabsorb fluid; in the absence of antidiuretic hormone, the kidneys excrete more fluid. By controlling fluid balance, antidiuretic hormone aids in the maintenance of blood pressure. Oxytocin, another hormone of the posterior pituitary gland, stimulates contraction of the uterus during delivery and ejection of milk from the breast during lactation.

The anterior pituitary produces many hormones: **Growth hormone** increases the rate of protein synthesis and aids in the transport of amino acids to cells. In adults, this hormone also participates in fat release from adipose tissue and the use of this fat as an energy source. **Thyroid-stimulating hormone** stimulates the normal growth and activity of the thyroid gland. Adrenocorticotropic hormone corticotropin stimulates the activity of the adrenal cortex. **Gonadotropic hormones** include follicle-stimulating hormone and **luteinizing hormone,** which are responsible for maturation and function of the gonads, and **prolactin,** which supports lactation.

Thyroid Gland

The **thyroid gland** surrounds the trachea and is located just below the larynx (voicebox). The major hormones produced by the thyroid gland are **thyroxin,** triiodothyronine, and **calcitonin.** The thyroid hormones triiodothyronine and thyroxin increase the rate of metabolism; regulate the metabolism of fat, carbohydrates, and protein in the cells; and increase body temperature. They also affect cardiac, neurologic, and musculoskeletal function. The function of calcitonin is to keep calcium and phosphate within the bone matrix.

Parathyroid Glands

The **parathyroid glands** are located on the posterior surface of the lobes of the thyroid gland. **Parathyroid hormone,** an antagonist of calcitonin, stimulates the movement of calcium and phosphorus from the bones into the blood.

Pancreas

The **pancreas** is both an exocrine and an endocrine gland. It functions as an exocrine gland in digestion and is discussed in detail in Chapter 8. The endocrine secretions of the pancreas are produced by α and β cells in the islets of Langerhans. The α cells produce glucagon, which stimulates the liver to convert glycogen to glucose. The β cells produce **insulin,** which increases the permeability of cell membranes and enables the cells to use glucose, amino acids, and fatty acids.

Adrenal Glands

The **adrenal glands** are located on the top of each kidney. The **adrenal medulla** is the inner portion of the gland, and the **adrenal cortex** is the outer portion. The adrenal medulla secretes **epinephrine** and norepinephrine, which are the major neurotransmitters of the sympathetic portion of the autonomic nervous system. Thus hormone release from the adrenal medulla has effects similar to those of the sympathetic nervous system. These hormones help the body cope with stressors by decreasing functions that are not required for the fight-or-flight response and by increasing cardiac activity, blood pressure, release of energy reserves, and other functions necessary for survival when faced with danger.

The adrenal cortex releases **mineralocorticoids, glucocorticoids,** and small amounts of sex hormones. The mineralocorticoid aldosterone is important in the regulation of fluid and electrolyte balance and the maintenance of blood pressure. The glucocorticoid **cortisol** is involved in the conversion of glycogen to glucose and in antiinflammatory activities.

Ovaries and Testes

The **testes** and **ovaries** secrete the hormones that are involved in sexual maturation and function. The primary hormones secreted by the ovaries are **estrogen** and progesterone. These hormones are responsible for maturation of the ova, stimulation of the uterine endometrium, and development of the secondary female sexual characteristics. The testes secrete the major male sex hormone, **testosterone,** which is responsible for maturation of sperm and for development of the secondary male sexual characteristics.

NORMAL AGE-RELATED CHANGES

With aging, a variety of changes occur in endocrine function (Table 3-12). The pituitary gland continues to produce adequate levels of critical hormones throughout life. It produces less growth hormone as we age, leading to a decrease in muscle mass. In recent studies, growth hormone was administered to elderly men,

TABLE 3-12

Endocrine Changes Associated with Aging

Physiologic change	Results
Decreased pituitary secretions (growth hormone)	Decreased muscle mass
Decreased production of thyroid-stimulating hormone	Decreased basal metabolic rate
Decreased production of parathyroid hormone (seen with osteoporosis)	Increased blood calcium levels

who then showed significant increases in muscle mass. Growth hormone is very expensive, may have undesirable side effects, and is currently an investigational drug.

A decrease in production of thyroid-stimulating hormone is seen in some elderly individuals. Basal metabolic rate begins to decrease in young adulthood and continues to decrease gradually throughout the remainder of life. Because lean body mass also decreases, the overall metabolic rate does not change significantly. In response to decreased thyroid function, some elderly people become more sensitive to cooler temperatures.

Studies of parathyroid function reveal conflicting information. Parathyroid hormone appears to decrease with age, except in cases of osteoporosis where it appears to increase. Elevated levels of parathyroid hormone may lead to increased blood calcium levels. This is of concern particularly for elderly women, who may manifest symptoms of confusion, kidney stones, and osteoporosis.

Pancreatic function appears to decrease with aging; however, barring the onset of some form of DM, its function remains adequate to meet normal body functioning.

Adrenal function is not altered significantly with advancing age. Adequate hormone levels are produced to meet bodily needs.

The levels of gonadotrophic hormones decrease more significantly in women than in men. After menopause, estrogen and progesterone production drop significantly. As the production of female sex hormones decreases with aging, some changes in secondary sexual characteristics may be observed such as the development of facial hair and genital atrophy. Studies indicate that estrogen depletion in postmenopausal women has negative effects on bone density, cardiovascular function, memory, and cognition. Because production of the male hormone testosterone decreases gradually with aging, changes are gradual and often undistinguishable.

CONDITIONS COMMON WITH AGING

Diabetes Mellitus

The incidence of **diabetes mellitus** increases with age. The likelihood of becoming diabetic doubles with each decade of life. Studies have shown that up to 20% of persons over 70 years of age have problems with glucose regulation. DM is a disease with multiple causes that is characterized by abnormal metabolism of carbohydrates, protein, and fats, resulting in elevated plasma glucose levels. Long-term complications include retinopathy (resulting in loss of vision), nephropathy (resulting in renal failure), peripheral neuropathy (resulting in foot ulcers, amputation), autonomic neuropathy (resulting in GI, genitourinary, and cardiovascular symptoms and sexual dysfunction), atherosclerotic vascular problems (resulting in an increased incidence of cardiovascular, cerebrovascular, and peripheral vascular disease), hypertension, and periodontal disease.

The most current classification system categorizes DM according to its etiology, or cause. The first category, **type 1** DM, is defined as a result of either autoimmune destruction of the β cells of the pancrease or unknown idiopathic causes. The second category, **type 2** DM, results from a combination of resistance to insulin action and inadequate compensatory insulin secretion. In the third category, **other specific types** of DM are identified by their unique etiologies, including genetic defects or syndromes, exocrine diseases of the pancreas, diseases of the endocrine system, drugs or chemicals, infections, or other uncommon immune-mediated disorders. A fourth category, **gestational** DM, exists only during pregnancy. This system replaces the older classification system (insulin-dependent diabetes mellitus, or IDDM, and non–insulin-dependent diabetes mellitus, or NIDDM), which was based on the treatment method used.

Diagnosis of DM is made based on symptoms and on the determination of elevated plasma glucose levels. A casual (no specific relation to meals) plasma glucose level of 200 mg/dl or higher, particularly when symptoms are present, warrants further testing. This can be done using the oral glucose tolerance test or the fasting plasma glucose (FPG) level (no calorie intake for at least 8 hours). The FPG level is the more commonly accepted test because it is less costly and less time-consuming. FPG levels less than 110 mg/dl are classified as normal. FPG levels between 110 and 126 mg/dl are classified as impaired fasting glucose. FPG levels of 126 mg/dl or higher warrant a provisional diagnosis of diabetes. Abnormal results must be confirmed on a subsequent day to make the diagnosis.

Type 1

Type 1 DM can occur at any age, but its onset usually is before age 25. Approximately 10% to 15% of the total diabetic population has type 1 DM.

Type 1 DM typically has a sudden onset, but it may occur slowly depending on the rate at which the pancreatic β cells are destroyed. People suffering from type 1 DM produce little or no insulin because of β-cell destruction. Absolute lack of insulin production results in excessively high levels of glucose in the blood (hyperglycemia) and leads to the classic symptoms of diabetes. Symptoms include **polyuria** (excessive and frequent urination), **polydipsia** (excessive thirst), and **polyphagia** (excessive appetite). Even with increased food and fluid intake, the person with type 1 DM may lose weight.

The type 1 diabetic is prone to further metabolic problems. When the body is unable to use glucose because of inadequate insulin production, starvation at the *cellular* level occurs. The body may attempt to meet cell needs by using fat or muscle as a source of fuel. This results in an accumulation of **ketones** (by-products of incomplete metabolism of fatty acids) in the bloodstream. As the blood ketone level increases, the acid–base balance is altered, the blood becomes too acidic, and a condition called **ketoacidosis** occurs. The body attempts to maintain acid–base balance through the compensatory systems of the kidneys and lungs. When a severe imbalance occurs, **ketonuria** may occur, and acetone or "apple pie" breath may be detected. Severe acidemia can result in a deep and rapid pattern of breathing called **Kussmaul's respirations.** If not recognized and treated, type 1 DM will result in death.

Type 1 DM requires continuous, careful monitoring and medical supervision. Treatment involves a careful balance of diet, insulin therapy, exercise, and stress management. Each diabetic requires an individualized program that meets his or her particular needs.

Changes in diet or activity, infections, and stress can easily cause problems for the type 1 diabetic. The plasma glucose levels of a diabetic receiving insulin therapy must be monitored closely. Plasma glucose levels may be determined by the laboratory or by a variety of self-testing devices. Any significant changes in plasma glucose levels should be reported to the physician promptly.

Type 1 diabetics who live independently must be taught the importance of following the prescribed balance of diet, insulin, and exercise. They should be strongly urged to call the doctor *immediately* if they have any signs of infection, particularly any infection that results in vomiting. Special medical identification bracelets or necklaces are advisable. Such devices can help ensure that proper care is provided in emergency situations.

Type 2

The form of DM that is most often observed in the elderly is type 2 DM; this form comprises 85% to 90% of the diabetic population and is more commonly observed in individuals who are over 40 years of age, who are obese, or whose family history includes type 2 DM. The symptoms of type 2 DM are usually mild and unrecognized by an aging person. Diagnosis often occurs during routine medical visits or when the person seeks medical attention for visual disturbances,

delayed wound healing, or recurrent vaginal or yeast infections.

With type 2 DM, the individual may have normal or even elevated levels of insulin. Despite these normal levels, glucose does not enter the cells normally. It is suspected that a problem with the receptor sites on the cells prevents normal cellular functioning in these individuals.

Physicians prefer to control type 2 DM by dietary means. Weight loss is encouraged because it often results in a spontaneous decrease in plasma blood glucose levels. If diet alone is not successful, oral hypoglycemic agents may be prescribed. When under physical stress due to infection or surgery, persons with type 2 DM may experience abnormally high plasma glucose levels. In these cases, the classic symptoms of DM may occur and the person may require insulin administration to maintain normal plasma glucose levels. Once these levels are normal and the stressor is removed, insulin administration is typically discontinued. Plasma glucose levels should be monitored frequently to ensure that they remain within normal limits.

Hypoglycemia

Hypoglycemia is a potentially serious problem for people receiving insulin or oral hypoglycemic agents. Classic signs of hypoglycemia include headache, nausea, weakness, tremors or trembling sensations, pallor, anxiety, irritability, tachycardia, sweating, and hunger. Many of these symptoms can be easily missed or misinterpreted in the elderly population. If hypoglycemia is suspected, the plasma glucose level should be measured promptly. Treatment is based on the specific plasma glucose level. Those with levels of 40 to 60 mg/dl respond best to foods such as milk and crackers, and those with levels of 20 to 40 mg/dl respond best to refined carbohydrates such as honey, juice, or sugar. If unconscious, the patient is treated with an intramuscular injection of glucagon or an intravenous infusion of 50% glucose. Individuals who are prone to hypoglycemia should be taught to carry a carbohydrate source, such as hard candy or glucose tablets.

Hypothyroidism

Reduced function of the thyroid gland, called **primary hypothyroidism,** is more common in older than in younger persons. The symptoms of hypothyroidism include cold intolerance, dry skin, dry and thin body hair, constipation, depression, and lack of energy. Because many of these changes are commonly observed with aging, the symptoms may not be recognized as signs of hypothyroidism. Diagnosis is made by means of blood tests. Treatment of hypothyroidism with very high levels of thyroid hormone have been shown to reduce bone density in elderly women but not in elderly men.

THE REPRODUCTIVE AND GENITOURINARY SYSTEMS

In both men and women, the genital and urinary systems are located close to each other. As mentioned previously, many structures in men are used for both the sexual and elimination functions. In women, the structures of elimination are completely separate from those of reproduction.

NORMAL STRUCTURE AND FUNCTION

Female Reproductive Organs

The primary female sexual organs include the **ovaries, fallopian tubes, uterus,** and **vagina.** These structures, which are necessary for normal human reproduction, are located in the pelvic cavity between the bladder and the bowels. It is important to visualize their location to understand the symptoms that may occur if the size, shape, or position of these organs changes. During the reproductive years, the ovaries produce the hormones estrogen and **progesterone.** Under the influence of these hormones, the **ova** mature in the ovaries, and the endometrium of the uterus changes in vascularity to support a possible pregnancy. When a woman reaches menopause (sometime between 45 and 60 years of age), the hormonal function of the ovaries decreases and then ceases. This physiologic timing of the end of reproduction probably developed because it increased the likelihood that the mother would live to see her children reach maturity. Recent technology and extensive medical intervention can allow pregnancies to occur after menopause, but the number of women who will choose to become pregnant this late in life is probably not significant. Most women reach menopause either resigned or delighted to reach the end of the reproductive stage.

Male Reproductive Organs

The male organs of reproduction consist of the **testes,** a series of ducts and glands, and the **penis,** which contains the passageway by which **sperm,** the male sex cells, leave the body in the **ejaculate.** The testes are suspended in a tissue sac called the **scrotum,** which

hangs between the thighs. The testes produce the hormone **testosterone,** which is responsible for the production and maturation of sperm. Testosterone is also responsible for the secondary sex changes in the men, including body hair patterns, voice changes, and muscle development. A series of ducts and glands provides additional fluid volume to the ejaculate and adds nutrients needed for sperm maturation and development. The **prostate gland** is located just below the urinary bladder. The prostate produces an alkaline secretion that increases sperm motility and also contracts to aid in the ejaculation of sperm.

NORMAL AGE-RELATED CHANGES

Several significant changes occur with menopause (Table 3-13). Production of progesterone and estrogen diminishes. There is no longer the need to produce ova to be fertilized, and there is no need to prepare a site to support a pregnancy. Other changes related to the decline in hormones are not as desirable. Along with other body tissue, the tissues of the external female reproductive organs atrophy as a result of vascular changes. The tissues of the reproductive organs become less elastic, and the amount of subcutaneous tissue decreases. This results in a flattening of the tissue of the external genitalia, or labia, and frequently the amount and distribution of pubic hair decreases. Vaginal epithelial tissue becomes thinner and less vascular. The tissue of the vagina is drier and more alkaline, and fewer **rugae** (folds) are present within the vagina. The uterus, cervix, ovaries, and fallopian tubes decrease in size and may be difficult to palpate on examination. The decrease in hormone production and resulting tissue changes may lead to more fragile, more easily irritated vaginal tissue. Decreased vaginal secretions may lead to **vaginitis,** which can cause vulvar soreness and pruritis or painful intercourse (called **dyspareunia**). Once menopause has occurred, vaginal bleeding is considered abnormal. Older women who receive estrogen supplements may experience fewer reproductive tissue changes, and in some cases the lining of the uterus responds to these supplemental hormones. Vaginal bleeding may occasionally be observed in these women.

The breasts are part of the secondary female sexual organs. As a result of the decrease in hormones with aging, breast tissue atrophies. As supporting muscle tissue atrophies, the breasts tend to sag and decrease in size.

Male age-related changes in the reproductive system are less noticeable because testosterone continues to be produced into old age, although the amount tends to decrease. Men even in their late eighties have successfully fathered children.

TABLE 3-13

Reproductive Changes Associated with Aging

Physiologic change	Results
FEMALE	
Decreased estrogen levels	Decreased vaginal secretions
Decreased tissue elasticity	Decreased pubic hair; increased vaginal tissue fragility; increased tissue irritation; decreased size of uterus; decreased vaginal length and width; decreased size of vaginal opening; increased pain with intercourse (dyspareunia); decreased breast tissue mass
Increased vaginal alkalinity	Increased risk of infection
MALE	
Decreased testosterone levels	Decreased amount of facial and pubic hair
Decreased circulation	Decreased rate and force of ejaculation; decreased speed gaining an erection

With aging, there is some change in the size and firmness of the testes. The penis retains the ability to become erect, although it may take longer and require more stimulation. Once achieved, erection may last longer than at a younger age. Ejaculations tend to be slower and less forceful in aging men and may not occur during each sexual encounter, particularly if intercourse is frequent.

Enlargement of the scrotum may indicate problems with the testes or part of the duct system. The penis should remain free from any tissue changes, and the presence of ulcers, nodules, or other changes is abnormal. The prostate gland commonly enlarges with age. Most aging men experience some degree of prostate enlargement. The signs and symptoms most often experienced include urinary frequency, hesitancy, dysuria, decreased force when voiding, dribbling, nocturia, increased incidence of urinary tract infections, and decreased force during ejaculation. In cases of **benign prostatic hyperplasia,** surgical intervention such as a **transurethral prostatectomy** may help reduce the symptoms.

CONDITIONS COMMON WITH AGING

Uterine Prolapse

Prolapse of the uterus (into the vagina) is frequently observed in elderly women. This is particularly a problem for those who have had many pregnancies or for those who delivered children with little medical assistance. Most often the first signs of uterine prolapse involve changes in either urine or bowel elimination. Urinary frequency, urinary retention, recurrent urinary tract infections, back pain, and constipation may be symptomatic. In some cases, the cervix and uterus may prolapse through the vagina and be observed protruding outside of the vulva. Surgical correction of this condition may be required.

Vaginal Infection

Change in vaginal pH may lead to increased incidence of vaginal infections, particularly **yeast** infections. This is most often manifested by increased vaginal discharge, irritation, odor, and itching.

Breast Cancer

The risk of **breast cancer** does not disappear with increased age. Breast cancer continues to be a major cause of cancer deaths in women, and the incidence of this form of cancer continues to increase with age. It is important that regular breast examinations (including mammography) continue as a woman ages. Any sign of dimpling; masses; nipple retraction; or breast drainage, discharge, or bleeding is suspicious and requires further medical attention.

Prostate Cancer

There are no obvious changes in function to indicate the presence of prostate cancer. Therefore, it is important for aging men to have regular medical examinations. A skilled physician who palpates the prostate may detect changes that indicate malignancy. Prostatic cancer is a major cause of death in aging men.

SUMMARY

Nurses must possess knowledge about the normal structures and functions of all of the body systems so that deviations from the norm can be detected. All of the body systems are affected to a greater or lesser degree by aging. Although these changes are normal and should be expected, they can have a significant impact on the older person's functional ability, self-image, and lifestyle. In addition to normal, age-related changes, a variety of diseases are increasingly common in the aging population. Nurses must be careful to distinguish between normal physiologic changes and abnormal alterations that indicate the need for prompt medical attention.

READINGS AND REFERENCES

Barrett-Connor E, Palinkas LA: Low blood pressure and depression in older men: a population based study, *BMJ* 308:446, 1994.

Eaglstein WH, McKay M, Pariser DM: The problems that plague aging skin, *Patient Care* 28:89, 1994.

Ebersole P, Hess P: *Toward healthy aging, human needs and nursing response,* ed 5: St Louis, 1998, Mosby.

Gunby P: Graying of America stimulates more reserach on aging-associated factors, *JAMA* 272:1561, 1994.

Lueckenotte A: *Gerontologic nursing,* St Louis, 1996, Mosby.

Martini FH, et al: *Fundamentals of anatomy and physiology,* ed 3, Englewood Cliff, NJ, 1995, Prentice Hall.

Mayo Foundation for Medical Education and Research, Topics in Geriatrics, www.mayo.edu/geriatrics.

Mulrow CD, Cornell JA, Herrera CR: Hypertension in the elderly: implications and generalizabilitiy of random trials, *JAMA* 272:1932, 1994.

Schneider DL, Barrett-Connor EL, Morton DJ: Thyroid hormone use and bone mineral density in elderly men, *Arch Intern Med* 155:2005, 1995.

Sweeting JG: *Normal effects of aging.* In *Columbia University College of Physicians and Surgeons complete home medical guide,* ed 2, 1989.

Sweeting JG: *Common complaints of aging.* In *Columbia University College of Physicians and Surgeons complete home medical guide,* ed 2, 1989.

Sweeting JG: *Major illness affecting the aging.* In *Columbia University College of Physicians and Surgeons complete home medical guide,* ed 2, 1989.

Thibodeau GA, Patton KT: *Structure and function of the human body,* ed 10, St Louis, 1997, Mosby.

University Hospital: The aging eye, *University Health Quarterly,* www.umdj.edu/univhosp, 1996.

VanderSchaaf R: Body audit: is your body older than your chronological age? *Weight Watchers Magazine* 10:28, 1996.

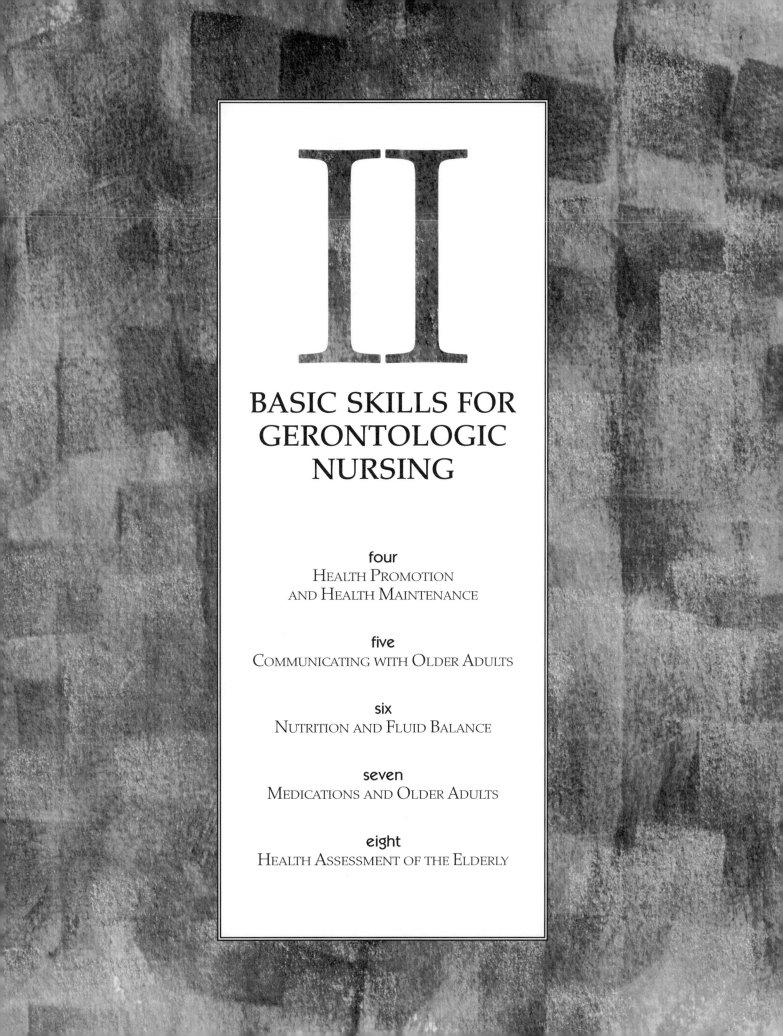

II

BASIC SKILLS FOR GERONTOLOGIC NURSING

chapter four

4

HEALTH PROMOTION AND HEALTH MAINTENANCE

LEARNING OBJECTIVES

1. Describe recommended health maintenance practices and explain how they change with aging.
2. Discuss the relationship of culture and religion to health practices.
3. Identify how perceptions of aging will affect health practices.
4. Describe how health maintenance is affected by cognitive and sensory changes.
5. Discuss the impact of decreased accessibility on health maintenance practices.
6. Describe methods of assessing health maintenance practices.
7. Identify older adults who are most at risk for experiencing health maintenance problems.
8. Identify selected nursing diagnoses related to health maintenance problems.
9. Describe nursing interventions that are appropriate for older adults experiencing alterations in health maintenance.

As people live longer and the percentage of elderly in the population increases, society faces several major challenges. One of the most significant of these challenges involves meeting the health care needs of the aging population.

Today's elderly are generally healthier than were the elderly of previous generations. Improvements in sanitation, public health, and occupational safety implemented during the 20th century have helped to raise the age at which a person can expect to experience a life-threatening disease.

The elderly can and do experience acute, life-threatening, medical conditions just as younger persons do, but acute episodes in the elderly are more likely to be associated with chronic conditions. Either an acute condition is caused by a chronic problem, or a chronic problem persists after an acute episode. It is estimated that 80% of the elderly live with chronic conditions such as arthritis, hypertension, diabetes, heart disease, and vision or hearing disorders. Most of those with chronic illness are able to meet their own needs; only about 25% require any special type of care. Both acute and chronic health care are expensive.

Although the elderly comprise only about 12% of today's population, they account for more than a third of all health care expenditures. By and large, today's elderly population has benefited from improvements in medical care. Advances in surgery, technology, and pharmacology have enabled us to prolong life in situations that even a few years ago would have been impossible.

This level of care is not without substantial cost. Because a significant portion of the elderly's health care expenses are covered by Medicare and Medicaid, the burden on the younger members of society is becoming overwhelming. Predictions indicate that despite steady increases in payroll taxes on the working population, Medicare will be operating at a deficit by the start of the 21st century. Because there is a limit to how much taxpayer money is available, society must identify appropriate and acceptable ways to control health care costs.

One way of dealing with a steady increase in demand for health care services involves rationing the type and amount of care provided to the elderly. This approach would prohibit or severely limit the type of care provided, particularly in cases in which the potential for significant improvement in health status is limited. For example, some of the more costly treatments and procedures (e.g., renal dialysis, bypass surgery) could be refused if the person was over a predetermined age. This method has been adopted in some countries but is unpopular in the United States. To avoid rationing health care, we must find ways to maximize the effectiveness of our health care expenditures.

Most studies reveal that it is more cost-effective to prevent problems than it is to attempt to cure or treat them. Therefore, more health care providers and the public (including the elderly) are beginning to recognize the need to devote more attention to health promotion and health maintenance.

Health promotion is not a new concept. For decades, health care providers have stressed the importance of good nutrition, exercise, and regular medical care. Although most of this information was directed toward younger people, many older people who desired to live longer, healthier lives also paid attention. As the benefits of healthy lifestyle choices became obvious, television, radio, and other media joined health care providers in promoting health awareness. Awareness of the importance of good health maintenance practices increased. Many individuals have modified their lifestyle and health care practices to improve their overall health and quality of life. Those who are unaware or are unwilling to heed this advice persist in risky, health-threatening behavior. Nurses need to be aware of the health promotion and maintenance practices that will most benefit the elderly. They also need to understand why some elderly people choose to adopt positive health behaviors while others persist in seemingly self-destructive behavior.

RECOMMENDED HEALTH PRACTICES FOR THE ELDERLY

Diet

The elderly should consume a well-balanced diet based on the food pyramid and recommended daily allowances of nutrients. Some changes in caloric intake and protein and vitamin needs appear to be desirable with aging (see Chapter 6).

When special diets are indicated, the elderly need to learn how to read and interpret the information provided on packaging labels. This is particularly important with sodium-restricted diets because sodium is common in foods that do not necessarily taste salty. Because food labels are often printed in very small type, the elderly should be sure to bring their eyeglasses or a magnifying glass when they go shopping. If someone else shops for them, that individual needs to know how to shop wisely.

Exercise

Regular exercise should be a part of any daily plan for the elderly (Fig. 4-1). Exercise can help keep the joints flexible, maintain muscle mass, control blood glucose levels and weight, and promote a sense of well-being. Exercise does not need to be aerobic to benefit the el-

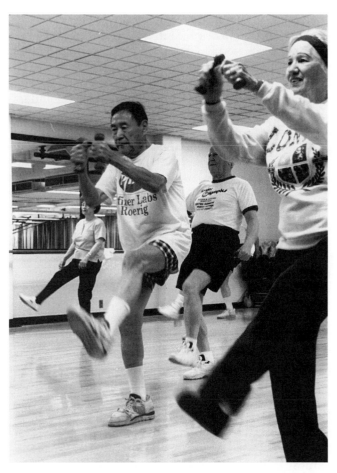

FIG. 4-1   Older adults in exercise class: practicing health promotion. (Courtesy of Ursula Ruhl, St Louis.)

derly. Walking, swimming, golf, housekeeping, and active lawn work or gardening are all considered exercise. To be of most benefit, at least 30 minutes of continuous activity are necessary. The type, level, and amount of exercise that is most beneficial will differ for each person and should be based on physician recommendations.

Tobacco and Alcohol

It is never too late to stop smoking. Even the body of an elderly person can repair damage once smoking is discontinued. This may be difficult when smoking has been a longstanding habit, but various aids are now available to help smokers quit. Before using any of these aids, the elderly should seek guidance from their physicians because there may be some special precautions related to existing health problems.

Excessive consumption of alcoholic beverages is never recommended. Alcoholism is an all too frequent problem in the elderly population—both men and women—because alcohol may be used as a means of coping with depression, sleep disorders, or other

problems. Occasional or moderate alcohol consumption by the elderly is usually not prohibited or restricted unless there is some medical condition or medication that precludes its use. Some physicians even recommend a glass of wine or beer as an appetite enhancer in certain situations.

Physical Examinations and Preventive Overall Care

The elderly should be examined at least once a year by their physicians, and more often if known health problems exist. Some elderly resist this because of the cost or of fear about what the physician may find. Cost is a real concern to many elderly people, but inadequate health maintenance should be of more concern. A delay in the recognition of problems may make them more difficult and more costly to treat. Physical examinations provide an opportunity for the physician to detect problems before they become more serious, to monitor and treat chronic conditions, and to prevent some health problems.

Physical examinations in the elderly should include evaluations of height and weight, blood pressure, and blood cholesterol levels as well as a rectal examination. In addition, women should have a pelvic examination, mammogram, and PAP test. Elderly men will need a prostate examination and blood tests to rule out prostate cancer. Persons with identified risk factors for colon cancer will require occult blood screening and possibly colonoscopy.

Evaluation of joints, feet, and gait should be part of the physical examination. Problems with the knees and shoulder joints can cause pain, limitation of activity, poor sleep, and decreased overall function. Some problems require surgical correction, whereas others can be treated more simply using analgesics, antiinflammatory medications, or physical therapy. Inspection of the feet often reveals problems. One study in England found that about 75% of the elderly had difficulty caring for their toenails because of poor vision, an inability to reach the feet, or hypertrophic nail changes. Bunions, calluses, and corns also cause problems for the elderly. Neglecting the feet can lead to discomfort, restricted mobility, and a poorer quality of life. If the feet are not properly cared for the risks for infection and even amputation increase, particularly in elderly individuals with compromised circulation. The elderly should be encouraged to wear properly fitted shoes that provide good support. Regular visits to a podiatrist can significantly reduce foot problems. Joint or foot problems, illness, pain, and other conditions commonly seen with aging can contribute to gait changes that are likely to result in imbalance or falls. When gait problems are identified, physical therapy for gait retraining and strengthening exercises, use of assistive devices, and environmental modification are appropriate (see Chapter 9).

Vision should be checked on a yearly basis to monitor for glaucoma or other eye problems. Refractive examinations can detect the need for a change in eyeglass prescription. Hearing examinations need not be done on a yearly basis unless a problem is suspected. When signs of diminished hearing are present, audiometric testing is appropriate.

Blood tests for hypothyroidism, diabetes, or cholesterol levels; electrocardiograms; and other diagnostic tests are not routinely part of the physical examination. The elderly should be aware of the need to communicate any symptoms they experience so their physicians can determine the need for additional testing.

In addition to regular physical examinations, the elderly should be sure to obtain immunization against diseases such as pneumonia and influenza that are more common in the elderly than in younger adults. The pneumonia vaccine is given once, usually at 65 or 70 years of age and Medicare now covers the cost of this immunization. The influenza vaccine must be obtained on a yearly basis, usually in the fall, because the strain of the virus changes frequently. "Flu shots" can be obtained from private physicians or from clinics that are available in most communities. The need for the hepatitis B immunization is based on individual risk factors and should be discussed with a physician. The need for tetanus immunizations for the elderly is somewhat controversial: Recommendations for tetanus boosters range from once every 10 years to a single booster given at age 65.

Prophylactic use of medications such as aspirin (to prevent cardiovascular disease) and the hormones estrogen and progesterone (to prevent coronary artery disease and osteoporosis) are gaining increased acceptance in the medical community. The elderly should be encouraged to discuss the possible benefits of this type of therapy with their physicians and then follow the recommendations.

Use of prescription and over-the-counter medications is common in the aging population. Elderly people with medical conditions must understand the reasons for and the importance of their treatment plans. They should keep a record card listing all of their medications and the name of the physicians who prescribed them. This card should be shown to all licensed professionals they see in order to prevent serious drug interactions. They must know how and when to take prescribed medications, how to use over-the-counter medication safely, how to store their medications, and when to report side effects. Sharing prescription medications with friends or neighbors is dangerous and should be avoided. Medications can be

confusing and even overwhelming to many elderly persons. Additional precautions regarding medications are discussed in Chapter 7.

In order to keep track of medical appointments, elderly persons should have a calendar or datebook where they can record all appointments or reminders for things such as immunizations. They should also be aware of signs and symptoms that indicate a need to seek medical attention above and beyond routine yearly examinations. Signs and symptoms indicating the need for prompt medical attention are listed in Box 4-1.

Elderly people who have health problems or allergies, those taking medications such as heparin, and those with implanted medical devices such as pacemakers are advised to wear a Medic Alert–style bracelet or necklace. If they do not wish to wear such a warning device, these individuals should at least carry a card in their wallets or purses to provide the necessary health information.

Dental Examinations and Preventive Oral Care

Dental examinations should be obtained and inspection of the oral cavity performed on a regular basis (at least once a year). Today's elderly are keeping their natural teeth longer than previous generations were able to, probably because of better nutrition and improved prophylactic dental care. Gum disease and

---

BOX 4-1

Signs and Symptoms Indicating a Need for Prompt Medical Attention

- Severe pain; radiating or crushing chest, neck, or jaw pain; severe unremitting headache
- Difficulty breathing
- Loss of consciousness
- Loss of movement or sensation in any body part or parts
- Sudden vision changes
- Unusual drainage or discharge from any body cavity
- Wounds that do not heal
- Nausea or vomiting that persists for 24 hours or longer
- Elevated body temperature
- Inability to urinate
- Swelling of the lower extremities
- Excessive (>10%) weight gain or loss
- Sudden or dramatic behavior changes

tooth decay are major causes of tooth loss. To prevent or slow the progress of these dental problems, the elderly should brush their natural teeth at least daily using a fluoride toothpaste and should floss carefully between the teeth. Mouthwash may help refresh the breath, but it cannot replace regular brushing.

It is recommended that the elderly use soft-bristle brushes to clean all tooth surfaces. Elderly persons, particularly those suffering from arthritis, may have difficulty holding a standard toothbrush. Enlarging the brush handle using tape, wide rubber bands, sponges, or polystyrene or lengthening the brush by attaching a wood or plastic strip may make it easier to hold. Some elderly prefer an electric toothbrush that provides the movement.

Circular or short back and forth brushing works best to clean the teeth. Close attention should be paid to removing all plaque from along the gumline. Red, swollen, or bleeding gums indicate the need to see a dentist. People should have their teeth professionally cleaned at least once a year to remove stains and other debris missed by routine brushing.

Elderly people who wear dentures still need regular oral examinations because people over 65 years of age account for more than half of the new cases of oral cancer each year. Good oral hygiene is also necessary. Dentures must be brushed or cleaned at least once a day to remove food debris, bacteria, and stains and to prevent gum irritation or bad breath. Some denture wearers prefer to brush the dentures using a special dentifrice, whereas others prefer to use a soaking solution that works overnight. Either cleansing method is appropriate, but the chemicals should be rinsed thoroughly from the denture before it is put back into the mouth.

An elderly person wearing dentures for the first time needs to become adept at inserting and removing them. Wearing dentures is often awkward, necessitating some relearning in order to chew effectively. Taking smaller pieces of soft, nonsticky foods and chewing more slowly are recommended. Because dentures make the mouth less sensitive to heat, cold, and foreign objects such as bone fragments, special care is required when eating.

Poorly fitting dentures are a major reason that some elderly fail to wear them regularly. This contributes to problems with nutrition and digestion. A few extra appointments with the dentist are often necessary to help fit the dentures properly. These adjustments are important because poorly fitting dentures can cause irritation to the gums or mucous membranes of the mouth. Additional adjustments may be needed when the denture wearer gains or loses weight.

Other changes in the oral cavity (e.g., dryness) are also common with aging. Although saliva production does not decrease in all elderly people, a variety of medical conditions, medications, and treatments can cause or contribute to dry mouth. Dry mouth can best be relieved by drinking more water. Excessive use of "hard candy," caffeine beverages, alcohol, or tobacco increases dryness of the mouth.

Maintaining Healthy Attitudes

There are strong connections between the mind and body. Elderly people who maintain a positive outlook on life tend to follow good health practices and remain healthier longer.

Regular interaction with other people of all age groups helps maintain a positive attitude toward life. It is recommended that the elderly get out of the house as often as possible, even if just for shopping or dinner. Keeping in touch with family and friends is important. When spouses or friends are lost through death or relocation, the elderly will benefit from attempting to establish new relationships by joining church or community social groups. Volunteering in hospitals, schools, literacy centers, or other community agencies is a popular and desirable activity because it helps to promote a sense of values and self-worth. Nurses cannot force an individual to participate beyond his or her wishes, but a little encouragement and information about options can help stimulate the elderly person's interests.

FACTORS AFFECTING HEALTH PROMOTION AND MAINTENANCE

The actions taken to promote, maintain, or improve health are based on that individual's perception of his or her health. Health perceptions influence day-to-day choices regarding hygiene practices; nutrition; exercise; use of alcohol, drugs, and tobacco; accessing health care; and many other activities. Health maintenance practices include safety precautions taken to prevent injury from automobile accidents, falls, poisoning, and other hazards. Health perceptions and health maintenance practices in the elderly are influenced by personal beliefs, religious and cultural beliefs, socioeconomic status, education, and life experiences.

As people mature, they establish a set of beliefs, perceptions, and values related to health. These perceptions include basic ideas regarding what health is and how to best maintain it. These beliefs form the foundation for each person's health practices. Based on their unique beliefs, most people perform activities that they perceive to be helpful in maintaining their health and avoid activities they perceive as harmful. It is very difficult to change the health practices of a lifetime. Only those who are highly motivated to change are likely to be successful.

Religious beliefs contribute to an individual's perceptions. These beliefs can promote health maintenance or interfere with good health practices and result in increased health risks. For example, some religions teach that the body is a temple, stressing the importance of avoiding alcohol, tobacco, and other behaviors that are harmful to health. Individuals with these religious beliefs tend to live longer, healthier lives than do people who do not share these values. Other persons, whose religions teach that illness is a punishment for sins, may feel that they are not worthy of health and must endure illness as atonement for things they have done wrong in their lives.

Cultural beliefs and practices also play a significant role in health perception and health maintenance. For example, reliance on home health remedies is common in many cultures. Some home remedies are harmless, whereas others are quite dangerous. Problems can occur when home remedies are used in place of conventional medical care or when their use results in delayed care, which can be serious or even fatal if the illness is a serious one. Culture also plays a significant role in the selection of food and the methods used for food preparation. These preferences and practices play a significant role in health promotion and maintenance. Diets that consist mainly of fruit, vegetables, and grains are common in some cultures, whereas diets high in fat and sodium are prevalent in others. These variations can contribute to the good health of some ethnic populations or to the health problems seen in others.

As our society becomes increasingly diverse, nurses need to become more aware of the religious and cultural factors that affect the health maintenance practices of all persons. Information about the beliefs and practices of organized religions and major cultural groups is available through sources such as textbooks on transcultural nursing. Although nurses can gain valuable insight from such sources, we must be careful not to generalize. It is common for two individuals from very similar religious and cultural backgrounds to have widely disparate perceptions and practices. Although a general understanding of cultural factors is important, the best source of accurate information about a person's beliefs and practices is that individual. An overview of common health practices will help nurses understand the underlying values and beliefs that motivate each individual.

Factors other than religious and cultural beliefs also play a part in health perceptions and health maintenance practices. Knowledge plays a key role in maintaining health and promoting safety; knowledge of recommended health practices is essential in order to make good choices. Health and safety teaching must start early and be reinforced throughout life. Whenever there is a significant change in a person's health status, additional teaching is necessary to ensure the safety and highest possible level of wellness of that individual. People cannot make informed decisions regarding their health and safety unless they know the ramifications of various behaviors. Individuals experiencing cognitive changes due to disease processes or chemical dependence may not be able to understand the need for safety or health maintenance practices despite repeated teaching. People with severe cognitive or perceptual problems are very likely to experience injuries and alterations in health maintenance practices.

Health maintenance requires motivation in addition to knowledge. People experiencing grief, depression, hopelessness, or low self-esteem may not be motivated to maintain good health practices. Motivating individuals to maintain health is often difficult. All of the teaching in the world will not replace the desire to live a healthy life.

Even people who are knowledgeable and motivated to maintain their health may have trouble if they cannot obtain the goods or services they need. People with limited physical mobility, transportation, or money are likely to experience difficulty. A person who knows the importance of nutritious food but who cannot get to a store or afford the food will have difficulty maintaining good health. A person who knows it is important to see a physician but who can neither get to the office nor pay for medical care is similarly at risk.

Assessment of the values, perceptions, knowledge level, motivations, and lifelong health practices of individuals provides an understanding of the likelihood of problems with health maintenance. Previous behavior is a good indicator of future practice and motivation.

Importance of Aging

Many beliefs about health and health maintenance are formed early in life. The longer a belief is held, the harder it is to change that belief. Hence it is often difficult to change the health behaviors of older adults.

Perceptions of good health and good health practices vary widely among the aging population. Older adults have their own beliefs about what is normal and expected with aging. Some are willing to accept declining health as a normal part of aging, whereas others are not. Those who perceive a decline in health as normal and expected with aging may do little to prevent loss of function, simply accepting the changes. "Why should I bother to see the doctor? It's just old age" is a common sentiment. Some elderly people frequently ignore early signs of illness or attribute them to aging. This often results in a delay before seeking medical care. Others, particularly those who have followed good health practices throughout their lives, believe that old age is not synonymous with disease or loss of function. They continue to follow high-level health maintenance practices in all aspects of their lives, including diet, exercise, rest, and medical attention.

Perceptions regarding aging greatly affect a person's motivation and willingness to participate in health maintenance activities. A person who feels capable and in control of his or her life is more likely to be willing to change behaviors and to work at maintaining health. Elderly persons who feel useless, helpless, or without purpose, particularly the newly widowed or those who are estranged from their families, are less likely to be motivated to maintain their health.

Impact of Cognitive and Sensory Changes

Cognitive and sensory changes related to aging or disease can lead to problems with health maintenance. Even the normal sensory changes of aging can increase the risks of personal neglect or injury. When significant cognitive or perceptual problems occur, the risks are even greater.

An elderly person with changes in vision and smell may have body odor or wear soiled clothing because he or she cannot see or smell soiling. Changes in vision, hearing, smell, sensation, taste, and memory can also lead to decreased awareness of normal environmental hazards. Sensory changes increase the risk of injuries from falls, poisoning, fire, and other traumatic events. Vision changes can cause the elderly person to miss the edge of a step or a curb and result in a fall. Changes in smell and taste can result in consumption of spoiled, unsafe food. Changes in sensation can lead to the use of overly hot bath water, resulting in burns. Changes in the sense of smell can cause the older adult to not perceive a burning odor, resulting in the increased likelihood of injury from fire.

Elderly people who are seriously impaired either perceptually or cognitively commonly lack awareness of their own needs. They may ignore parts of their hygiene or may completely forget to perform routine health maintenance activities such as bathing, eating, or taking medication. Common health practices may be neglected even though the person is physically capable of performing the activities.

Cognitively impaired elderly persons are at serious risk of injury because they are unable to recognize the danger of their actions or lack of actions. They may forget to turn off the burner on the stove, forget to put on a coat when going outside in winter, turn up the furnace instead of turning it off, or walk into a busy street without looking for traffic. Severely impaired persons are at great risk of experiencing problems related to safety and health maintenance, often requiring some form of supervised living or institutional care for their own protection.

Impact of Changes Related to Accessibility

Aging persons are likely to experience more problems accessing goods and services than are younger people. Access may be limited by decreased physical mobility, lack of transportation, or limited finances. If more than one of these factors is present, the risk of altered health maintenance increases dramatically.

Physical limitations, including loss of motor skills, decreased strength and endurance, and the presence of disease, make health maintenance activities more difficult. Decreased physical strength and agility can interfere with normal health maintenance practices. Simple acts such as bathing, cooking, and cleaning can be too physically demanding for some elderly, who may be too fatigued to even attempt normal self-care activities. This lack of strength or energy often results in poor health maintenance practices.

Transportation difficulties present many problems for the elderly. Simply getting to the grocery store, pharmacy, or physician's office when necessary can be a major impediment to health maintenance. Even if the elderly desire to practice good health maintenance, they may be hindered by a lack of transportation.

Finances cannot be ignored when discussing health maintenance. Although Social Security, Medicare, and Medicaid offset some financial concerns, they do not cover the entire cost of health care prescriptions or meals. The lack of these resources may cause the elderly to limit medical care. Many elderly persist in trying to treat themselves before seeking medical attention. They may try to stretch the time between medical visits or take less than the prescribed amount of medications to conserve money. Financial constraints can also affect ability of the elderly person to purchase special foods and equipment necessary to promote or maintain health.

Finances can also impact safety. Many elderly people live in older housing, which is more likely to contain safety hazards such as poor electric wiring, steep stairwells, and inadequate lighting. High crime rates in poorer areas make the elderly who live there particularly vulnerable to rape, mugging, and theft.

Even if these factors are not a problem, simple home maintenance can increase the risk of injury. Because it is costly to hire people to do even routine home maintenance chores, many elderly people attempt these tasks alone. Some fall from chairs or ladders while trying to paint walls, clean windows, or hang pictures. Many injure themselves trying to shovel snow or mow a lawn.

NURSING PROCESS
ALTERED HEALTH MAINTENANCE

Assessment of health perception and health maintenance takes into account the unique problems, beliefs, and perceptions of the aging person. It is important to assess both past and current health management practices because they are good predictors of future health practices.

Assessment of Health Perceptions and Health Maintenance

- How does the person rate his or her current health?
- Does the person feel in control of the conditions that affect his or her health?
- What does the person routinely do to maintain his or her health?
- How does the person manage illnesses?
- What are the person's religious or cultural beliefs regarding health and health practices?
- How do the person's health practices compare with recommended health practices?
- How often does the person see a physician, dentist, or other health professional?
- Does the person undertake high-risk behaviors such as smoking, excessive alcohol intake, or drug consumption?
- Does the person have adequate financial resources to maintain his or her health?
- Does the person have access to the goods and services necessary to maintain health?
- Is the person's knowledge adequate to make informed decisions regarding his or her health?

See Box 4-2 for a list of the characteristics of older persons who are at risk for alterations in health maintenance.

Nursing Diagnosis

Altered health maintenance

Nursing Goals/Outcomes

The nursing goals for an elderly person demonstrating altered health maintenance are to verbalize appropriate health maintenance practices; demonstrate adequate health maintenance practices; and identify community resources that can assist in health maintenance.

Nursing Interventions

The following nursing interventions for altered health maintenance should take place in hospitals or extended-care facilities:

1. **Assess the person's ability to resume normal health maintenance practices.** After hospitalization or rehabilitation in an extended-care facility, the elderly must be assessed carefully to determine whether they are capable of returning home and resuming normal health maintenance practices. Ideally, discharge from the facility should be delayed until the nurse can be reasonably sure that the patient is ready to take responsibility for his or her own health care needs. If possible, an assessment of the home environment should also be made before discharge. If necessary, the environment should be modified to promote health maintenance and safety. A referral for a follow-up visit after discharge will help ensure that the elderly person is safe and able to meet his or her health maintenance needs.
2. **Teach the skills required to monitor health status if and when the patient returns home.** Before discharge from a health care institution, the elderly should have a thorough explanation of what they need to do to maintain health, including when to call or see the physician; what medications are required and when they should be taken; how to per-

---

BOX 4-2

Characteristics of Older Adults Likely to Experience Alterations in Health Maintenance

- Lack of adequate knowledge of recommended health practices
- Physical limitations
- Limited financial resources
- Altered cognitive or perceptual function
- Difficulty accessing health-related goods or services
- Loss of motivation because of grief, hopelessness, or powerlessness

form home screening procedures (e.g., blood glucose monitoring, daily weights); and how to keep records and monitor their health condition.

3. **Consult with the social worker or with agencies that can assist with health maintenance practices.** The community social worker or social agencies may be able to help the elderly meet their health maintenance needs by providing transportation, delivering food or groceries, assisting with home maintenance, or offering other services.

The following interventions should take place in the home:

1. **Assess the existing health maintenance practices.** The nurse should assess the elderly person's knowledge of the factors that promote health. Any problem areas should be examined in greater detail. The nurse should also determine what motivates the person to maintain his or her health because these motivators may be valuable if modifications in health care practices become necessary.

2. **Explain and reinforce positive health maintenance behaviors.** The nurse should review health practices regarding diet, safety, stress management, exercise, elimination, and sleep. It is important to review when and how to contact a physician, particularly in cases of serious illness or emergency. If the elderly are receiving treatment for any health problems, they should know what health care behaviors are recommended in order to maintain the highest level of wellness (Box 4-3). They should know what medications to take and when to take them as well as how to perform any special care or treatments.

3. **Assist in identifying family or community resources that will promote health maintenance.** Individuals living in their homes may be unaware of services that are available to provide help. Often a little assistance is all that is needed to enable an elderly person to live a healthy, independent lifestyle. If assistance is delayed, health maintenance

may deteriorate to a point at which hospitalization or institutional placement is required. These services should be identified before they are required in order to avoid delays or waiting lists for the services.

4. **Use any appropriate interventions that are used in the institutional setting.**

NURSING PROCESS
NONCOMPLIANCE

A person is said to be noncompliant when he or she fails to follow through with recommended health practices. Failing to take prescribed medications, failing to attend scheduled medical appointments, and failing to follow prescribed diets are examples of noncompliant behaviors. Many factors may be related to noncompliance: cognitive impairment, inadequate knowledge, inadequate resources, lack of transportation, fear, anger, decreased self-esteem, substance abuse, and conflict of beliefs or values. Noncompliance should be suspected when a person does not show the expected amount of progress toward wellness, when a person gets worse instead of better, or when a person develops repeated or unexpected complications.

Assessment of Risk for Noncompliance

- Does the person verbalize unwillingness or inability to follow through with the necessary health maintenance or medical care recommendations?
- Does the person verbalize a conflict between personal beliefs or values and the treatment plan?
- Are there unexpected relapses, or do the health problems appear to be getting worse instead of better?
- Does the person often miss medical appointments? What reasons does he or she give?
- Is there more medication left in the bottle than would be expected if it were taken properly?
- Are there signs of the presence of prohibited foods (e.g., candy for diabetics, salt shaker for persons with sodium restriction)?

See Box 4-4 for a list of the characteristics of older persons who are at risk for noncompliance.

Nursing Diagnosis

Noncompliance

BOX 4-3

Recommended Health Practices to Maintain Wellness

- Eat a well-balanced diet.
- Establish a regular exercise program.
- Quit smoking.
- Consume alcohol in moderation.
- Get routine immunizations as recommended.
- Stay involved in activities and with others.
- Keep a healthy attitude.
- See the dentist and physician regularly.

BOX 4-4

Characteristics of Older Adults Likely to Be at Risk for Noncompliance

- Cognitive or perceptual problems
- Lack of adequate financial resources
- Poor self-esteem or altered body image
- Lack of a support system of friends and family
- Substance abuse problems
- Negative past experiences with the health care system
- Differing cultural or religious beliefs

Nursing Goals/Outcomes

The nursing goals for an elderly person demonstrating noncompliance are to identify factors that contribute to noncompliant behavior and demonstrate the acceptance of treatment.

Nursing Interventions

The following nursing interventions for noncompliance should take place in hospitals or extended-care facilities:

1. **Identify the reasons for noncompliant behavior.** There are many reasons a person may not comply with recommended health maintenance practices. Unless the nurse can determine the specific reasons why the person is not following the recommended practices, interventions are likely to be inappropriate and unsuccessful. If the person does not take medication because of forgetfulness, more teaching will not help. If the person refuses medication because he or she feels unworthy of living, no amount of reminders will help. Interventions must address the root problem. Forgetful people need a system of reminders; persons with poor self-esteem need to feel valued before care is accepted.

2. **Provide care in a nonjudgmental manner.** The values and beliefs of the elderly are often different from those of their caregivers. If the nurse indicates verbally or nonverbally that the elderly person's beliefs and practices are in some way inferior, the nurse is not likely to be able to convince the person to comply with the desired health practices.

3. **Actively include the patient in planning care, and adapt or modify the care plan so that it is more acceptable to the patient.** Develop all plans *with* not *for* the elderly person. Each individual can then incorporate his or her unique culture, beliefs, and values into the plan that is developed. This enables the elderly to retain control and responsibility for their own health care. When they "own" the plan

and determine the goals, they are more likely to be compliant.

4. **Emphasize the benefits of compliant behavior.** Many aging persons do not comply with recommended health care practices because they do not really believe that compliance will help. If the person has the opportunity to benefit when he or she is compliant, active involvement in care is more likely. For example, if a diabetic continually sneaks extra food and thus frequently has high blood glucose levels, the nurse can demonstrate how much lower the blood glucose level is when the person follows the prescribed diet. If less insulin or fewer injections would be required when the blood glucose level is controlled, these benefits should be stressed. Unfortunately, it is not always possible to see any obvious immediate benefits from compliant behavior.

5. **Acknowledge the aging person's right not to comply with the plan of care.** If an alert elderly person chooses not to comply with the plan of care despite explanations, teaching, and reminders, the nurse must recognize that this is in fact a right of the individual.

The following interventions should take place in the home:

1. **Assess the support system.** In the home setting, it is particularly important to identify the strengths of the elderly person and the amount of support he or she receives from friends and family. The likelihood of achieving compliance is far greater when the person is willing to learn and to modify his or her behavior and when he or she has others who are willing to help. The individual who resists intervention and receives little support is likely to continue to have problems with compliance.

2. **Help structure the environment to promote compliance.** Many individuals are noncompliant simply because they are confused or forgetful. Memory devices can catch their attention and verify that critical actions take place. For example, if the person forgets to eat meals, a checklist for the days of the week and the three basic meals can be posted on the refrigerator door. Each time the person fixes a meal, the box is checked. Likewise, special divided containers are available for people who have trouble remembering to take their medication. Medication for an entire week can be prepared by a responsible assistant or nurse. A simple glance in the box lets the person know whether he or she has taken the right medication at the right time. Bold markings on a calendar, preferably one with large print, can be used to mark special events. Signs in bold letters can be posted in appropriate places. For example, "take a drink" can be posted over the sink of a person whose fluid intake is inadequate.

NURSING CARE PLAN

HEALTH MAINTENANCE

Mrs. Fisher is an alert, well-groomed 82-year-old who lives alone in an apartment. She has a history of type 2 diabetes mellitus. Her blood glucose levels, which you test weekly, are consistently 200 mg/dl or higher. Her physician has prescribed a 1200-calorie diabetic diet and an oral hypoglycemic medication.

When you arrive early for a home visit, you find an open box of ginger snaps next to the chair where she was sitting. She says, "I like to sit around most of the day and read or watch TV." You ask about the cookies and she replies, "They're not very sweet; I need to have some food that I enjoy. I won't live forever, you know." You check the bottle of oral hypoglycemic medication and find that she has taken only two tablets in the past week. She states, "I forget to take them. They don't help anyway and they cost too much."

NURSING DIAGNOSIS

Noncompliance

DEFINING CHARACTERISTICS

- Consistently elevated blood glucose levels
- Failure to take prescribed medications
- Failure to follow prescribed diet
- Complaints of lifestyle changes in conflict with personal values

GOALS/OUTCOMES

Mrs. Fisher will
- follow her prescribed diet.
- increase her activity level.
- take her prescribed medications.
- achieve blood glucose levels of less than 120 mg/dl.

NURSING INTERVENTIONS

1. Assess Mrs. Fisher for any signs of tissue breakdown or other problems related to hyperglycemia.
2. Allow her to verbalize feelings and problems experienced with activity, diet, and medications.
3. Review her daily food intake.
4. Explain the importance of following her prescribed diet.
5. Set up a reminder system for daily medications.
6. Explore ways of increasing her physical activity.
7. Encourage her to comply with the plan of care.
8. Praise positive health care behaviors.
9. Continue to monitor her blood glucose level and notify the physician if it remains elevated.
10. Arrange a consultation with the dietitian at her next physician's office visit.

EVALUATION

At the next home visit a week later, you find that Mrs. Fischer's blood glucose level is 174 mg/dl. She states proudly that with the new medication system she has remembered to take six of her oral hypoglycemic tablets and only forgot one day. She further states that she has taken four short walks with her neighbor. After providing positive feedback on these signs of improved health maintenance, you discuss diet with her. Mrs. Fischer states that she has tried to be more careful, but because she still likes an occasional cookie she will limit herself to one or two at most a day. Improvement is demonstrated, but Mrs. Fischer's goals are only partially met. You will continue with the plan of care and reassess her again in 1 week.

3. **Enlist the help of family, friends, and neighbors to provide reminders.** Reminder phone calls from friends or family are useful for less frequent occasions such as doctor visits. It is wise for the friend or family member to call the person the day before the appointment and then again on the day of the appointment to ensure that he or she has not forgotten. Even better is for a responsible friend or family member to transport the person to the medical appointment. Responsible friends and family members can also provide help in setting up the weekly pillbox and preparing other reminders around the home.

4. **Involve social service agencies in promoting compliance.** If the person is noncompliant because of financial or transportation problems, a social worker or social service agency may be able to provide assistance that enables the person to comply with the care plan.

5. **Use any appropriate interventions that are used in the institutional setting.**

A nursing care plan for health maintenance in the elderly is presented on p. 83.

SUMMARY

A large percentage of today's aging population continues to live independently despite a variety of chronic health problems. Health maintenance is an ongoing challenge for these people, their families, and health care providers. Careful assessment of the aging person's perception of his or her health, health practices, and knowledge of safety factors is an important part of nursing care in all settings. Early detection of problems and early intervention can prevent more serious complications and enable older adults to maintain the highest possible level of wellness and function.

READINGS AND REFERENCES

AARP Web site: *Health promotion,*www.aarp.org/programs/healthpro, 1995.

Administration on Aging, National Institute on Aging Age Web site: *Taking care of your teeth and mouth,*www.aoa.dhhs.gov/aoa/pages/teethmou.html.

Ebersole P, Hess P: *Toward healthy aging: human needs and nursing responses,* ed 5, St Louis, 1998, Mosby.

Gurland BJ, Chachkes EE: Involving the elderly in their own health care. In *Columbia University College of Physicians and Surgeons complete home medical guide,* ed 2, 1989.

Gunby P: Graying of America stimulates more research on aging-associated factors, *JAMA* 272:1561, 1994.

Koch AL, Williams SH, Hylton HC: Marketing prevention to elderly. In Lueckenotte A: *Gerontologic nursing,* St Louis, 1996, Mosby.

Medicare beneficiaries enrolled in an HMO: the San Diego Medicare preventive health project, *Health Care Mktg,* 13:46, 1993.

Mayo Foundation for Medical Education and Research Web site: *Topics in geriatrics: preventative medicine,* www.mayo.edu/geriatrics, 1996-1997.

COMMUNICATING WITH OLDER ADULTS

1. Identify communication techniques that are effective with elderly persons.
2. Define empathetic listening.
3. Identify the significance of nonverbal communication with the elderly.
4. Discuss the verbal communication techniques used when sending and receiving messages.
5. Differentiate between social and therapeutic communication.

EFFECTIVE COMMUNICATION

Nursing Process and the Care of Older Adults

Communication is the process of exchanging information (i.e., sending messages back and forth between individuals or groups of people). Problems between individuals, families, or groups or difficulties on the job or in society are often the result of poor communication. Each of us who participates in communication is a unique individual with our own personal values, beliefs, perceptions, culture, and understanding of how the world operates. This is particularly important to remember when working with the elderly. The elderly of today formed their opinions, values, and beliefs in a very different society than ours today. Most of today's elderly grew up during the Great Depression when men sold apples on street corners and searched for pieces of coal in railroad yards to survive. They lived through a major world war and witnessed the beginning of the Nuclear Age when the first atomic bomb was dropped. They grew up in a world without many of today's conveniences, including televisions and private telephone lines. Today's elderly have experienced many good and bad times. It is not easy for a younger person to understand the experiences that made the elderly who they are today. The most effective way to bridge the gulf between the generations is good communication.

Effective communication is not easy even among people of the same age group and background. Communication among people with these differences can be even more difficult. Effective communication requires the desire to share knowledge with someone else. In order to want to communicate with the elderly, one must realize that there is value and merit in what elderly people have to say. Although effective communication does not mean that we must agree with everything that other people say, we should respect their right to think and say it. This atmosphere of mutual respect and understanding is called **rapport.**

For effective communication, one must learn to identify the barriers that can interfere with an exchange and the methods that will help overcome these barriers. Effective communication is not easy. Conscious, ongoing effort is required to become an effective communicator (Fig. 5-1).

Empathetic listening

In order to communicate effectively, one must first learn to listen actively and empathetically. Listening is more than simply hearing. Hearing involves the ability of the ears to detect sound, whereas listening involves interpretation—that is, figuring out what the sounds mean. One has not really listened until he or she understands for certain what was intended by the speaker. We cannot simply listen to the words; we must listen for the *meaning* of the words.

Empathy is defined as the willingness to attempt to understand the unique world of another person. It is the ability to put oneself in another person's place, and to understand what he or she is feeling and thinking in various situations. Empathetic listening involves actively trying to understand the other person, not just knowing a lot of facts about that person.

Active listening skills are needed in all areas of nursing, but particularly in dealing with the elderly. Empathetic listening requires sensitivity to the strengths and limitations of the aging individual (e.g., hearing changes, vision changes, fatigue, pain). It involves patience when an elderly person needs extra time to voice a response and includes a willingness to spend time getting to know the elderly person better as a human being—not just another body in need of skilled physical care. Too often we as nurses provide excellent physical care to people we have not taken the time to know. Empathetic listening requires the ability to focus on the aging person, not simply on the tasks at hand.

More than just the ability to talk to someone, communication involves all of the ways that we send messages to someone else, including nonverbal ways. Communication makes use of all of the senses. Hearing and vision are the senses used most frequently in communication, but touch, smell, and even taste also play a part in the relay of messages. It is important to remember this when communicating with the elderly because their perceptions may be altered by the physiologic changes that occur with aging. The diverse social and cultural backgrounds of the elderly and the

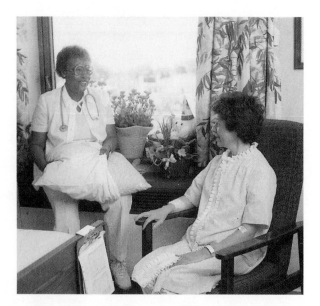

FIG. 5-1 Nurses integrate therapeutic communication skills into all aspects of care. (From Potter PA, Perry AG: *Basic nursing: theory and practice,* ed 3, St Louis, 1995, Mosby.)

physiologic changes that occur with aging make the area of communication a challenge for nurses (see the following clinical situation box).

Nonverbal Communication

Research has shown that only 7% of communication comes from the actual words we use; 93% is nonverbal. About 38% of communication is transmitted by para-linguistic cues (i.e., tone, pitch, and volume of voice), and 55% is transmitted by body cues. The importance of understanding nonverbal communication can be summed up in the statement: "What you are saying [nonverbally] is so loud I can't hear you." Because so much of our communication is nonverbal, it is essential that we examine each aspect of nonverbal communication to see its effect on our interactions with the elderly person.

Symbols

If two people entered a room—one wearing a white lab coat with a stethoscope around her neck and the other wearing a clerical collar and a cross—what message would you receive? Would these people have to *say* anything for communication to take place? What is being communicated? What we wear or carry (e.g., clothing, jewelry, stethoscopes, masks, gowns, gloves) sends messages; we use these symbols to communicate something about who we are. Distinctive uniforms are worn to make people identifiable: police-officers, flight attendants, clergy, and nurses wear uniforms so they can be recognized even in a crowd.

In health care settings, uniform styles and colors help patients distinguish the various caregivers. Many patients, particularly older adults, were unhappy when nurses stopped wearing caps. The white uniform and cap were symbols that helped the elderly easily distinguish nurses from other caregivers. For this reason, nurses in some nursing homes continue to wear white uniforms and caps. In other settings nurses may not wear any distinguishing uniform. Street clothes or

a navy blue outfit with an identifying name tag are preferred in some agencies, particularly in home care or public health. This can be confusing to the elderly because such clothing is not distinctive enough to identify the individual as a nurse, and many elderly cannot read the small print on name tags. The elderly have been heard to say to caregivers, "Who are you and what are you going to do to me?" Although nurses may not place much importance on wearing a uniform, it does play a part in communication.

Tone of voice

Think of the sound of a whisper, shout, or whine. Try saying "I don't want to do that" in a whisper, shout, and whine and then in a normal speaking voice. Was your understanding of the message the same in each situation? Probably not. In order to survive, we learn very early in life to understand that tone of voice is a fairly reliable way of judging a person's emotions. Because the nonverbal message is so strong, we typically respond to the emotion we perceive from the tone of voice and may not even hear the words. When a person shouts at us, we normally shout back. Shouting is often associated with anger or displeasure, yet many people shout in an attempt to communicate with someone who is hard of hearing. Shouting is not an appropriate way to deal with hearing problems because our tone of voice may lead the hearing-impaired person to think we are angry with them when this is not the case. Speaking in a low tone of voice close to the person's good ear is much more effective. Use of other nonverbal methods of communication, such as communication boards or gestures, can also help.

Body language

You walk past a room and observe a nurse standing in the doorway, with his or her head sticking into the room and body still in the hallway. The nurse's mouth is saying, "Can I help you?," but the body is saying, "I'm in a hurry; you really don't want anything, do you?" We communicate many things by how we move, stand, sit, and position our bodies. In dealing with all patients, but particularly the elderly, it is important that we be aware of what we are communicating through our body language.

In situations in which the words and body language are conveying two different messages, most people will respond to the body language. Standing at the door, hurrying down the hallway, sitting behind the nurses' station, and working in the medication or treatment room all communicate that the nurse is busy and does not want to be interrupted. Many older adults and their families are intimidated by this body language and may hesitate to interrupt, even to report serious concerns. Nurses must be careful not to create barriers

---

CLINICAL SITUATION

A doctor and a clergyman happened to arrive in an elderly patient's room at the same time. The patient became very anxious and started to cry. The physician and the clergyman were taken aback because the patient was doing well and was ready for discharge. After much time was spent calming the patient and listening carefully, they realized that she responded as she did because she thought the doctor was going to tell her that she was dying, and the clergyman was there to console her.

between themselves and their patients. Going *into* the rooms to talk with patients, sitting down at eye level with residents, and spending time in the lounge with visitors are all ways of nonverbally communicating that you are truly interested and concerned.

Another part of nonverbal communication involves watching for the messages that patients are communicating to us through their body language. For example, patients who slump down or slouch in their chairs may be communicating fatigue or physical weakness, or they may be communicating lack of interest, sadness, defiance, or a number of other things. Turning away from the nurse could indicate anger, fear, or lack of interest. When body language says something different than the words, believe the body language. Explore the situation using techniques such as reflective or open-ended statements. (These techniques will be clarified later in the chapter.)

Space, distance, and position

Physical space, distance, and position are other ways we communicate. The study of use of personal space in communication is referred to as **proxemics.** Personal space refers to how close we allow someone to get to us before we feel uncomfortable. The amount of space that separates two individuals when they communicate is significant. In the traditional American culture, most people are comfortable when strangers are 12 feet or more away. This is considered **public space;** at this distance, there is no real positive or negative connection with the other person. Between 4 and 12 feet is considered **social space.** This is a comfortable distance for a casual relationship in which communication is at an impersonal level. If a nurse stays this far away from his or her patients, the message being communicated is indifference. A distance of 18 inches to 4 feet is considered **personal space.** This is the optimal distance for close interpersonal communication with another person. A nurse who communicates from within this space is usually viewed as concerned and interested. The space within 18 inches of the body is considered **intimate space.** Most people allow only trusted individuals to get this close. Entering the intimate space without permission is usually perceived as a threat.

A nurse or other caregiver may approach an elderly person to provide care or treatment and without thinking enter this intimate space too quickly. (Because of the nature of their work, nurses and other caregivers are used to entering a person's intimate space and they think nothing of it.) An elderly person who has poor vision or hearing, who has been sleeping, or who is not totally alert may be startled by the nurse's approach. He or she may not be able to recognize the nurse as a trusted person at first and may

strike out verbally or physically. This response results from fear of physical attack. It is essential that nurses recognize the importance of personal space and attempt to get the elderly individual's attention and (if possible) permission before attempting to perform any physical care.

Gestures

Gestures are a specific type of nonverbal communication intended to convey ideas. Gestures are highly cultural and generational; those that are acceptable in one culture may be considered offensive in another. Some gestures that are accepted today as commonplace were once considered crude or insulting. Gestures that have a certain meaning in one culture may have a different meaning in another. For example, nodding the head up and down means yes in most cultures, but to some Eskimo tribes it means no. Before using gestures, it is wise to determine that both parties have the same understanding of just what a particular gesture means.

Gestures are helpful for people who cannot use words. After a stroke, many individuals suffer from a condition called **aphasia.** Because of brain damage, these individuals may not be able to recognize words or to "find" the words they want to use. This inability to communicate wants, needs, and feelings is often very frustrating to the affected person and the use of gestures and other nonverbal forms of communication can be effective.

Facial expressions

Facial expressions are yet another form of communication. The human face is most expressive, and facial expressions have been shown to communicate across cultural and age barriers. Smiles, frowns, and grimaces appear to have the same meaning whether you are in the outback of Australia or a board room on Wall Street. Humans respond to facial expressions from the time they are born. We tend to mirror the expressions of the person with whom we are communicating: Smiles tend to elicit smiles, and frowns elicit frowns. Fear, anger, joy, and a wide variety of other emotions can be conveyed by a simple change in facial expression. Nurses need to be aware of this fact and ensure that their expressions communicate what is intended. Too often nurses are preoccupied while interacting with an elderly person. A frown may lead the individual to think that he or she has done something wrong. A wrinkled nose, particularly when cleaning up an episode of incontinence, could be viewed as lack of acceptance. A smile when listening to serious concerns may make the person wonder whether the nurse really cares about what is being said.

Eye contact

"Look me in the eye" is a phrase many white Americans have heard. Looking someone in the eye is perceived in our and other cultures as a measure of honesty. Yet in some cultures (e.g., African-American and some parts of Southeast Asia), averting the eyes communicates respect. When dealing with the elderly, it is important to be sensitive to the meaning of eye contact for them. Face-to-face, eye-to-eye contact can be helpful when communicating with the elderly, providing this does not frighten or intimidate them. Face-to-face contact also maximizes the chance that an elderly person with hearing problems can lipread if necessary.

Pace or speed of communication

Nurses tend to be substantially younger than the aging people they serve. The resulting difference in rate of speech and movement can be overwhelming and frustrating to the elderly. Many choose not to respond or interact with younger nurses because they feel they are being hurried. Nurses have often been observed completing sentences for elderly persons when they should have the patience to wait for the individuals to organize their thoughts and speak. Many times nurses complete the communication according to their own way of thinking rather than waiting to hear what the elderly person wants to say. Patience and active listening are greatly needed skills when working with the elderly. "Slower is better" should be the motto impressed in the mind of anyone who chooses to work with the elderly.

Time and timing

Timing is related to the pace of communication, but it has other distinct implications as well. The amount of time a person must wait after seeking attention is important. If a nurse delays in responding, the person who sought the attention may communicate anger, displeasure, anxiety, fear, and many other feelings. Studies have shown that nurses take longer to respond to terminally ill patients. Nurses also tend to give delayed responses to demanding individuals. This can set up a vicious cycle because the longer a person waits for a response, the greater his or her anger, fear, and anxiety becomes. This only increases the demanding behaviors, which often occur in an attempt to reduce fear. If the elderly person's needs are dealt with promptly, the number of demands tends to *decrease,* not increase. Making the elderly wait unnecessarily constitutes a subtle form of abuse.

Many elderly individuals have an altered sense of time. A message that is communicated too early may lead to either forgetfulness or to repeated questions of whether "it's time yet." A message that is communicated too late may lead to distress and frustration. Older adults often need more preparation time than younger individuals need to get ready for an activity such as going to the bathroom or getting necessary items together. Communicating an exciting message late in the evening (whether it is good or bad news) may disturb the elderly to the point that they are unable to sleep. Nurses need to be aware of these issues so they can choose the proper time to communicate.

Touch

Caring touch is a basic need of all humans, and many elderly suffer from touch deprivation. Many elderly people, particularly those who have lost their spouses and have little contact with children or other family, have no one to meet this need. Research shows that psychotic patients and the elderly are touched the least by caregivers. Those who most need physical contact and the comfort provided by touch receive the least.

Touch is the most elementary form of communication. No words are required, and there is no need for high-level sensory or cognitive functioning. When all else fails, touch is left.

Use of touch as a method of communication is often difficult and uncomfortable, particularly for young or inexperienced nurses. Touching is a very personal form of communication. Affection, understanding, trust, hope, and concern can be communicated by a hand placed on a shoulder, a stroke of the forehead, or a frail hand held by another stronger one. Touch is a common method of expressing concern and caring. People who are emotionally close hold hands and touch and hug one another. High on the list of things lonely elderly people say they miss are hugs and touching. Empathetic use of touch is a much-needed skill when working with the elderly. When words do not work, touch often does.

Therapeutic touch, a specific and focused form of touching or "laying on of hands," is designed to provide compassionate help to another person. Therapeutic touch has been gaining popularity and acceptance in recent years. Research shows that this form of touch helps reduce pain, decrease anxiety, promote sleep, reduce depression, and enhance feelings of well-being in the elderly. Even increased hemoglobin levels, reduced edema, and more rapid wound healing have been attributed to therapeutic touch.

Whereas appropriate use of touch is of great benefit to the elderly, inappropriate touching can be equally destructive. Touch is inappropriate when it is used to communicate anger or frustration. Rough handling, slapping, pushing, or otherwise communicating displeasure constitutes patient abuse and is inappropriate at all times.

Silence

Saying nothing is also saying something. At times words can be intrusive; they can interfere with true communication. Many times the elderly require more time to compose their thoughts. At times no words are necessary. During intense grief, pain, or anxiety, simply *being there* without saying or doing anything may be the most appropriate form of communication nurses can give. The simple presence of another human in case he or she is needed expresses true concern and can be worth more than all of the words in the world.

Verbal Communication

Verbal communication involves sending and receiving messages by means of words. Some verbal communication is formal, structured, and precise; some is informal, unstructured, and flexible. Formal communications have a specific intent and purpose. Informal or social conversations are less specific and are used for socialization. Both have a place in nursing. Nurses must be effective in both formal and informal communication and must know when to use each type.

Effective communication starts with proper introductions. Nurses should determine how the elderly they meet wish to be addressed. It is presumptuous for nurses to become too familiar with the elderly by addressing them by their first names. It is better to start by using the elderly person's proper title and name (e.g., Mrs. Quinn, Dr. Jones) and then clarifying which form of address the person prefers. Patronizing "baby talk" names such as "sweetie" or "honey" demean the elderly and are inappropriate in a clinical setting.

Whether in a formal or informal situation, when communicating verbally nurses should know as much as possible about the others involved. Age, marital status, educational background, interests, and ability to hear and see will influence the communication techniques used and the words chosen. Many aging persons experience changes in hearing that can interfere with their understanding of speech. Nurses must know which of these changes are present in an individual before starting any type of verbal exchange.

Knowledge of the individual's educational background and interests provides nurses with a starting point for conversation. Social discussions often center around past employment, family, or other interests. Increased knowledge of the individual enhances the nurse's ability to respond empathetically. Effective verbal communication requires the ability to use a variety of techniques when sending and receiving messages.

Informing

Informing uses direct statements regarding facts. A good information statement is clear, concise, and expressed in words the patient can understand. When informing, the nurse is active and the patient is passive. Informing is the least effective form of communication because the patient is not actively involved. When nurses give information, they should ask their patients to restate what they understand using their own words.

Direct questioning

Direct questioning is helpful when nurses need to obtain specific information. Direct questions tend to include the words *who, what, when, where, do you,* and *don't you.* Direct questioning is appropriate when information must be obtained quickly; if overused, however, patients can become defensive. Many students and new nurses approach patient assessment with a list of 50 questions that must be answered. After the first 10 questions, the patients begin to feel like they are on trial and communicate the bare minimum of information. Direct questions tend to yield brief answers and often a simple *yes* or *no.*

Open-ended techniques

Open-ended communication techniques include open-ended questions, reflective statements, clarifying statements, and paraphrasing. These techniques allow the patient more leeway to respond and establish a more empathetic climate. The patient is more likely to feel that the nurse is interested in him or her personally and not just trying to fill out a stack of forms. Examples of open-ended responses include "And after you moved to the nursing home, what happened?," "And then?," "That must have been frightening!," "What I hear you saying is . . . ." Open-ended techniques allow patients to express more about their feelings and perceptions. They also allow nurses to verify that the information being relayed is accurate.

Confronting

Confronting is used when there are inconsistencies in information or when verbal and nonverbal messages appear contradictory. Confrontation is one of the most difficult communication techniques to use and should only be used after good rapport has been established. It is never advisable to confront a highly agitated or confused person because conflict and a breakdown in communication will result. Confrontation should only be used when there is adequate time to explore the problem and come to some form of resolution.

TABLE 5-1

Communication Do's and Don'ts When Working with the Elderly

Do	Don't
Identify yourself.	Assume that the person knows who you are.
Address the person using the name he or she desires (e.g., Mr. Smith or Mary).	Use "baby talk" or patronizing names such as "sweetie" or "honey."
Speak clearly and slowly in a low tone of voice.	Shout.
Get to know the person.	Make generalizations about elderly people.
Listen empathetically.	Pay too much attention to tasks and forget the person.
Pay attention to body language—yours and theirs.	Be afraid to use touch as a method of communication.
Use touch appropriately and frequently.	

Social communication

Simple chitchat has a place in nurse-patient communications. If nurses only talked about things related to health treatment, they would know very little about their patients. Small talk; pleasantries; and conversations about the weather, a favorite television show, or the latest news can demonstrate that the nurse thinks of the patient as a real person, not just a patient. This is particularly important in extended-care facilities because the nursing staff often becomes the "family" for the aging person.

Communication with Visitors and Families

Nurses must be prepared to interact with their patients' friends, families, and other visitors. These people make up the older adult's social network and support system. Families and friends are interested and concerned about what is happening to their loved ones. Not only do they turn to nurses for information and reassurance, but they can also be a good source of information for the nurse.

These **significant others,** as they are often called, can help in many ways if nurses are responsive to them. Many of the elderly person's significant others are themselves senior citizens. Nurses must be aware that communication with these individuals may also require special attention and the use of special techniques. It is important to take the time to develop good rapport with your patients' significant others. Good communication with these important people can do a great deal to facilitate care. Because they have known the patient longer and better than the nursing staff has, they are often able to detect subtle changes before trained nurses can. Many times nurses need to rely on

the significant others to interpret the behaviors and communications of the elderly. Listen to what they have to say.

SUMMARY

Keys to effective communication include knowledge about the other person and respect for their uniqueness. In order to develop rapport and communicate effectively with elderly persons, nurses must identify sensory changes that can interfere with the transmission of messages and cultural or age-related values that can result in misunderstandings. Nurses must accurately recognize and interpret both verbal and nonverbal messages being sent by the elderly, their families, and their friends, and nurses must also be aware of the messages they themselves are sending. The desire to interact effectively with others, patience, empathy, and the use of appropriate communication techniques are an essential part of effective nursing practice (Table 5-1).

READINGS AND REFERENCES
Cole G: *Fundamental nursing concepts and skills,* ed 2, St Louis, 1996, Mosby.
Ebersole P, Hess P: *Toward healthy aging: human needs and nursing responses,* ed 5, St Louis, 1998, Mosby.
Lueckenotte A: *Gerontologic nursing,* St Louis, 1996, Mosby.
Mandel E, Shulman MD, Begany T: Overcoming communication disorders in the elderly, *Patient Care* 31:55, 1997.
Martin R, Web site: *KU researcher studies how people talk down to the elderly,* www.urc.ukans.edu/News/96N/NovNews/Nov20,1996.
Sieh A, Brentin LK: *The nurse communicates,* Philadelphia, 1997, WB Saunders.
Simington JA: The elderly require a "special touch": touching expresses caring, and the quality of care improves, *Nursing Homes* 42:30, 1993.

NUTRITION AND FLUID BALANCE

LEARNING OBJECTIVES

1. Identify the various types of nutrients.
2. Identify the components of a healthy diet for the elderly.
3. Describe age-related changes in nutritional and fluid requirements.
4. Identify age-related changes that affect nutrition, digestion, and hydration.
5. Discuss how emotional, social, and cultural factors affect nutritional status.

Nutrition plays an important role in health maintenance, rehabilitation, and prevention and control of disease. When dealing with nutritional issues, nurses who work with older adults must consider the following: (1) the basic components of a well-balanced diet for the elderly; (2) how the normal physiologic changes of aging will change nutritional needs; (3) how the normal physiologic changes of aging may interfere with the purchase, preparation, and consumption of nutrients; and (4) how cognitive, psychosocial, and pathologic changes commonly seen in aging will impact the aging individual's nutritional status. More information regarding meeting nutritional and fluid needs of the elderly is presented in Chapter 10.

NUTRITION AND AGING

Nutritional needs do not remain static throughout life. As with other needs, the nutritional needs of the elderly are not the same as those of younger individuals. An understanding of the nutritional needs of the elderly is essential to providing good nursing care. In order to assess nutritional adequacy and select interventions that promote good nutrition, nurses must be knowledgeable about basic nutrition and diet therapy.

Caloric Intake

Calories are units of heat that are used to measure the available energy in consumed food. Because people's energy requirements differ widely, the number of calories they require will differ significantly. Many factors influence how many calories will be used by a person: activity patterns, gender, body size, age, body temperature, emotional status, and the temperature of the climate in which they live. Generally, when a person's caloric intake is in balance with the energy needs of the body, his or her weight will remain constant. When caloric intake exceeds energy needs, the excess is converted into adipose (fat) tissue for storage and the individual gains weight. When caloric intake is less than the energy needs, the person loses weight (Table 6-1).

Various nutrients provide different amounts of calories. Fats, which can come from either plant sources (e.g., oleomargarine) or animal sources (e.g., butter), yield 9 calories per gram. Proteins and carbohydrates yield 4 calories per gram. Vitamins, minerals, and water yield no calories. Alcohol yields 7 calories per gram without contributing any nutritional value.

Studies have shown that caloric needs in healthy in-

dividuals decrease at a rate of approximately 5% for each decade between age 55 and 75 and 7% percent for each decade after age 75. The body's muscle and lean tissue masses decrease with aging, and adipose tissue increases. As the proportion of muscle and fat changes, the **basal metabolic rate** (the rate at which the body uses calories) decreases. The normal decrease in physical activity commonly seen with aging further slows the rate at which the body burns calories. Healthy individuals who maintain an active lifestyle that includes exercise may see little need to change their caloric intake. Inactive individuals may need to restrict caloric intake significantly. The lowest recommended daily intake to adequately meet nutritional needs is 1200 calories.

When determining the adequacy of caloric intake, disease processes must be considered. Diseases that result in restricted mobility and physical activity (e.g., arthritis, stroke) are likely to decrease caloric needs. Other disease processes (e.g., infections, various forms of cancer) actually increase the body's caloric requirements. Individuals suffering from diabetes mellitus require special diets, which are prescribed by a physician. Diet plays an important role in the medical management of diabetes and is used to control and treat the disease. The diabetic diet will normally include calorie restrictions and will be specially balanced with regard to the percentage of fats, proteins, and carbohydrates.

Nutrients

Although caloric needs often decrease with age, the need to include all of the various nutrients does not. Therefore, foods high in nutritional value and relatively low in calories must be selected in order to maximize the amount of nutrients the body receives while reducing the number of calories (Table 6-2).

Vital nutrients needed by all humans include carbohydrates, protein, fats, vitamins, minerals, and fluids. The adequacy of a persons diet and nutritional intake is determined by comparing their intake to accepted standards (Table 6-3). The most common standard for measuring the balance of a diet plan is the food pyramid (Fig. 6-1). The accepted standard for measuring nutritional adequacy of a diet is the recommended daily allowance (RDA). Because the RDA standards were established for all adults over 50 years of age, however, some questions are arising about its appropriateness for the older age groups in this population. Significant research is taking place in this area.

TABLE 6-1

Average Weight of Older Adults per Inch of Height

Height (inches)	Weight (lb)					
	Age 65-69	Age 70-74	Age 75-79	Age 80-84	Age 85-89	Age 90-94
WOMEN						
58	133	125	123	—	—	—
59	134	127	124	116	110	—
60	135	129	126	118	113	—
61	137	131	128	121	116	—
62	139	134	131	124	120	119
63	141	137	134	128	124	119
64	144	140	137	132	133	120
65	147	144	140	136	138	124
66	151	147	143	140	142	129
67	155	151	146	144	—	—
68	159	155	—	—	—	—
69	164	160	—	—	—	—
MEN						
61	142	139	137	—	—	—
62	144	141	139	135	—	—
63	146	143	141	136	133	—
64	149	146	143	138	135	—
65	151	149	145	141	139	130
66	154	152	148	144	142	133
67	156	155	151	147	145	136
68	159	158	154	150	148	140
69	163	162	158	154	152	144
70	167	165	162	159	156	149
71	172	169	166	164	160	154
72	177	173	171	170	165	—
73	182	178	175	—	—	—

From Loftis P, Glover T: *Decision-making in gerontologic nursing,* St Louis, 1993, Mosby.

TABLE 6-2

Mean Heights and Weights and Recommended Energy Intakes for Adults

Gender	Age (years)	Weight		Height		Energy Needs (with Range)
		(kg)	(lb)	(cm)	(in)	(kcal)
Male	23-50	70	154	178	70	2700 (2300-3100)
	51-75	70	154	178	70	2400 (2000-2800)
	76+	70	154	178	70	2050 (1650-2450)
Female	23-50	55	120	163	64	2000 (1600-2400)
	51-75	55	120	163	64	1800 (1400-2200)
	76+	55	120	163	64	1600 (1200-2000)

Adapted from Food and Nutrition Board, Committee on Dietary Allowances, *Recommended dietary allowances,* ed 4, Washington DC, 1980, National Academy of Sciences. In Burke MM, Walsh MB: *Gerontological nursing: care of the frail elderly,* St Louis, 1992, Mosby.

TABLE 6-3

Present and Probable Future Recommended Daily Allowance (RDA) Recommendations for Older Adults

Nutrient	RDA Recommendations	
	1989	**Future**
Riboflavin	1.4 mg (men), 1.2 (women)	Same or higher
Vitamin B$_6$	2.0 mg (men), 1.6 (women)	Higher
Folic acid	200 μg (men), 180 μg (women)	Higher
Vitamin B$_{12}$	2.0 μg	Higher
Vitamin D	5 μg	Higher
Calcium	800 mg	Higher
Vitamin A	100 RE (men), 800 RE (women)	Same or lower

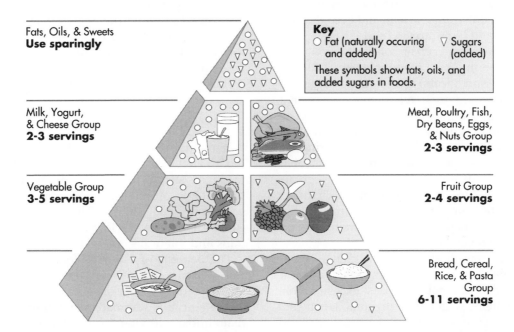

FIG. 6-1   Food guide pyramid. (Courtesy of the United States Department of Agriculture.)

Carbohydrates

Carbohydrates include the familiar sugars and starches that compromise approximately half of the standard American diet. A ready source of energy for the body, carbohydrates are usually divided into two categories: simple and complex. Simple carbohydrates are used most readily by the body because their simple bonds are easily broken. Table sugar, honey, syrup, and candy are examples of simple carbohydrates.

Complex carbohydrates must be broken down into simple sugars before they can be used by the body. This breakdown requires time and energy. Foods such as vegetables, grains, and fruits contain complex carbohydrates. Foods that contain complex carbohydrates usually also contain other nutrients (e.g., minerals and vitamins), making them more nutritious

than foods containing simple carbohydrates. In addition, complex carbohydrates usually contain significant amounts of soluble fiber, which aids bowel elimination. The American Heart Association recommends that 55% to 60% of calories should come from carbohydrates with an emphasis on complex carbohydrates. This recommendation appears to be appropriate for the aging population.

A diet high in complex carbohydrates is recommended as part of the control of many disease processes. The soluble fiber in complex carbohydrates has been shown to reduce blood cholesterol levels, which is helpful for individuals who are at risk of coronary artery disease. Complex carbohydrates also play an important role in the control of diabetes because they effectively meet energy needs without causing rapid increases in blood glucose levels the way simple sugars do.

Proteins

Proteins are composed of **amino acids,** which are essential for tissue repair and healing. The need for protein remains constant or may increase slightly with aging to compensate for the loss of lean body tissue. The RDA of protein for women over 50 years of age is 50 grams per day; for men over age 50 the RDA is 65 grams per day. Data from the National Health and Nutrition Examination Survey reveal that 10% to 25% of women over age 55 consume less than half of the recommended daily amount of protein. Protein consumption in the elderly can be affected by many factors, including the ability to procure and prepare food, the cost of foods containing protein, and even the ability to chew common high-protein foods.

Tissue replacement and repair continue throughout life. Any condition in which tissue integrity is altered (e.g., surgery, pressure ulcers) increases the amount of protein needed to aid in tissue repair. Red meats, poultry, fish, eggs, and dairy products are good sources of **complete proteins,** which contain all of the amino acids necessary for making and repairing tissues. Plant foods such as legumes (peas and beans), nuts, and cereals (whole grains and rice) contain smaller amounts of incomplete proteins, which do not individually contain all of the necessary amino acids. Incomplete proteins must be combined carefully in order to meet protein needs.

Some foods that are high in protein such as steak, ham, organ meats, egg yolks, hard cheese, and whole milk also contain large amounts of fats. Excessive consumption of proteins with a high fat content can contribute to elevated blood levels of cholesterol and triglycerides, which in turn contribute to plaque formation and atherosclerotic changes in the blood vessels. Atherosclerosis frequently results in hypertension and heart disease. For this reason, many physicians and dietitians recommend that high-fat protein foods be restricted. A person who is on a fat-restricted diet should consume low-fat proteins such as fish and lean poultry as well as protein from plant sources such as peas and beans.

Fats

It is recommended that fats be limited to approximately 25% to 30% of the total daily caloric intake. This recommendation does not change with aging. A certain amount of fat is necessary and desirable in the diet to aid in the absorption of fat-soluble vitamins and to provide adequate amounts of essential fatty acids. Fat is desirable because it adds flavor to food

and provides a sense of fullness with a meal. Foods with no fat would be unappealing, poor tasting, and not very satisfying.

When considering fat intake in the diet, it is important to watch the type of fats ingested. The body incorporates fats into substances called **lipoproteins,** which contain cholesterol and proteins. There are three important types of lipoproteins: high-density lipoprotein (HDL), low-density lipoprotein (LDL), and very-low-density lipoprotein (VLDL). LDL is composed primarily of cholesterol and is believed to contribute to blood vessel disease. VLDL is composed primarily of triglycerides and may contribute to vessel disease but not as significantly as does LDL. HDL, the so-called healthy fat, is composed primarily of protein that appears to protect against blood vessel disease.

Some individuals who have been eating high-cholesterol foods for their entire lives may be reluctant to change their eating habits as they age. They may find it difficult or unpleasant to shop for and prepare foods in new ways. Others can successfully alter their dietary intake to avoid foods high in these substances.

Vitamins

Vitamins are organic compounds found naturally in foods. They can also be produced synthetically. Vitamins are needed for a wide variety of metabolic and physiologic processes. Vitamins are classified as fat soluble or water soluble. The fat-soluble vitamins include vitamins A, D, E, and K. The B-complex vitamins and vitamin C are water soluble (Box 6-1).

The benefits of vitamins for the elderly are being closely examined. Some researchers who subscribe to the free radical theory of aging are studying the effects of the so-called antioxidant vitamins. It is theorized that antioxidant vitamins can block or neutralize free radicals and prevent cell damage, thereby slowing the effects of aging and preventing a number of diseases such as cancer and heart disease. Although research into this area is promising, many experts are not yet convinced of the effectiveness of antioxidant vitamins or satisfied that we have an adequate understanding of their method of action, therapeutic dosage, or long-term effects. Vitamins A, C, and E are considered antioxidants.

Vitamin deficiencies have been connected to a variety of problems experienced by the elderly. Vitamin D deficiency is more common in the elderly due to less exposure to the sun, reduced capacity of the skin to synthesize the vitamin, and decreased dietary intake. Because vitamin D is required for calcium absorption, a deficiency can contribute to excessive bone demineralization or osteoporosis. Adequate intake of vitamin D and calcium supplements can help prevent or even reverse the severity of this problem.

BOX 6-1

Summary of Essential Vitamins

FAT-SOLUBLE VITAMINS

Vitamin A	Found in milk, butter, cheese, fortified margarine, liver, green and yellow vegetables, and fruits
	Promotes healthy epithelium, ability to see in dim light, normal mucus formation
	Many elderly people may be deficient in vitamin A due to chronic conditions that interfere with fat absorption such as gallbladder disease and colitis
Vitamin D	Found in fortified milk and margarine, cod liver oil, fatty fish, and eggs
	Promotes absorption of calcium
	May contribute to skeletal changes with aging
Vitamin E	Found in corn and safflower oils, margarine, seeds, nuts, and leafy green vegetables
	Promotes integrity of red blood cells
Vitamin K	Found in leafy green vegetables and liver; synthesized by bacteria in the colon
	Essential for formation of prothrombin, which is necessary for blood clotting

WATER-SOLUBLE VITAMINS

Vitamin B_1 (thiamine hydrochloride)	Found in organ meats, pork, legumes, and whole grains
	Essential for carbohydrate metabolism
Vitamin B_2 (riboflavin)	Found in milk, cheese, eggs, organ meats, legumes, leafy green vegetables
	Essential for normal tissue maintenance and tear production
Niacin	Found in lean meats, liver, whole grains, legumes
	Essential for energy release from fats, carbohydrates, and proteins
Vitamin B_6 (pyridoxine hydrochloride)	Found in whole grains, vegetables, legumes, meats, and bananas
	Acts in the processes of protein synthesis and amino acid metabolism
	May interact with levodopa taken by patients with Parkinson's disease
Folacin (folic acid)	Found in whole wheat, legumes, and green vegetables
	Important in hemoglobin synthesis and in metabolism of amino acids
	Common deficiency in the elderly
Vitamin B_{12} (cyanocobalamin)	Found in muscle and organ meats, eggs, shellfish, and dairy products
	Requires production of intrinsic factor by the stomach for absorption; inadequate absorption can result in **pernicious anemia**
	Needed for maturation of red blood cells
	Deficiency is commonly seen with folacin deficiency
Vitamin C (ascorbic acid)	Found in citrus fruits, tomatoes, cabbage, melons, strawberries, green peppers, and leafy green vegetables
	Important in the formation and maintenance of collagen structure of connective tissue
	Promotes healing and elasticity of capillary walls

Vitamin B_{12} deficiency can be related to inadequate protein consumption or physiologic changes in digestion. Normal aging changes result in decreased production of gastric acid and pepsin, which are necessary for protein digestion. When less protein is digested, less B_{12} is available for absorption. Vitamin B_{12} deficiency can result in neurologic changes that affect sensation, balance, and memory. If detected early and treated with supplements, some of the symptoms of vitamin B_{12} deficiency may be reversible.

Vitamin B_6 deficiency, also common in the elderly, is believed to be correlated with neurologic and immunologic problems. Supplements of vitamin B_6 help reverse these problems.

Vitamin E appears to play a role in maintaining immune function in the elderly and has recently been connected to delaying the onset of symptoms in Alzheimer's disease. The exact dose required to obtain maximum benefits is under study.

Older adults who consume well-balanced diets may not require supplemental vitamins. Those with increased risk factors such as gastrointestinal (GI) problems or inadequate nutritional intake may benefit from selective vitamin supplements. Supplements should be used with caution under the direction of a physician or dietitian. Excess amounts of the water-soluble vitamins are quickly eliminated from the body and pose few risks. Excess amounts of the fat-soluble vitamins (A, D, E, and K) are retained in fatty tissue or stored in the liver. Overconsumption of these vitamins can lead to toxic symptoms and even permanent liver damage.

Minerals

Minerals are inorganic chemical elements that are required in many of the body's functions. Minerals make up a small proportion of total body weight, yet a slight mineral imbalance can have serious effects.

Calcium, the most abundant mineral in the body, is necessary for bone and tooth formation, nerve impulse transmission and conduction, muscle contraction (including cardiac function), and blood clotting. The main dietary sources of calcium are milk and dairy products. Calcium is normally retained in bone, with only a small amount (1%) found in the tissues and blood. With aging and with immobility the bones tend to lose calcium, resulting in osteoporosis. In certain disease states, abnormal amounts of calcium leave the bone, enter the bloodstream, and cause **hypercalcemia,** which is an elevated level of calcium in the blood. Hypercalcemia is seen with hyperparathyroidism, disuse atrophy, metastatic bone tumors, and vitamin D excess.

Individuals experiencing hypercalcemia may manifest symptoms including confusion, abdominal pain, muscle pain, weakness, and anorexia. These symptoms may be easily missed in elderly individuals because they are vague and common to many other conditions. Extremely high levels of calcium in the blood can result in shock, kidney failure, and even death. When the kidneys attempt to rid the body of excess calcium, hypercalciuria (increased calcium in the urine) results and the risk of renal calculi (kidney stone) formation is increased.

Adequate calcium intake is important throughout life, but it is particularly important for those at risk of developing osteoporosis, especially postmenopausal women. Calcium may arrest the progress of osteoporosis. Vitamin D aids in the absorption of calcium. For this reason, vitamin D is added to milk products and fortified margarine.

Phosphorus is needed for normal bone and tooth formation, activation of some B vitamins, normal neuromuscular functioning, metabolism of carbohydrates, regulation of acid-base balance, and other physiologic processes. Inadequate nutritional intake of phospho-

rus can result in weight loss or anemia. The typical dietary sources of phosphorus compounds are dairy products, meat, egg yolks, peas, beans, nuts, and whole grains. Because of its wide availability, meeting the dietary requirements of this mineral is normally not a problem unless the individual is on a highly restricted diet.

Iron is found in the center of the **heme** portion of hemoglobin. Hemoglobin in the red blood cells transports oxygen to and removes carbon dioxide from the cells. Without adequate amounts of iron, the body cannot produce enough hemoglobin. When hemoglobin levels fall below the normal range, anemia results. Individuals suffering from anemia may manifest many symptoms depending on the severity of the condition: fatigue, exertional dyspnea, tachycardia, palpitations, headache, insomnia, vertigo, pallor (particularly of the mucous membranes), and cool extremities. The normal changes of aging or other disease processes may resemble these symptoms and prevent recognition of anemia. Laboratory tests for hemoglobin level are required to determine whether anemia is present (Table 6-4). Two forms of nutritional anemia are commonly seen in the elderly: iron-deficiency anemia and pernicious anemia.

Iron-deficiency anemia results from inadequate intake of dietary iron. Rich sources of dietary iron include red meat, particularly organ meats like liver; shellfish; egg yolks; leafy green vegetables; and dried fruits. Red meat is expensive and, unless properly prepared, can be difficult for the elderly to chew. Many people do not like the taste of liver and organ meats and refuse to eat them. In addition organ meats and egg yolks are high in cholesterol, which is often re-

TABLE 6-4

Laboratory Values Used to Assess Nutritional Adequacy in the Elderly

Diagnostic test	Appropriate range
Hemoglobin	14-18 g/dl (men)
	12-16 g/dl (women)
Hematocrit	40%-51% (men)
	38%-44% (women)
Blood urea nitrogen	10-30 mg/dl
Creatinine	0.5-1.0 mg/dl
Albumin	3.5-5.0 g/dl
Calcium	9-11 mg/dl
Folic acid	3-25 mg/dl
Glucose (fasting)	70-120 mg/dl

Data from Lewis SM, Collier IC, Heitkemper MM: *Medical-surgical nursing: assessment and management of clinical problems,* ed 4, St Louis, 1996, Mosby.

stricted from the diet. This can make meal planning difficult.

Pernicious anemia is caused by a deficiency in intrinsic factor secreted by the stomach. Without this factor, vitamin B_{12}, which is required for red blood cell maturation in the bone marrow, is not absorbed. In addition, there are fewer white blood cells and there may be cellular changes in the existing cells. Individuals suffering from pernicious anemia may manifest weakness, numbness, or tingling in the extremities; anorexia; or weight loss. Treatment typically consists of cyanocobalamin injections and oral folic acid and iron supplements.

It should be remembered that a concentrated iron formulation (liquid or solid) administered orally can irritate the GI tract. To reduce GI irritation, iron supplements should be taken during or after meals. Iron solutions can stain the teeth, so a straw should be used with liquid iron preparations. If iron is given by injection, it is important to use the Z-track method for deep intramuscular administration. Foods rich in vitamin C should be given in conjunction with iron to enhance its absorption. Patients should be told that iron will probably turn the stool a dark green or black color, and nurses should keep this in mind when assessing the stool of individuals receiving iron supplements. Concentrated iron supplements can also cause diarrhea.

Sodium is a very commonly occurring mineral and is one of the important elements in the body. Sodium ions are involved in acid-base balance, fluid balance, nerve impulse transmission, and muscle contraction. Sodium is mostly found in extracellular fluid. Sodium levels are regulated by the kidneys, which retain or eliminate sodium according to the body's needs. Sodium interacts with potassium as part of the fluid exchange through cell membranes. Sodium is naturally present in many foods. The most common, most familiar concentrated form is sodium chloride, or table salt, which is used to flavor and preserve food. The typical American diet tends to be higher in sodium than is nutritionally required. Many elderly people use excessive amounts of salt to compensate for the decreased ability to perceive the taste of foods. Excessive blood levels of sodium, or hypernatremia, can cause fluid retention, which in body tissue is manifested as edema. People with hypertension, renal failure, or cardiac conditions are often placed on sodium-restricted diets, and many (especially the elderly) report that food is less appetizing when prepared with reduced amounts of sodium. With less appetite, they may eat less.

Potassium is the major intracellular ion in the body. Potassium ions play an important role in acid-base balance, fluid and electrolyte balance, and (with sodium) normal neuromuscular functioning. Potassium is not as abundant in the diet of the elderly as are some of the other minerals. Dietary sources of potassium include citrus fruits, milk, bananas, and apple juice. Potassium deficiency, or hypokalemia, is a common problem in the elderly. Many diuretic and antihypertensive medications deplete the body of potassium, as can prolonged or frequent diarrhea. Symptoms of hypokalemia include muscle weakness, anorexia, apprehension, irritability, drowsiness, depression, and disorientation. Severe muscle weakness is the most common observation related to decreased potassium levels. Hypokalemia with digitalis therapy is often a cause of cardiac arrhythmias. Because not all patients who have decreased levels of potassium will demonstrate observable symptoms, nurses must check laboratory studies to verify levels of the electrolytes. Supplements are frequently prescribed to increase low blood potassium levels.

Zinc is a trace mineral that plays a role in protein synthesis. In adults, insufficient zinc may result in delayed wound healing, diminished sense of smell and taste, and decreased appetite. Certain conditions, including some that are common in the elderly, may result in zinc deficiency (e.g., cirrhosis of the liver, kidney disease, malignant cancers, and alcoholism). Supplemental zinc may be administered. Dietary sources of zinc include meat, shellfish, and nuts.

Trace elements such as magnesium, copper, iodine, fluorine, chromium, selenium, nickel, and sulfur are necessary in very small amounts for normal body functioning. Selenium is gaining importance as an antioxidant mineral and is credited with decreased risk of cancer and improved tissue elasticity.

Water

Water is essential for life. Humans can survive for many days without food but not without water. Water plays a role in many aspects of normal body functioning. Water is necessary for the formation of many of the body's secretions, including tears, perspiration, and saliva. Water aids in digestion and in transportation of electrolytes and nutrients. Water facilitates elimination of waste products and plays an important role in temperature regulation.

Approximately 60% of the average adult body is composed of water, with adult men having slightly more body fluid than women. Elderly individuals typically have less body fluid than do younger adults. The total amount of body fluid decreases by approximately 8% in the elderly. The amount of water in the bloodstream remains relatively constant with aging, but older adults tend to have less fluid in the intracellular and interstitial spaces than do younger people. This fluid decrease results in loss of skin turgor and leads to the wrinkled appearance that is common with aging. Decreased fluid increases the risk of fluid imbalances such as dehydration. Most adults require 2000 to 3000 ml of fluid each day. Most of this is consumed as beverages such as water, tea, coffee, and juice. Solid foods, particularly fruits and vegetables, contain significant amounts of water.

Water is normally lost through urination, perspiration, respiration, and defecation. Abnormal fluid loss occurs with diarrhea, vomiting, diaphoresis, gastric suctioning, and wound drainage; essential minerals are often lost along with the water.

The amount of fluid taken into the body should be in balance with the amount eliminated from the body. This is referred to as **fluid balance.**

MEETING THE NUTRITIONAL NEEDS OF INDEPENDENT OLDER ADULTS

Studies have shown that a majority of elderly Americans believe that nutrition is important for good health but that they do not always follow good nutritional practices (Fig. 6-2). Information from the National Council on Aging reveals that the elderly have a dis-

The Warning Signs of poor nutritional health are often overlooked. Use this checklist to find out if you or someone you know is at nutritional risk.

Read the statements below. Circle the number in the yes column for those that apply to you or someone you know. For each yes answer, score the number in the box. Total your nutritional score.

DETERMINE YOUR NUTRITIONAL HEALTH

	YES
I have an illness or condition that made me change the kind and/or amount of food I eat.	2
I eat fewer than 2 meals per day.	3
I eat few fruits or vegetables, or milk products.	2
I have 3 or more drinks of beer, liquor or wine almost everyday.	2
I have tooth or mouth problems that make it hard for me to eat.	2
I don't always have enough money to buy the food I need.	4
I eat alone most of the time.	1
I take 3 or more different prescribed or over-the-counter drugs a day.	1
Without wanting to, I have lost or gained 10 pounds in the last 6 months.	2
I am not always physically able to shop, cook and/or feed myself.	2
TOTAL	

Total Your Nutritional Score. If it's—

0–2   **Good!** Recheck your nutritional score in 6 months.

3–5   **You are at moderate nutritional risk.** See what can be done to improve your eating habits and lifestyle. Your office on aging, senior nutrition program, senior citizens center or health department can help. Recheck your nutritional score in 3 months.

6 or more **You are at high nutritional risk.** Bring this checklist the next time you see your doctor, dietitian or other qualified health or social service professional. Talk with them about any problems you may have. Ask for help to improve your nutritional health.

These materials developed and distributed by the Nutrition Screening Initiative, a project of:

 AMERICAN ACADEMY OF FAMILY PHYSICIANS

 THE AMERICAN DIETETIC ASSOCIATION

 NATIONAL COUNCIL ON THE AGING, INC.

Remember that warning signs suggest risk, but do not represent diagnosis of any condition. Turn the page to learn more about the Warning Signs of poor nutritional health.

FIG. 6-2   Checklist of warning signs of poor nutrition. (Courtesy of the Nutrition Screening Initiative, Washington, DC.)

proportionately high risk for poor nutrition, which in turn has a negative effect on their health.

Estimates of the elderly who actually suffer from some degree of poor nutrition or malnutrition range from 15% to 50%; with the risk for nutritional inadequacy even higher. Data collected by the Elderly Nutrition Program of the Older Americans Act revealed that approximately 75% of the elderly are considered to be at moderate to high nutritional risk.

The nutritional status of elderly living in the community is affected by personal, economic, social, and physiologic factors.

Personal factors that influence nutritional status include general health status, dentition, and emotional status. A person who does not feel well, cannot chew effectively, or is experiencing depression or cognitive changes is unlikely to have much of an appetite. Overall nutritional status will be affected if any of these problems persists for a significant period of time. The cost of food, the availability of food, the ability of the elderly to read food labels, transportation, and difficulties with food preparation and storage are all factors that must be considered when assessing nutritional status in the elderly.

Foods rich in protein such as meats and dairy products tend to be costly. Fresh vegetables and fruits that are rich in vitamins and minerals may also be costly, depending on the season and locale. Many older adults have limited incomes and may not purchase these more costly items even though they know their nutritional value and importance. Meat, milk, and fresh produce are susceptible to spoilage and must be properly refrigerated, cooked, and eaten within a short period of time. Older adults with altered senses of taste and smell may not be able to detect the changes that indicate spoilage. If spoiled food is eaten, the risk of GI infection or upset is increased.

Obtaining an appropriate variety and sufficient amount of food can be difficult for an elderly person or couple. Most foods are packaged in sizes appropriate for families of four or more. Although some manufacturers are responding to the needs of single and elderly people by packaging smaller servings, the cost is often higher per serving. The elderly individual must decide whether thrift or variety is more important.

Preparing food for one or two people is also more difficult. Most recipes are intended for four, six, or eight servings. If one of these recipes is used, the food must either be eaten day after day or wasted. Some farsighted elderly prepare their favorite meals and then package and freeze individual servings so they can have variety and avoid waste. Unfortunately, not everyone has a freezer and not all foods can be frozen.

Elderly or debilitated individuals, particularly those living alone, face additional problems. The simple act

of getting to a store may be difficult. Trends toward large-chain grocery stores have forced many smaller neighborhood grocery stores to close. These large stores are often located in shopping plazas that are far away from home. Even if there is a nearby neighborhood grocery or convenience store, its prices must be higher for it to stay in business. Either situation presents problems for the elderly person. Without a car, a homebound elderly person may find it difficult to obtain groceries, medicine, or other necessities. Many times, family members or friends drive the elderly person to the store to shop or pick up their groceries. As a courtesy to busy or elderly customers, more stores are offering call-in and delivery services for an added fee. Some communities offer scheduled transportation from senior citizen housing to grocery stores. Others provide volunteers to shop for homebound elderly people (Fig. 6-3).

Shopping requires physical exertion. Acts that a young, healthy person does not think about such as lifting cans from a top shelf, reaching for something near the floor, or moving groceries into and out of a store cart can physically exhaust an infirm or elderly person. Although store personnel or other shoppers would probably help with these activities (Fig. 6-4), the elderly are often too embarrassed or proud to ask for help.

Reading small print on labels can be difficult for an

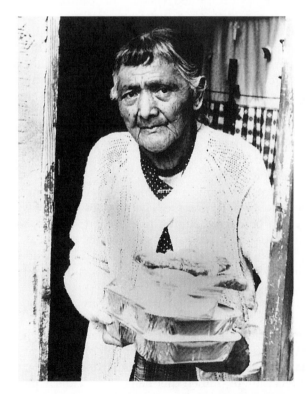

FIG. 6-3 A Meals-on-Wheels recipient. (Photographer unknown. Courtesy of the American Society on Aging.)

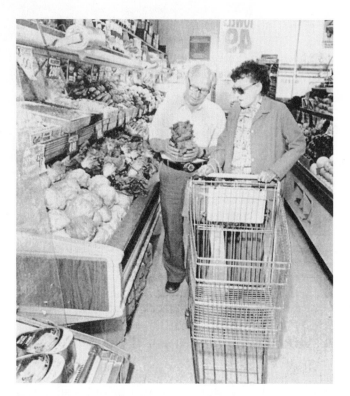

FIG. 6-4   Shopping for produce. (Photograph by Don Coyro. Courtesy of the American Society on Aging.)

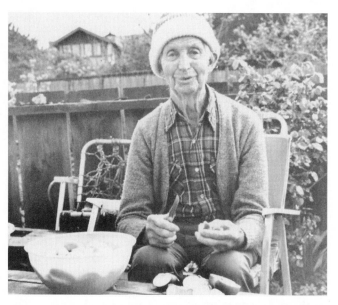

FIG. 6-5   Good nutrition at any age. (Photograph by Marianne Gontarz. Courtesy of the American Society on Aging.)

individual with limited vision. This can be problematic for someone on a restricted diet who needs to read the label to choose foods that are permitted. Once food is purchased and taken home, the task of food preparation remains. Opening cans, unsealing jars, and dealing with the ubiquitous plastic wrappers on food can all present insurmountable obstacles to the aging individual. Think of the problems that a young, healthy person has with current packaging, and then imagine performing the same tasks with decreased muscle strength, arthritis, or other age-related problems.

Even if packaging problems can be overcome, the food must still be prepared. Because the effort of cooking can be overwhelming to the aging person, meal after meal may consist of sandwiches or cereal. All of these food-related factors must be considered when working with elderly persons in a home setting (Fig. 6-5).

Problems related to poor nutrition are not limited to elderly residing in the community. Nutritional problems are also an area of concern for seniors who reside in institutional settings. Even though most institutions maintain well-staffed dietary departments under the supervision of trained dietitians, many elderly people do not consume the nutrients that are available to them. This may be due to a variety of external or personal factors. Some external factors that influence nutrition include the repetitive nature of institutional meals, problems maintaining the temperature and appearance of food while serving many people, environmental concerns such as odors or the behavior of others, and the inability of an institution to meet the specific cultural preferences or general likes and dislikes of a large number of people.

Social and Cultural Aspects of Nutrition

Food is more than a means of meeting nutritional needs. Food is also used as part of religious ceremonies, in social interactions, and as a means of cultural expression.

Throughout history, food has been linked to the gods. Many major religions such as Islam, Judaism, and Catholicism include some dietary restrictions. These religions may require avoidance of certain foods, fasting, or special methods of food preparation for all members of the faith. Although most religions have more lenient restrictions for the elderly and infirm, many older adults—especially those with great religious faith—want to comply with their religious teachings. Violating dietary rules may deeply upset them. This presents a challenge to caregivers, who are more concerned about adequate nutrition than about religious beliefs. If such a situation arises it would be appropriate for the nurse to consult with a dietitian or with the rabbi, minister, priest, or spiritual leader of

Text continued on p. 106

TABLE 6-5

Characteristic Food Patterns of Some Cultures

Ethnic group	Milk group	Protein group	Fruits and Vegetables	Breads and Cereals	Concerns Related to Ethnic Diet
Native American (many tribal variations; many Americanized)	Fresh milk Evaporated milk for cooking Ice cream Cream pies	Pork, beef, lamb, rabbit, fowl Fish Eggs Legumes Sunflower seeds Nuts: walnut, acorn, pine, peanut butter Game meat	Green peas, beans, beets, turnips, squash, peppers, leafy green and other vegetables	Refined bread Whole wheat Cornmeal Rice Dry cereals "Fry" bread Tortillas	Obesity, diabetes, alcoholism, nutritional deficiencies expressed in dental problems and iron deficiency anemia Inadequate amounts of all nutrients Excessive use of sugar
Middle Eastern* (Armenian, Greek, Syrian, Turkish)	Yogurt Little butter	Lamb Nuts Dried peas, beans, lentils Sesame seeds	Peppers, tomatoes, cabbage, grape leaves, cucumbers, squash Dried apricots, raisins, dates	Cracked wheat and dark bread	Fry many meats and vegetables Lack of fresh fruits Insufficient foods from milk group High consumption of sweetenings, lamb fat, and olive oil
African-American	Milk† Ice cream Cheese: longhorn, American	Pork: all cuts, plus organs, chitterlings Beef, lamb, chicken, giblets Eggs Nuts Legumes Fish, game	Leafy vegetables, green and yellow vegetables Potato: white, sweet Stewed fruit Bananas and other fresh fruit Rice	Cornmeal and hominy grits Biscuits, pancakes, white breads	Extensive use of frying, "smothering" in gravy, or simmering Fats: salt pork, bacon drippings, lard, and gravies High consumption of sweets Insufficient citrus fruits Vegetables often boiled for long periods with pork fat and much salt Limited amounts from milk group†
Chinese (Cantonese most prevalent)	Milk: water buffalo	Pork sausage‡ Eggs and pigeon eggs Fish Lamb, beef, goat Fowl: chicken, duck Nuts Legumes Soybean curd (tofu)	Many vegetables Radish leaves Bean, bamboo sprouts	Rice/rice flour products Cereals, noodles Wheat, corn, millet seed	Tendency of some immigrants to use large amounts of grease to cook Limited use of milk, milk products Often low in protein, calories, or both

Continued

TABLE 6-5

Characteristic Food Patterns of Some Cultures

Ethnic group	Milk group	Protein group	Fruits and Vegetables	Breads and Cereals	Concerns Related to Ethnic Diet
Polish	Milk Sour cream Cheese Butter	Pork (preferred), chicken	Vegetables, cabbage, roots Fruits	Dark rye	May wash rice before cooking, removing vitamins added in fortification Soy sauce (high sodium) Sodium in ham, sausages, pickles High consumption of sweets Tendency to overcook vegetables Limited fruits (especially citrus), raw vegetables, and meats
Puerto Rican	Limited use of milk products Coffee with milk (café con leche)	Pork, poultry Eggs (Fridays) Beans (habichuelas)	Avocado, okra, eggplant, sweet yams, starchy vegetables and fruits (viandas)	Rice, cornmeal	Small amounts of pork and poultry Extensive use of fat, lard, salt pork, and olive oil Lack of milk products
Scandinavian: Danish, Finnish, Norwegian, Swedish	Cream Butter Cheeses	Wild game, reindeer Fish (fresh or dried) Eggs	Berries Dried fruit Vegetables: cole slaw, roots	Whole wheat, rye, barley, sweets (cookies and sweet breads)	Insufficient fresh fruits and vegetables High consumption of sweets, pickled, salted meats, and fish Liberal use of fat
Southeast Asian: Vietnamese, Cambodian	Generally not consumed Coffee with condensed cow's milk Plain yogurt Ice cream (rare) Soybean milk	Fish (daily): fresh, dried, salted Poultry/eggs: duck, chicken Pork, beef (seldom) Dried beans Tofu	Seasonal variety: fresh or preserved Green, leafy vegetables, yams, corn	Rice: grains, flour, noodles French bread "Cellophane" (bean starch) noodles	Fresh milk products generally not consumed Poultry/eggs may be limited Meat considered "unclean" is avoided Preference for a diet high in salt and pepper as well as rice and pork High intake of MSG and soy sauce
Jewish: Orthodox*	Milk§ Cheese§	Meat (bloodless; Kosher prepared): beef, lamb, goat, deer, poultry (all types); no pork Fish with fins and scales only No crustaceans	Wide variety	Wide variety	High intake of sodium in meat products

TABLE 6-5

Characteristic Food Patterns of Some Cultures

Ethnic group	Milk group	Protein group	Fruits and Vegetables	Breads and Cereals	Concerns Related to Ethnic Diet
Filipino (Spanish-Chinese influence)	Flavored milk, milk in coffee Cheese: gouda, cheddar	Pork, beef, goat, deer, rabbit, chicken Fish Eggs, nuts, legumes	Many vegetables and fruits	Rice, cooked cereals Noodles: rice, wheat	Limited use of milk and milk products Tendency to prewash rice Tendency to have only small portions of protein foods
Italian	Cheese Some ice cream	Meat Eggs Dried beans	Leafy vegetables, potatoes, eggplant, tomatoes, peppers Fruits	Pasta White breads, some whole wheat Farina Cereals	Prefer expensive imported cheeses; reluctant to substitute less expensive domestic varieties Tendency to overcook vegetables Limited use of whole grains High consumption of sweets Extensive use of olive oil Insufficient servings from milk group
Japanese (Isei, more Japanese influence; Nisei, more Westernized)	Increasing amounts being used by younger generations	Pork, beef, chicken Fish Eggs Legumes: soya, red, lima beans Tofu Nuts	Many vegetables and fruits Seaweed	Rice, rice cakes Wheat noodles Refined bread, noodles	Excessive sodium: pickles, salty crisp seaweed, MSG, and soy sauce Insufficient servings from milk group May prewash rice
Hispanic, Mexican-American	Milk Cheese Flan, ice cream	Beef, pork, lamb, chicken, tripe, hot sausage, beef intestines Fish Eggs Nuts Dry beans: pinto, chickpeas (often eaten more than once daily)	Spinach, wild greens, tomatoes, chilies, corn, cactus leaves, cabbage, avocado, potatoes Pumpkin, zapote, peaches, guava, papaya, citrus	Rice, cornmeal Sweet bread, pastries Tortilla: corn, flour Vermicelli (fideo)	Limited meats primarily because of cost Limited use of milk and milk products Large amounts of lard Abundant use of sugar Tendency to boil vegetables for long periods

From Lowdermilk: *Maternity and women's health care*, ed 6, St Louis, 1997, Mosby.

* Religious holidays may involve fasting, which is believed to increase the likelihood of premature labor, but the fasting requirement may be waived during pregnancy.
† Lactose intolerance is relatively common in adults.
‡ Lower in fat content than Western sausage.
§ Milk and milk products not eaten with meat; milk may be consumed before the meal or 6 hours afterward; different sets of dishes and silverware are used to serve milk and meat products.
MSG, Monosodium L-glutamate.

the specific religious group to seek clarification and guidance. Many times the spiritual counselor can provide reassurance to the elderly person and guidance to the health care team.

Cultural influences in food are also significant. The foods we eat in our homes from early in life reflect our culture. Some people are happy to eat a wide variety of foods; others prefer to eat only foods with which they are familiar. Various cultures ascribe certain powers to foods. The culture may dictate what, when, or how foods should be eaten. An older adult from such a cultural background may find it difficult to understand or accept mainstream American nutrition practices. It is important to remember that good nutrition can be achieved within any culture (Table 6-5). Special planning with the dietitian is often necessary to achieve adequate nutrition and meet cultural preferences within an institutional setting. Family members and significant others from the same culture may be willing to provide special foods and assist in meeting the nutritional needs of the institutionalized elderly.

Food is often tied to social events. When people visit friends' homes, they are often served food. Food is served at parties, weddings, and wakes. People on dates go out to eat. Eating alone is often described as one of the worst things about being single or widowed. A common notion is that food eaten alone does not even taste the same. Nurses should remember this when working with the elderly.

Many elderly people like to go out to eat in restaurants. Eating out has many benefits, including a change of scenery, a wider choice of foods, and the opportunity for social interaction. Most elderly prefer restaurants with table service rather than buffets or fast-food establishments because they tend to be less noisy and do not require a person to balance trays of food.

Eating out is an occasional treat for some elderly, but it is a way of life for others. Elderly who eat out regularly should consider their choices and use care to avoid the high-fat, high-sodium items that are common restaurant fare. Many restaurants that cater to the elderly offer heart-healthy items and senior portions often at discounted prices.

Older adults who live in long-term or assisted-living settings are usually served one or more meals in a dining room. Most people tend to eat better when dining with others than when they are left to eat alone in a room or apartment. Snacks served during group or social activities tend to be consumed more readily.

SUMMARY

Indicators of nutritional and metabolic alteration are most commonly observed in the skin, mucous membranes, hair, and nails. Good nutrition has been shown

to be one of the most significant factors in the prevention of skin breakdown. Assessment of these structures can tell nurses a great deal about an aging person's nutritional status and fluid balance. Other signs and symptoms of poor nutrition such as confusion, weight loss, lethargy, and lightheadedness are mistakenly attributed to an illness or medication reaction rather than to the underlying nutritional problem.

A good understanding of nutrition and the nutritional needs of the elderly requires knowledge of a wide range of facts and concepts. This text only addresses the basics. For greater understanding, texts that specialize in geriatric nutrition should be consulted.

READINGS AND REFERENCES

American College of Gastroenterology Website: *Digestive health tips,* http//www.acg.gi.org/digest/tips/3di.-xiii/ htm.

American Dietetic Association: Position of the American Dietetic Association: nutrition, aging, and the continuum of care, *J Am Diet Assoc,* 96:1048, 1996.

Catalano CB, DeBruyne LK, Whitney LN: *Nutrition and diet therapy,* ed 4, St Paul, Minn, 1995, West Publishing.

Chandra RK: Nutrition and the immune system: an introduction, *Am J Clin Nutr* 66:460S, 1997.

Connor JR, Beard JL: Dietary iron supplements in the elderly: to use or not to use? *Nutr Today* 32:102, 1997.

Coulston AM, Graig L, Voss AC: Meals-on-wheels applicants are a population at risk for poor nutritional status, *J Am Diet Assoc* 96:570, 1996.

Dawson-Hughes B, et al: Effect of calcium and vitamin D on bone density in men and women 65 years of age or older, *N Engl J Med* 337:670, 1997.

Dudek SG: *Nutrition handbook for nursing practice,* ed 2, Philadelphia, 1993, JB Lippincott.

Evans WJ, Cyr-Campbell D: Nutrition, exercise, and healthy aging, *J Am Diet Assoc* 97:632, 1997.

Fishman P: Healthy people 2000: what progress toward better nutrition? *Geriatrics* 51:38, 1996.

Grodner M, Anderson SI, DeYoung S: *Foundations and clinical applications of nutrition,* St Louis, 1996, Mosby.

Gray-Donald K: The frail elderly: meeting the nutritional challenges, *J Am Diet Assoc,* 1995.

Greeley A: Nutrition and the elderly, *FDA Consumer,* October 1990.

Havala S Website: *A senior's guide to good nutrition,* enviroling. org/arrs/VRG/seniors. html#intro,1997.

International Food Information Council Foundation: Better eating for better aging, *Food Insight,* May/June 1990.

Johnson RM, et al: Maintaining good nutrition in the elderly, *Patient Care* 29:46, 1995.

Kurtzwell P: Growing older, eating better, *FDA Consumer,* March 1996.

Marwick C: NHANES III health data relevant for aging nation, *JAMA* 277:100, 1997.

Neyman MR, Zidenberg-Cherr S, McDonald RB: Effect of participation in congregate-site meal programs on nutritional status of the healthy elderly, *J Am Diet Assoc* 96:475, 1996.

Prince RL: Diet and the prevention of osteoporotic fractures, *N Engl J Med* 337:701, 1997.

Russell RM: New views on the RDAs for older adults, *J Am Diet Assoc* 97:515, 1997.

Ryan C, Shea ME: Recognizing depression in older adults: the role of the dietitian, *J Am Diet Assoc* 96:1042.

Sahyoun NR, et al: Nutrition screening initiative checklist may be a better awareness/educational tool than a screening one, *J Am Diet Assoc* 97:760, 1997.

Wardlaw GM, Insel PM: *Perspectives in nutrition*, ed 3, St Louis, 1996, Mosby.

MEDICATIONS AND OLDER ADULTS

LEARNING OBJECTIVES

1. Identify factors that increase the risk of medication-related problems.
2. Discuss the reasons why each of these factors increases health risks for the aging person.
3. Describe how pharmacokinetics is altered with aging.
4. Discuss the pharmacodynamic changes observed in the aging person.
5. Explain specific precautions that are necessary when administering medication to the elderly in an institutional setting.
6. Identify the risks related to aging and pertinent nursing observations for specific drug categories.
7. Discuss how medications fit into the nursing plan of care.
8. Describe specific nursing interventions and modifications in technique that are related to medication administration to the elderly.
9. Describe the elderly person's rights as they relate to medication administration.
10. Identify information that should be provided to the elderly regarding medications.
11. Discuss the impact of age-related changes on self-administration of medications.
12. Describe nursing interventions that can reduce problems related to self-administration of medication in the home.

Problems related to medications are common in the elderly, and they are costly in terms of both time and money. Medications can alter an aging person's ability to perform normal functions, can result in behavior changes, and can be life-threatening.

Adverse reactions to medications are common in the elderly. Studies have revealed that as many as 17% of hospitalizations of persons over 66 years of age were related to adverse drug reactions. In addition, one in three elderly persons is likely to develop iatrogenic (treatment related) complications secondary to medications taken during a hospital stay. Adverse drug reactions have also been linked to an increased risk of falls and automobile accidents. Studies show that the resulting hospitalizations cost the elderly and taxpayers several billion dollars each year.

Estimates indicate that the average person older than 65 years of age takes three or more prescription medications each day. In addition, the average older person takes three or four nonprescription medications obtained over the counter (OTC). The cost of these medications exceeds 3 billion dollars per year.

Considering these numbers it is no surprise that use, misuse, and abuse of medication present serious threats to the aging population. Medications are potent substances. For every desired effect, many side effects and untoward effects are likely to occur. Although often useful or necessary to maintain health, medications present risks to people of all ages, and the elderly are at even greater risk than the younger population (Box 7-1).

RISKS RELATED TO DRUG-TESTING METHODS

The methodology used to test drugs and to establish therapeutic dosages generally does not take into account the unique characteristics of the elderly. Most

---

BOX 7-1

Factors That Increase the Risk of Medication-Related Problems

- Drug-testing methodology
- Physiologic changes related to aging
- Use of multiple medications
- Cognitive and sensory changes
- Knowledge deficits
- Financial concerns

---

drug testing is performed on healthy, young adult men. Because older adults normally have had some changes in body function and are more likely to suffer from at least one disease process, they are not physiologically the same as young adults. It seems obvious that an 80-year-old, 94-pound woman with heart disease should not be expected to respond in the same way that a healthy 35-year-old, 200-pound man would. The drugs and dosages that are appropriate for one may be unsuitable for the other. No medical professional would think of giving an adult dose of medication to a child, yet the same consideration is not always given to the unique situation presented by the elderly. **Geropharmacology,** the study of how the elderly respond to medication, is a new but growing area. Until all physicians recognize the uniqueness of the elderly and modify treatment accordingly, overmedication is likely to occur.

RISKS RELATED TO THE PHYSIOLOGIC CHANGES OF AGING

All individuals do not experience age-related physiologic changes at the same rate. When considering the responses of the elderly to medication, it is more important to consider physiologic age than chronologic age. The more physiologic changes experienced, the greater the risk will be of an altered response to medications. Even the most common physiologic changes of aging can have a significant effect on pharmacokinetics and pharmacodynamics (Table 7-1).

Pharmacokinetics
Drug absorption

Most medications are taken orally and are absorbed through the gastrointestinal tract. Gastric acid secretion decreases as we age, resulting in an increased gastric pH. When the concentration of acid is lower than normal, drug absorption is reduced. Decreased acidity also affects the breakdown of capsules and tablet coatings in the stomach, resulting in a variable absorption rate depending on the way a drug is manufactured.

Decreased gastric motility and a slower emptying rate of the stomach are common with aging. These can increase the amount of time that the medication is in contact with the gastric mucosa and can lead to increased absorption. Decreased peristalsis can also affect the speed at which enteric medication reaches the intestine. It may take longer for a drug to reach its site of absorption; hence its onset of action may be delayed. Changes in the ability of the cells in the gastrointestinal tract to absorb and transport the drug can further influence its absorption. If medication is not transferred effectively through the cell membrane, the amount of absorption will be decreased.

Drug distribution

With aging there is typically a decrease in total body mass, lean body mass, and total body water and an increase in total body fat. These changes can significantly alter the distribution of medications.

Because there is less total body water, water-soluble drugs such as gentamicin, histamine-receptor blockers, and lithium tend to remain in higher concentrations in the bloodstream. This results in increased blood concentration levels of these drugs. An elderly person who is dehydrated is at even greater risk of reaching excessive blood levels of water-soluble drugs.

As muscle mass decreases and the percentage of adipose tissue increases, fat-soluble drugs such as phenobarbital and the benzodiazepines become trapped in the fatty tissue, resulting in abnormally low blood levels. If the dosage is increased based on these blood levels, an excessive amount of medication may be administered. Because fat-soluble drugs continue to be released slowly from the fat into the bloodstream, elderly persons may exhibit delayed or "hangover" effects. The half-life of a single dose of diazepam, which is 36 hours in a young adult, may extend to as much as 100 hours in an elderly individual.

TABLE 7-1

Factors Affecting Drug Response in the Elderly

Effect	Cause
Decreased drug absorption	Decreased hydrochloric acid; altered gastrointestinal motility
Altered drug distribution	Storing of fat-soluble drug in fatty tissue; decreased serum albumin for binding of drugs
Altered drug metabolism	Decreased enzyme activity in liver
Decreased drug excretion	Decreased renal blood flow; decreased glomerular filtration rate; decreased number of functional renal tubules

From Wolanin MO: *Geriatr Nurs* 4:227, 1983.

A decrease in hemoglobin and the plasma protein albumin is common with aging. This results in fewer available sites for protein-bound drugs such as warfarin, phenytoin, theophylline, salicylates, and tolbutamide. The danger of adverse or toxic reactions is high even with smaller doses because unbound *active* drug still circulates in the bloodstream. The risk for toxicity is greater in malnourished elderly. Aging persons who consume high-carbohydrate, low-protein diets are more likely to develop toxicity than are aging persons who consume a well-balanced diet. Because not all of the serum drug assay tests can distinguish between free and bound medications, these tests may not provide reliable measures of toxicity.

Drug metabolism

The liver is the primary site of drug metabolism. Aging often results in decreased activity of liver cells, decreased metabolic enzymes, and decreased cardiac output, which results in reduced blood flow to the liver. By 65 years of age, the liver has only 55% to 65% of the perfusion of a young adult. This reduction in perfusion decreases the liver's effectiveness in metabolizing drugs. When drugs are not metabolized effectively by the elderly liver, the risk of toxicity increases. Toxicity is always a concern with medications commonly prescribed for the elderly, including digoxin, β-blockers, calcium-channel blockers, and tricyclic antidepressants.

Drug excretion

Aging kidneys are significantly less effective at removing waste products, including the byproducts of medications. As the kidneys become less effective in excreting drugs, more drug remains in the circulation, leading to elevated drug levels and symptoms of drug toxicity. Circulatory changes that reduce blood flow to the kidneys result in drug accumulation in the bloodstream and increase the risk of toxicity.

Because the changes in kidney function are accompanied by changes in lean body mass, serum creatinine levels often remain constant, masking the decline in function. When assessing the risks for toxicity, creatinine clearance tests provide a more effective measure of kidney function than does the serum creatinine level.

Medications such as aminoglycosides, digoxin, lithium, procainamide, and cimetidine are likely to reach toxic levels due to poor renal excretion. Nonprescription drugs such as alcohol and nicotine can also affect kidney function and cause changes in drug elimination in elderly persons.

Pharmacodynamics

Responses to medications are less predictable in the aging person. Pathologic changes in target organs may affect the response to medications. Receptor sites on the target organs may respond more or less sensitively to medications. The receptors may respond normally to some medications but not to others. Receptors may often be more sensitive to medications, placing the elderly at increased risk for toxic responses. Brain receptors are particularly sensitive, hence the very strong response of most elderly persons to psychotropic medications. When the receptor sites are less sensitive, the individual may require larger-than-normal doses to achieve therapeutic effects. If receptor sites in the myocardium are affected, elderly persons may require higher doses of common medications such as propranolol and lidocaine. Administration of these higher doses increases the risk of toxicity.

RISKS REALTED TO USE OF MULTIPLE MEDICATIONS

Polypharmacy, the prescription, administration, or use of more medications than are clinically indicated, is a common problem in the elderly (Fig. 7-1). According to many studies, the elderly ingest a far greater number of medications than do younger persons. A recent survey revealed that the average institutionalized elderly person takes 7.5 medications. Nearly 10% of those living independently take as many as 12 prescription drugs. This number does not include OTC medications that may be taken with or without a physician's recommendation or knowledge. It is estimated that the elderly purchase 40% of all nonprescription medications. The more medications

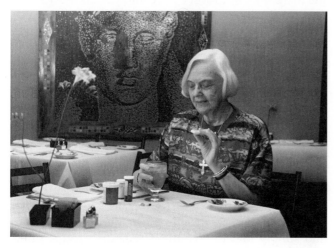

FIG. 7-1   Older adults' concurrent use of many prescription medications can lead to polypharmacy. (Courtesy of Loy Ledbetter, St Louis.)

taken, the greater the risk of untoward reactions, drug interactions, and drug toxicities will be. Drug interactions and toxicities in the elderly are likely to result in behavioral or cognitive changes, which are often mistaken for dementia.

Many factors contribute to the increased usage of medication among the elderly, including an increased likelihood of multiple acute or chronic disease conditions, increased availability of a wide variety of prescription and OTC medications, changes in patient expectations, and changes in the health care delivery system.

Newer, better, and more potent medications are developed every day. Medical conditions of the elderly that were once considered untreatable are now treated routinely using medications. Because the elderly tend to have more physical complaints or diseases than younger individuals, medication usage increases exponentially.

The elderly seek medical intervention for many reasons. Some live with their problems and only seek medical attention when they have serious concerns. By the time such a person seeks medical attention, his or her condition may have seriously deteriorated, requiring the prescription of multiple medications. Other elderly persons make frequent visits to their physicians, seeking reassurance that nothing is seriously wrong. Rather than spending the time needed to reassure the elderly, some physicians issue a prescription as a way to terminate the visit. This poor medical practice unfortunately occurs too often and can result in the elderly taking unnecessary or marginally necessary medications.

Still other elderly persons expect their physicians to be able to eliminate all of their problems and ailments with medications. Every television show, magazine article, or recommendation from a friend extolling the benefits of a new medication sends some elderly to their doctor's offices to request or even demand the new medicine. They expect the physician to provide a medication to relieve their ailments, and they often perceive that the physician is not doing anything for them unless some medication is prescribed. Some elderly will even go from doctor to doctor until they find one who will give them what they want. Under these pressures, some physicians prescribe medications that they otherwise would not have ordered.

Changes in health care delivery, particularly increased medical specialization, have contributed to medication-related problems. It is increasingly common for an elderly person to have two or more physicians providing their care. When more than one physician writes prescriptions, the risk of medication reactions and overmedication increases dramatically. If a physician does not know what drugs the person is already taking, he or she cannot take the drugs into account when determining the safety of another prescription. Every physician providing care to an elderly person must be aware of all medications that person is taking, no matter who prescribed them (see the clinical situation box on this page).

RISKS RELATED TO COGNITIVE OR SENSORY CHANGES

Cognitive and sensory limitations increase the risks of medication errors in the elderly. Cognitive problems come in several forms, including a lack of the literacy skills needed to read the labels and directions, the inability to understand and comply with directions, and the inability to make correct judgments about medications. In severe cases of cognitive impairment, elderly individuals may not even recognize that they have to take medication. If they do attempt to take medication, serious and potentially harmful errors are often made. Cognitively impaired elderly people should not be responsible for medicating themselves but should be supervised by a family member or nurse.

Sensory changes, particularly visual and to a lesser extent hearing changes, present problems for the elderly. When vision changes render an elderly person unable to read a medication label or to recognize the different sizes, shapes, or colors of the various medications, serious problems can arise. Many elderly essentially *guess* about what medications they are taking, frequently taking the wrong medication at the wrong time and in the wrong amount because they are unable to read the directions. Liquid medications, particularly injectables such as insulin, are frequently overdosed or underdosed because of poor vision. Many of these risks can be reduced by adequately assessing the

person's ability to read labels accurately, by proper teaching, and by using special labels or magnifying devices that facilitate safe administration.

RISKS RELATED TO INADEQUATE KNOWLEDGE

Inadequate knowledge about medications can result in serious problems for the elderly. This lack of knowledge, which can relate to both prescription and nonprescription medications, has many causes and manifests in different ways.

One common sign of lack of knowledge involves sharing medications with friends or relatives. This practice is common and persists because many of the elderly are unaware of the dangers. When one elderly person finds a medication that makes him or her feel better, he or she often may attempt to share it with friends who have similar problems. The intention of helping friends is good, but the consequences can be serious and even fatal. All people, particularly the elderly, must be aware that it is not safe to take a medication prescribed for someone else. If a person feels that a certain medication will help, he or she should get the name of the medicine and then contact the physician. The physician—not a friend—is best able to determine whether the drug will be safe and beneficial.

Many elderly people have misconceptions about OTC preparations. It is estimated that 60% to 70% of the elderly use at least one OTC preparation. Many do not feel that OTC medications are "real" because no prescription is needed to purchase them. Because they do not consider OTC medications to be real drugs, the elderly are not likely to consult with a physician, pharmacist, or nurse regarding their use. They simply go to the drug store or grocery store and purchase whatever preparation looks like it might help. This uneducated use of OTC drugs can be hazardous to the elderly, particularly those who are also taking prescription medications. OTC medications are capable of potentiating or interfering with the effects of prescription medications, possibly resulting in serious harm. OTC drugs can also create or mask symptoms of disease. Use of these drugs can make it difficult for the physician to recognize changes in health status. The elderly must be taught to consult with their physicians or pharmacists before taking any OTC medication.

The elderly often lack adequate knowledge regarding their prescription medications as well. Frequently elderly persons are given one or more prescriptions and simply told to take them according to the directions. The directions provided may be very clear to a knowledgeable health care professional, but they are often misunderstood or misinterpreted by the elderly.

Even simple misunderstandings can lead to improper self-medication and result in serious consequences. To reduce the risks, the elderly often require additional instruction in order to take their prescriptions safely. Because this is a common problem among the elderly, self-administration of medication is addressed in greater detail later in this chapter.

RISKS RELATED TO FINANCIAL FACTORS

Medications are expensive. A single prescription can easily cost $50 or $100 a month. If the aging person requires more than one medication, the cumulative cost can be overwhelming. To save money, elderly people living on limited incomes may fail to take their medications or they may make changes in the amount or frequency in order to conserve their supply. Because these changes do not follow the recommended therapeutic schedule, all manner of untoward responses can occur.

A significant percentage of prescriptions written by physicians are never filled because of their cost. If the prescription is filled, the elderly person may skip doses or take only part of the prescribed dose to make the medication last longer. Some will get the prescription filled once to see if it's "worth the price." If the benefits gained from taking the medication are not readily obvious to the individual, he or she may not get the prescription refilled.

Because medications are expensive, many elderly will save medications that were prescribed in the past, even if the drugs are no longer part of their therapy. The elderly are often reluctant to discard costly medications, holding on to them "just in case" they are needed again. This practice can bring serious harm if the medications are kept long enough to become outdated. Outdated medications can undergo chemical changes that make them hazardous. Saving old medications also increases the risk of problems if the elderly person thinks the drug is appropriate and takes it without checking with the physician (see the clinical situation box on p. 112).

It is obvious that medications can present a wide range of problems for the elderly. Nurses who work with the elderly must consider each of these risks when determining a plan for safe administration.

MEDICATION ADMINISTRATION IN AN INSTITUTIONAL SETTING

Medication administration is a common part of nursing care of the elderly in hospitals, extended-care facilities, and home settings. Approaches and methods

CLINICAL SITUATION

A patient who was using timolol eyedrops that were prescribed by an ophthalmologist for glaucoma began to experience joint pain. Not seeing any connection between his eye problems and his aching joints, he sought the advice of his rheumatologist. Fortunately, the rheumatologist asked if he was taking any other medications. When timolol was identified, the rheumatologist recognized the possibility of a drug-induced problem and contacted the ophthalmologist, who then changed the medication. The joint pain disappeared without further medical intervention.

may vary according to the setting, but the safety of the older adult remains the primary concern. A great deal of nursing time in a hospital or extended-care facility is spent on medication-related activities. Because medications play a very important role in the health care of the elderly, nurses must take special precautions to ensure that drugs are administered safely.

Safe drug administration begins with a thorough knowledge and understanding of each medication. Any questions regarding medication therapy must be clarified and resolved *before* a medication is administered. Information regarding medications is contained in many reference books, which should be readily available to nurses. Before administering a medication, nurses should have the following information:
1. The therapeutic effects of the medication
2. The reasons this particular person is receiving the medication
3. The normal therapeutic dosage of the medication
4. The normal route or routes of administration
5. Any special precautions related to administration
6. The common side effects or adverse effects of the medication (see the clinical situation box on this page)
7. Signs of overdose and toxicity

NURSING ASSESSMENT AND MEDICATION

Nurse must be sure to thoroughly assess their elderly residents before administering any medications. After administration, nurses should monitor the residents continually to determine whether the medication is having the desired effect. This should be done after administering both scheduled and as-needed medications. Residents should also be observed for any untoward effects or significant changes in medical condition or behavior.

Because normal physiologic changes and the effects

of disease place the elderly person at increased risk for drug-related problems, nurses should be particularly watchful for any signs of overdose or toxicity. Special age-related risk factors and observations for the more common drug classifications are summarized in Table 7-2.

Implementation of computerized records as part of the Minimum Data Set 2.0 provides better linkage between nurses and pharmacists. This interdisciplinary approach to medication will hopefully promote early recognition of problems or areas of concern regarding the medication regimen.

MEDICATIONS AND THE NURSING CARE PLAN

Medications are only a part of the overall care of the elderly person and should be included as such. For example, the administration of laxatives should be only a part of a more comprehensive plan to assist bowel elimination, and administration of analgesics should be only a part of a larger nursing care plan for pain control.

Nursing interventions and precautions related to medications should be addressed in the plan of care. This could include use of safety devices, call signals, behavior monitoring, or any other specific precaution related to medications. The care plan should indicate when it is necessary to check vital signs, monitor laboratory values, or make any other special observations. All parameters specified by the physician should be readily identified. If ordered, for example, the care plan should indicate "hold digoxin if apical pulse is below 60" or "give 6 U regular insulin h.s. if the fingerstick blood glucose is over 150."

The care plan should indicate any individual preferences of the elderly person. Many elderly persons use a particular order or method to take their medication. This information should be in the care plan so that all staff nurses can be consistent.

Nursing Interventions Related to Medication Administration

It is often necessary to modify procedures and techniques of medication administration when working with the elderly. Despite modifications, the traditional "rights" of medication administration remain essential to the process.

Right resident

Proper identification of the resident or patient is an essential part of safe nursing care. This simple task can

be a challenge to nurses who work in extended-care facilities. Whenever a large number of residents are up and about, accurate identification becomes more difficult.

The most accurate way to verify identity is to compare the medication record to the identification bracelet (Fig. 7-2). Whenever possible, these bracelets should be used for identification checks. Not all long-term residents wear identification bracelets, however, and if they do wear them the bracelets are frequently old and blurred. When such bracelets are not available, alternative methods must be used.

Resident pictures are sometimes used as a means of identification. Pictures that are old or bear little resemblance to the individual are useless. Pictures used for identifications must be kept up-to-date and must be readily available when medications are distributed.

Identification can also be accomplished by asking the resident to state his or her name. Most people will respond promptly and appropriately with the correct name. A response to hearing the nurse call a name that involves a head shake or a "yes" from a patient is not enough to ensure identification. Many elderly people suffering from hearing or cognitive impairment will give some sort of response to *any* name. When an elderly person is not oriented to person, bracelets or pictures must be used (Box 7-2).

Attempting to identify a resident by room and bed number is not adequate because cognitively or perceptually impaired individuals often wander into the wrong room or lie down in someone else's bed. Nurses should be careful to avoid the trap of insisting that they "know the residents." Identification must be checked with each medication pass—no matter how long you have been caring for the patient. Serious mistakes can and do occur when nurses take shortcuts with safety procedures.

Right medication

Before administering a medication, the nurse must ensure that the drug provided by the pharmacy is in fact the correct one. This is not as easy as it seems. Because each medication has a generic name and one or more trade names and the appearance of a medication can vary widely depending on the manufacturer, nurses must use a reference source to verify that the right drug is in fact available. Physician's orders should be checked carefully and the pharmacy contacted if any questions arise. Many drug names look or sound alike; therefore, it is important to check spellings carefully.

If telephone medication orders are permitted, the nurse taking the order should repeat the complete order to the physician to avoid the possibility of error. Be sure to clarify the spelling of the drug.

TABLE 7-2

Common Drug Categories with Precautions Related to Aging

Type of medication	Risk factors	Observe for
Cardiac medications Digoxin, propranolol	Dehydration, hypothyroidism, decreased renal excretion, and hypoxia increase the risk of toxicity.	Visual spots, dizziness, headaches, fatigue, drowsiness, mental changes, numbness around lips or of hands, altered pulse rate or regularity, loss of appetite, nausea, vomiting, diarrhea, weight loss
Diuretics Bumetanide, furosemide, hydrochlorothiazide, chlorothiazide	May result in dehydration. May precipitate urinary incontinence or retention in elderly men with prostate hypertrophy. May result in altered electrolytes K^+ and Na^+, which predispose to digitalis toxicity.	Signs of dehydration, hypotension, weight loss, lethargy, and confusion
Antihypertensives Captopril, clonidine, hydralazine (HCl), methyldopa	High doses may aggravate existing problems in cerebral, coronary, and renal circulation. Hot weather, alcohol, and exercise are likely to increase the risk of hypotension.	Bradycardia, postural hypotension, weakness, headaches, palpitations, nausea, vomiting, diarrhea or constipation, difficulty urinating, and edema
Psychotropics (including antianxiety agents, antidepressants, and antipsychotics) Flurazepam, triazolam, diazepam, haloperidol, thorazine, mellaril	Elderly persons usually require smaller doses to achieve therapeutic response. Tardive dyskinesia is a significant risk with long-term therapy.	Apathy, confusion, drooling, lip smacking, grimacing, difficulty swallowing, decreased mobility, skin reactions, jaundice, impaired sense of balance, alteration in gait, falls, drowsiness, fainting, hypotension, palpitations, constipation, hypothermia and complaints of feeling cold
Antiinfectives Cephalosporins, penicillins, sulfanomides, tetracyclines	Standard dose may result in higher blood levels in the elderly. Increased risk of allergic reactions or superimposed yeast infections with aging. Damage to cranial nerve VIII particularly common in the elderly.	Nausea, vomiting, diarrhea, dehydration, signs of oral or vaginal yeast infection, urticaria, tinnitus
Nonsteroidal antiinflammatory agents Aspirin, ibuprofen, tolmetin, naproxen	Increased risk of gastrointestinal and central nervous system problems with aging.	Signs of gastrointestinal upset including nausea, vomiting, tarry stools, diarrhea or constipation, and occult blood loss; central nervous system side effects include dizziness, confusion, mood swings, depression, and tinnitus
Bronchodilators and spasmolytics Theophylline	Elderly taking allopurinol, propranolol, and cimetidine are at increased risk of toxicity.	Tachycardia, arrhythmias, anorexia, nausea, headaches or insomnia
Antiulcer medications Cimetidine, ranitidine, aluminum and magnesium hydroxide	May affect the absorption of other medications.	Confusion, dry mouth, gynecomastia, impotence, constipation, diarrhea

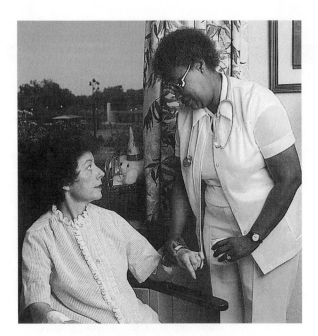

FIG. 7-2   Before administering any medication nurses should check the resident's identification bracelet to be sure the right person receives the right drug. (From Potter PA, Perry AG: *Basic nursing: theory and practice,* ed 3, St Louis, 1995, Mosby.)

Right amount

The goal of drug therapy in the elderly is to achieve the maximum therapeutic benefits while giving the smallest amount of medication necessary (Box 7-3). Therefore, the dosage prescribed for the elderly will frequently be lower than what would be prescribed for a younger adult (Table 7-3). To achieve therapeutic levels without overdosing the elderly person, the physician may order lower doses or less frequent administration of a medication. With lower doses it is imperative that the nurse verify the strength of the medications (checking decimal points closely). All measurements, particularly for liquids, must be made with great care. Decreased frequency in administration can result in medications that are administered every other day or every third day. Nurses must pay close attention when administering medication to avoid administering it on a day when the drug should be withheld. Any questions regarding the dosage should be clarified with an approved reference, the pharmacist, or physician before the medication is administered.

Right dosage form

Problems arise when the elderly person is unable to swallow tablets or cannot swallow at all and relies on a gastric or nasogastric tube for nourishment. In these cases, nurses must consider safe alternatives. If the medication is available in liquid form, the nurse

---

BOX 7-2

SAFETY ALERT

Identification must be checked (following agency policies) each time a medication is administered. Failure to do this can result in serious errors and harm to the elderly.

BOX 7-3

Guiding Rule for Medication Administration in Older Adults

To achieve the maximum therapeutic benefits while giving the smallest necessary amount of medication!

TABLE 7-3

Examples of Drug Dosages

Drug	Dosage for healthy adults* (mg)
Ibuprofen	200-800 three to four times/day
Indomethacin	25-50 three to four times/day
Naproxen	250-750 twice/day
Sulindac	150-200 twice/day
Piroxicin	10-20 once/day

From Ham RJ, Sloane PD: *Primary care geriatrics: a case-based approach,* ed 2, St Louis, 1992, Mosby.
*Older patients should generally be started on the lowest dose.

should discuss the possibility of an order change with the physician. Because liquids might be absorbed more rapidly than solids, all changes in medication form require a physician's order. Many times when the drug form is changed, the dosage is also changed. If a liquid form is not available, the tablet or capsule may have to be crushed or broken to facilitate swallowing. Not all medications can be crushed or broken because these activities can alter the action of the drug (Box 7-4). If there is any question of whether a medication should be crushed, the pharmacy should be consulted. Lists of common medications that should not be crushed or chewed are available from many sources and should be kept on the nursing unit as quick references.

Right route

Most medications are prescribed for oral administration. When administering an oral medication, the importance of the medication, the preferences of the elderly person, and his or her capabilities must be considered.

BOX 7-4

Medications That Should Not Be Chewed or Crushed

- Enteric-coated tablets
- Time-release tablets or capsules
- Sublingual or buccal tablets
- Medications that stain the mouth
- Medications that are extremely bitter or irritating to the oral mucosa

Many older adults receive numerous medications. Give the most important medications first so that if the person refuses to take them all, at least the most essential ones will have been administered. Whenever a person refuses to take his or her medication, it should be noted in the chart and the nurse in charge should be notified.

Some elderly are capable of and prefer swallowing several tablets at one time to "get it over with." If they experience no difficulty taking their medications this way, there is no reason to try to make them change their habits. Other people prefer to take their medications one tablet at a time. If this is their preference the nurse should oblige. Still others have trouble swallowing any solid medications.

Tablets, particularly large ones, are likely to cause the greatest problems. Dryness of the mouth related to aging often makes swallowing difficult and results in complaints of pills "sticking in the throat." Encouraging the elderly person to take a drink of water or some other beverage *before* he or she tries to swallow the tablet may make swallowing easier. Coating the tablet with a spoonful of pudding, ice cream, or applesauce might also help the patient swallow it more easily. Only small amounts of these foods should be used to facilitate swallowing.

Crushed medications should not be mixed into a serving of food during meal time. This practice is unsafe because it often results in a partial missed dose because the entire serving of food may not be consumed and because the nursing assistant assigned to feed the patient is not qualified to administer medications.

Administration of medication through a feeding tube is often necessary and must be done correctly. Liquid forms of a medication are preferable and should be requested when available. Large particles of a medication can block the feeding tube and necessitate tube replacement. To prevent blockage, each tablet should be finely crushed and then placed in a plastic medication cup, where it should be thoroughly dissolved in a small amount of warm water. Once completely dissolved, medications are administered through the feeding tube. Each medication should be administered separately. The feeding tube should be flushed with a small amount of water before giving the first medication, again after each medication, and before reconnecting the tube with the feeding solution. Medications should never be mixed together or with feeding solutions.

Medications with an unpleasant taste should be given after all other medications. Offering a sip of ice water before the medication or refrigerating bad-tasting liquid medications can make them more palatable.

When a parenteral medication is ordered, other precautions must be taken. Because older adult generally have less muscle mass and subcutaneous tissue than younger people, injection sites should be selected carefully. Intramuscular injections are best administered using the ventrogluteal site, which is easily accessible without excessive repositioning. It is free from any major nerves or blood vessels. This muscle remains large enough for injection even in very slender people and is well away from areas of contamination if the elderly person is incontinent.

The needle length should be chosen with caution, depending on the injection site. The deltoid muscle is usually a poor site for all but very infrequent administrations of very small volumes. To prevent striking the bone of an emaciated elderly person, a shorter-length needle (e.g., 1 inch instead of 1.5 inches) may be needed.

Right time

Some medications are more effective or better tolerated if given under specific conditions. For greatest effect, medications that are ordered before meals should be given when the stomach is empty. Because people produce less gastric acid as they age, a sufficient rate and amount of absorption may depend on having the stomach free of food. Medications that are ordered after meals should only be given after the person has eaten.

Activities of daily living can be affected by medications. Medications should be administered at times chosen so that the drugs interfere as little as possible with normal activities. For example, a diuretic should be given early in the day to prevent the elderly person from having to get up several times at night to urinate.

The timing of eyedrop administration becomes an issue when an aging person requires more than one type of medication in the same eye. Some eye medications are compatible and can be given together; others cannot. The timing and order of administration for eyedrops should be clarified with the pharmacy, and the schedule should be clearly stated in the medication administration record.

Right documentation

Care must be used when documenting medications. Facilities use a variety of different forms and records to document various aspects of care, including medication administration. To ensure that all medications are administered properly, the rules of charting must be followed.

Medications cannot be charted as having been administered *until they are actually taken*. This means that the nurse must stay in the room and watch the elderly person take the medication. It is not safe practice to leave medication at the bedside unless the resident has specific orders that permit self-medication.

Special observations regarding the patient's or resident's response should be included in the daily nursing notes and narrative summaries. The reasons for administration of as-needed medications should be identified each time one is administered, and the effectiveness of these medications should be documented. When a medication is refused or withheld, the reasons should be clearly documented and the physician notified so that the plan of care can be adjusted if necessary.

PATIENT RIGHTS AND MEDICATION

Elderly people have the right to know what medication they are receiving and why they are receiving it. Nurses should provide this information whenever questioned and whenever a new medication is prescribed.

The elderly also have the right to refuse to take medication. If a person refuses to take medication, nurses cannot use force. A positive attitude and encouragement may help persuade the individual to cooperate. However, when a medication is still refused, the reasons for refusal must be determined and documented, the nurse in charge notified, and any problems communicated to the physician.

The elderly person must be provided with privacy during injections or any other such procedure. Doors should be closed and curtains drawn. Failure to do this is a violation of resident rights.

The use of psychotropic drugs as chemical restraints presents a risk to the rights of the elderly, and their administration is strictly controlled by Omnibus Budget Reconciliation Act (OBRA) regulations. Nurses must carefully follow the very specific guidelines regarding the administration and monitoring of behavior when an elderly person is receiving a psychotropic medication. Each abnormal behavior that is an indication for administration of such drugs must be individually identified in the plan of care. During each shift, the nurse must document the number of times these identified behaviors occur. If no symptoms occur at a given dosage of psychotropic medication, the physician will attempt to decrease the dose. This process continues as long as the elderly person receives these medications.

SELF-MEDICATION AND OLDER ADULTS

In an Institutional Setting

Under OBRA legislation, residents of care facilities should have the option of self-medication if they are capable of doing so safely. A physician's order stating that self-medication is permitted is usually required.

Self-medication by a resident can be time consuming because the nurse remains responsible for monitoring the resident's compliance and response to the medications. When self-medication is anticipated, the nurse must assess the elderly person's ability to understand and comply with the medication regimen. This assessment should include the resident's ability to read labels, follow directions, and measure dosages accurately.

Once it has been determined that the person can safely assume responsibility for self-medication, the nurse should develop a plan, including (1) delivery of adequate amounts of medication, (2) safe storage of medications that will be kept at the bedside, (3) record keeping of medications taken, and (4) follow-up assessments of medication effectiveness or side effects.

In the Home

Taking medications correctly can be a complex problem for the elderly. Because medications are a significant part of the medical plan of care, older adults who live independently must learn to take them properly. The responsibility of assessing medication-taking behaviors and teaching safe self-administration often falls to the home health care nurse.

TEACHING OLDER ADULTS ABOUT MEDICATIONS

Elderly persons and their families or significant others should be given complete information about the prescribed medications and the proper method for taking them. Explanations should be given well in advance of leaving the office, clinic, or hospital. If possible, nurses should select a time when the elderly person's anxiety level is low because the individual will be more likely to remember the important points when he or she is calm. If the directions are complex, extra time may be needed to ensure that they are understood completely. Many times the elderly person will fail to ask questions because he or she is afraid of being judged as ignorant or bothersome. Consequently, this information should be reviewed and repeated if necessary at subsequent visits.

Most medications are taken orally, but an increasing number are delivered by alternative routes. When medication is taken in any way other than the oral route, the nurse should verify that the elderly person understands and is able to demonstrate safe self-administration. This includes transdermal patches, suppositories, eyedrops or eardrops, and injections. Remember that many things that seem obvious or simple to nurses are complex for others.

In addition to teaching independent elderly persons about their prescription medications, nurses should teach the importance of consulting with the physician or pharmacist before taking any OTC medications. Those individuals should also be reminded never to take medication prescribed for someone else without consulting the physician first.

Each elderly person who lives independently should have an up-to-date record that identifies his or her major physical problems, physician or physicians, any allergies, and all current medications. This list must be updated each time a medication is added or discontinued. If the person is not capable of keeping the record up-to-date, the nurse or family should provide assistance. This record should be taken along each time the individual receives health care services so that all care providers have the necessary information. A written record relieves the elderly person of the burden of trying to remember too many details, which is particularly difficult when the person is under stress.

Nurses can assist the elderly by preparing medication cards or sheets that identify and give the important information about each medication (Box 7-5). Teaching aids should be kept simple and clear. Writing should be large and legible so that the elderly person can read it with ease. Family members should be included in the teaching so that they are able to assist the elderly person if necessary.

Cognitive and sensory limitations increase the risk of medication errors. Keeping track of multiple medications can be confusing to anyone, but it is more likely to present problems for the elderly. One or two medications do not seem to cause many problems, but a significant number of elderly people become confused and noncompliant when three or more medications are ordered. Special precautions and complicated time schedules compound the problems. To reduce the risk of noncompliance, nurses should encourage the elderly to talk to the physician and/or the pharmacist to see whether there is any safe way to re-

---

BOX 7-5

Information to Include on Medication Teaching Sheets

- The name of the medication (trade and/or generic)
- The time or times when the medication should be taken
- Whether the medication should be taken before, with, or after meals
- Any precautions to take when preparing the medication
- How much of the medication to take
- The reason the person is receiving each medication (desired effects)
- The most common side effects
- What action to take if these side effects occur
- What to do if the person forgets to take a dose of the medication
- What to do if the person experiences nausea or vomiting and is unable to take oral medication

---

duce the number of medications or simplify the medication schedule.

Associating medication schedules with regular daily events such as meals or bedtime can help the elderly remember to take their medications. Additional teaching may be necessary if medications require special timing (e.g., before or after meals). Unless the elderly person is aware of the reasons and necessity for this schedule, he or she may not comply and therefore may experience untoward effects.

The elderly should be taught to prepare medication in a well-lit area. Poor lighting can further reduce vision in the elderly and increase the chance of making an error.

Visually impaired elderly people can continue to self-medicate if measures are taken to compensate for visual problems. Large, preferably upper-case or printed lettering should be used on all labels and teaching materials. All print or writing should be in dark, bold letters. If there is any risk of moisture spilling on the labels, they should be coated in clear plastic or otherwise protected. This will prevent blurring of the lettering, which can lead to errors.

Color codes, tape strips, pictures, or textures such as sandpaper can be applied to containers to help the elderly recognize them. For example, black could indicate medicine that is to be taken with breakfast, red could indicate medications for lunch, and a piece of sandpaper attached to the bottle could indicate bedtime medications. Yellow should be avoided because many elderly have difficulty distinguishing this color. Alternately, there could be one strip for morning administration, two strips for lunch, three strips for dinner, and four strips for bedtime. The nurse should ensure that the person understands whatever code is selected. Medication cups can be marked with dark lines or tape to improve accuracy when measuring liquids, and special magnifiers are available for insulin syringes.

Impaired physical function can interfere with self-medication. Many pill bottles routinely come with safety caps that the elderly cannot open. If requested, most pharmacies will provide containers that are easier to open.

If the elderly person is receiving both eardrops and eyedrops, these containers should be stored well away from each other and marked clearly with a large picture of an eye or an ear so that they are distinguishable. This is particularly important because many ear preparations can cause permanent damage to the eye.

The elderly should be taught how to store medications properly. Medications should be stored away from direct light and moisture, which can cause chemical changes. The tiny pill boxes used by many elderly can be dangerous and should be avoided. Pills left in the boxes may undergo chemical changes. Nitroglycerin can become totally ineffective if stored improperly. Once medications are removed from the prescription bottle, they cannot be readily identified and the elderly person can easily take the wrong pill. It is safest to leave medications in the pharmacy bottles even though they may be bulky.

When the elderly person are unable to keep their medication schedule straight using the bottles provided by the pharmacy, other approaches may be necessary. There are several ways nurses can help the elderly remember to take their medications. Medication reminder systems help some elderly people remember to take medications. These systems typically consist of divided containers that sort the medications by day of the week or by time. They can either be purchased or created using foam egg cartons labeled with the day and time. A simple check of the box reveals whether the medication was taken on time. Some individuals require more medication than fits conveniently into these standard containers or fear that they will drop the egg carton and mix everything up. These individuals may benefit from a system using small zip-closure baggies that are labeled (using masking tape) with the appropriate day and time.

It is not advisable for the elderly to keep any medications, particularly those taken to promote sleep, at the bedside. Sleepiness can interfere with the ability to read labels. If not completely awake, the person can easily take the wrong medication. Because sleeping pills dull the ability to perceive things accurately, those who have trouble getting to sleep can easily take extra doses of their medication and be seriously harmed.

The elderly can achieve maximum benefits from their medication when nurses pay careful attention to all aspects of medication administration. Careful assessment, good teaching, and well-planned interventions can enable many elderly to function independently.

SUMMARY

On average, elderly people take three or more medications each day not including OTC preparations. Drug use, misuse, and abuse present serious threats to the well-being of elderly individuals and increase the risk of hospitalization due to adverse drug reactions. The chance of adverse reactions is increased by the normal physiologic changes of aging, pathologic changes related to the higher incidence of acute or chronic diseases, and myriad other factors. We have long recognized that children require special considerations with regard to medication, and we are now aware that the aging population also requires special considerations. Geropharmacology, the study of how the elderly respond to medications, is an expanding area. Physicians who prescribe medication, pharmacists who dispense medication, and nurses who administer medication must continue to work together to understand the unique problems and needs of the elderly with regard to these potentially dangerous substances.

Nurses must work diligently to build a knowledge base of the medications administered to their patients or residents, know how to administer each medication safely, know how to assess the aging person's need for and response to each medication, and develop an appropriate plan of care that included safety concerns and teaching needs.

READINGS AND REFERENCES

Atkin PA, et al: Functional ability of patients to manage medication packaging: a survey of geriatric inpatients, *Age Aging* 23:113, 1994.

Bihm B: Psychotropic medications and the elderly, *Med Surg Nurs* 5:191, 1996.

Carlson JE: Perils of polypharmacy: 10 steps to prudent prescribing, *Geriatrics* 51:26, 1996.

Connolly MJ: Inhaler technique in elderly patients: comparison of metered-dose inhalers and large volume spacer devices, *Age Aging* 24:190, 1995.

Cooper JW: Drug-related problems in the elderly patient, *Generations* 18:19, 1994.

Corlett AJ: Aids to compliance with medication, *BMJ* 313:926, 1996.

Davant C: Taking the confusion and danger out of polypharmacy, *Med Ec* 70:125, 1993.

Dunne FJ: Misuse of alcohol or drugs by elderly people: may need special management, *BMJ,* 308:608, 1994.

Duxbury AS: Geriatrics: unmasking polypharmacy problems and adverse drug effects, *Consultant* 36:762, 1996.

Gambert SR, Grossberg GT, Morley JE: How many drugs does your aged patient need? *Patient Care* 28:61, 1994.

Gianfrancesco FD, Baines AP, Richards D: Utilization of prescription drug benefits in an aging population, *Health Care Financing Rev* 15:113, 1994.

Gorman C: Overdosing the elderly: many older Americans are taking the wrong drugs, *Time* 47, August 8, 1994.

Hanlon JT, et al: Is medication use by community dwelling elderly people influenced by cognitive function? *Age Aging,* 25:1996.

Ireland GA: Aging well with fewer medications, *Am Behav Scientist* 39:306, 1996.

Jaggar SF: Dangerous prescriptions for the elderly, *Consumers' Research Magazine,* p22, June, 1996.

Loughran S: Medication use in the elderly: a population at risk, *Med Surg Nurs* 5:121, 1996.

Mold JW, McCarthy L: Pearls from geriatrics, or a long line at the bathroom, *J Fam Pract,* 41:22, 1995.

National Institute on Aging Web site: *Safe use of medications by older people,* www.agepage.com/medicine.htm, 1997.

Rogers K: Seniors' hypertension therapy hurt by noncompliance, *Drug Topics* 138:35, 1994.

Struck AE, et al: Inappropriate medication use in community dwelling older persons, *Arch Intern Med* 154:2195, 1994.

Ukens C: Drug regimens go mostly unmonitored in Oregon program, *Drug Topics* 138:63, 1994.

Willcox SM, Himmelstein DU, Woolhandler S: Inappropriate drug prescribing for the community dwelling elderly, *JAMA* 272:292, 1994.

HEALTH ASSESSMENT OF THE ELDERLY

LEARNING OBJECTIVES

1. Identify different levels of assessment.
2. Describe the difference between subjective and objective data.
3. Discuss the importance of thorough assessment.
4. Describe appropriate methods for structuring and conducting an interview.
5. Identify approaches that facilitate a successful physical examination of the elderly.
6. Discuss the modifications used when preparing an elderly person for physical examination.
7. Describe the techniques used when performing a physical examination.
8. Explain the adaptations used when assessing vital signs in the elderly.
9. Discuss the significance of the Minimum Data Set as a tool for comprehensive assessment of the institutionalized elderly.

Health assessment of the elderly can be done on several levels ranging from simple screenings to complex in-depth evaluations. In order to perform assessments accurately, nurses and other health care providers who gather information regarding the elderly must possess the necessary knowledge and skill to perform the assessments correctly. They must know how to use diagnostic tools and equipment safely. Furthermore, they must be knowledgeable and sensitive to the unique needs and characteristics of the elderly.

HEALTH SCREENING

Health screenings are done to identify elderly individuals who are in need of further, more in-depth assessment. Screening for high blood pressure, hearing problems, foot problems, and problems with activities of daily living are commonly performed at senior citizen centers and health clinics. Screening services are often provided by medical and nursing schools or by other health groups committed to helping needy elderly persons. Many screenings are performed by lay individuals working under the direction of professionals. Special screenings for depression and suicide risk, although less common, are recommended for the elderly population.

Screenings are not designed to provide treatment; rather they are intended to identify elderly individuals with significant findings and refer them to the most appropriate health service provider (i.e., physician, social worker, dietitian, or nurse). Early screening and appropriate referral help ensure that elderly individuals who are most in need of care are seen in a timely manner. They also help to reduce frustration in the elderly and wasteful use of time and resources. Depending on what is being evaluated, health screenings may be conducted in person, by telephone, by telecomputer, or, less commonly, via mail surveys.

HEALTH ASSESSMENTS

In-depth health assessments are time consuming and must be performed by skilled professionals. Nurses perform health assessments of the elderly in the community, in clinics, and in institutional settings.

Health assessment includes collection of all the important health related data using a variety of techniques. **Data** are all of the information a nurse gathers about a person. This information will be used to formulate nursing diagnoses and plan patient care; there-

fore, it is essential that accurate and complete data be collected. Data can be either objective or subjective.

Objective data include information that can be gathered using the senses of vision, hearing, touch, and smell. Objective information is collected by means of direct observation, physical examination, and laboratory or diagnostic tests. Because objective data are concrete by nature, all trained observers should report very similar findings about a person or that person's behavior at any given point in time. Behaviors such as crying, limping, and clutching the abdomen can be verified by anyone who observes the patient. Rashes, skin lesions, and wound drainage are likewise observable to anyone. Objective data can be made more precise and specific by using meters, monitors, and other measuring devices. A blood pressure reading, a change in weight, the size of a wound, the volume of urine, and laboratory test results are all examples of specific objective data. Whenever possible, objective data should be stated using specific information because accurate and precise data enhance the nurse's ability to determine changes in a person's health status. For example, it is better to actually take a temperature reading than to touch the skin and determine that it feels warm. Both are objective observations, but one is more *precise* than the other.

Subjective data are information gathered from the elderly person's point of view. Fear, anxiety, frustration, and pain are examples of subjective information. Subjective data are best described in the individual's own words, such as "I'm so afraid of what is going to happen to me here" or "It hurts so much I could die!"

HEALTH ASSESSMENT AND THE ELDERLY

When performing a health assessment on an elderly person, nurses need to modify their usual approaches and techniques in order to make them more appropriate for older adults.

INTERVIEWING THE ELDERLY

Interviews such as those conducted during admission to a clinic or institution are likely to be planned and conducted in a formal manner. Other interviews may be spontaneous, informal, and based on an immediate need recognized by the nurse. Before beginning an interview with an elderly person, the nurse should plan ways to establish and maintain a climate that promotes comfort and develops trust. This includes preparing the physical setting, establishing rapport, and structuring the flow of the interview. During this planning phase, the nurse should take into consideration the unique needs of the elderly person.

Preparing the Physical Setting

The environment where the interview will take place should be chosen carefully. Distractions should be minimal; noise from televisions, radios, and public address systems should not be loud enough to distract the older adult or interfere with his or her ability to distinguish words and understand questions. Lighting should be diffuse because bright lights or glare may make it difficult for the interviewee to see clearly. Furniture should be comfortable. Privacy is very important. Conducting the interview in a room where there is little chance of interruption is ideal. If such a place is not available, the patient's room may provide sufficient privacy—draw the curtains and close the door. The room should be comfortably warm and should be free from drafts that might cause discomfort. Because many older adults experience urinary frequency or urgency, it is advisable either to assist them to the bathroom or to tell them that a bathroom is available nearby should they require it.

Establishing Rapport

It is most appropriate to begin the interview by greeting the elderly person and introducing yourself. During this first contact it is most appropriate to address the person using his or her formal name (e.g., "Mr. Smith" or "Mrs. Adams"). Appropriate use of names indicates respect and helps build rapport. Use of the individual's first name only without his or her consent is presumptuous and overly familiar. This familiarity may be resented by the elderly person whether or not it is verbalized. When there is any doubt as to the person's preference it is appropriate for the nurse to ask the person how he or she wishes to be addressed.

Briefly explain the purpose of the interview so that the individual will know what to expect. An explanation will help reduce anxiety that otherwise might interfere with understanding. Explain how long you expect the interview to last, and what will happen after it is completed.

Focus on and speak directly to the elderly person being interviewed (Fig. 8-1). This notion may seem obvious, but it is often disregarded in practice. Many times a younger family member present during the interview "takes over" the responses for the elderly person. The conversation then takes place between the

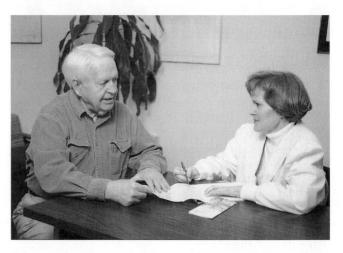

FIG. 8-1   Conducting an interview. (From Thompson JM, Wilson SF: *Health assessment for nursing practice*, St Louis, 1996, Mosby.)

nurse and the family member while the elder remains passive. An assertive elderly person might speak up and say "let me speak for myself," whereas a nonassertive elder may be left feeling frustrated and unimportant. The nurse should continue to direct the conversation to the elderly person and, if necessary, tactfully request that the family member allow the elder to respond first before he or she adds information. In situations in which the elderly person is confused, nonresponsive, or does not speak English the family member will, of necessity, need to be more actively included to translate or provide information.

Rapport is enhanced by determining and then focusing first on the problems or concerns that trouble the patient most. This helps reduce anxiety and increases the elderly person's perception that the nurse is truly concerned about him or her. Assessment should start with a look at the "whole person" before focusing on specifics.

Structuring the Interview

It is important to plan sufficient time for the interview. Elderly individuals typically have a long and complex life story to tell. Remember that the speed of recall and verbal responses may be slower with age. The individual may feel pressured or stressed if the pace of the interview is too rapid.

Try not to accomplish too much during a single interview. The effort involved in communication can be fatiguing to an elderly individual, particularly one with health problems. It is better to have several brief interactions lasting less than 30 minutes rather than one long one that leaves the patient exhausted. Be sure to stay alert for signs of fatigue (e.g., sagging head or shoulders, sighing, altered facial expression, irritability), which indicate the need to end the interview.

During the interview, use a variety of communication techniques to ensure that the patient accurately understands the information. Avoid using medical jargon, and use only words that the elderly person understands. Speak slowly and clearly and keep messages simple, but do not patronize the elderly. The fact that an elderly person requires extra time does not mean that he or she is in any way mentally impaired. Even if the elderly person has been diagnosed with a mental impairment, he or she deserves respectful and professional responses. Remain calm and empathetic. When the patient is speaking, do not interrupt. Listen to both the verbal and nonverbal messages being sent. Many elderly individuals tend to ramble in conversation and may need to be brought back on track. If this is necessary, a summary or restatement of the conversation is helpful. It is not appropriate to complete sentences for the elderly person. The nurse should remain attentive and patient and should allow the patient to complete his or her own sentences. Too often, the nurse's ending is considerably different from the patient's.

Try not to end an interview too abruptly. A statement such as "We're almost done for now" prepares the elderly person for the end of the interaction. Many lonely persons will try to extend the conversation beyond the time the nurse has available. Setting a time for further interaction by saying, "We'll talk again tomorrow morning" or "I'll set up another appointment so we can talk more" can help maintain rapport. It is essential that the nurse follow through as promised or the patient may lose trust and refuse to communicate freely in the future.

PHYSICAL ASSESSMENT OF THE ELDERLY

In the physical assessment, objective information is obtained that accompanies the subjective information offered by the elderly person. Objective information will further help the nurse determine the person's abilities and limitations. It may verify the subjective information given by the elderly person, and it may also reveal problems that were previously unrecognized. When assessing elderly persons, it is important that nurses pay close attention not only to obvious physiologic changes but also to changes in mood or behavior that may signal a change in condition. Seemingly small pieces of information can be important to the total assessment. Older adults have different physiologic responses than do younger persons. For example, a temperature change of just a few tenths of a

degree may indicate the onset of an infection in an elderly person. His or her temperature may not rise above the 100° F reading that is expected in younger people. Other changes can be equally meaningful and will be missed or ignored if nurses are not very careful.

Physical assessment should take place in a location that promotes physical comfort of the elderly person. Often this will be the person's room or a special examination room. Adequate privacy should be maintained by keeping doors and curtains closed. Care should be taken not to chill the elderly person while examining the body. Blankets and gowns that provide adequate warmth should be used to promptly cover the parts of the body not being assessed. If the examination is being done during physical care (e.g., during the bath), particular attention must be paid to prevent chilling due to evaporation.

Equipment such as a flashlight, measuring tape, scale, sphygmomanometer, stethoscope, and thermometer should be collected before beginning the assessment in order to convey a sense of competence and to allow the assessment to progress smoothly.

Complete physical assessment should be done in an orderly manner so that no important observations are missed. The most common method of physical assessment is a head-to-toe approach in which the entire body is assessed systematically. Other approaches such as body system or functional approaches are also viable. Later chapters provide guidelines for assessing safety needs, nutrition, skin, elimination, activity, sleep, cognitive function, and other areas in more detail.

When performing a physical assessment, nurses use a variety of techniques, including inspection, palpation, auscultation, and percussion.

Inspection

Inspection is the most commonly used method of physical assessment in which the senses of vision, smell, and hearing are used to collect data. Skill at inspection improves the more often inspection is done. Inspection requires that the nurse be totally active, alert, and aware of everything he or she sees, hears, or smells. Inspection begins the first time we see the older adult. Even during a brief interaction, skilled nurses should be inspecting the individual, looking for anything that may indicate a change in his or her condition.

Inspection can be both general and specific. General inspection is used to detect the need for more specific inspection. For example, if the nurse observes that the elderly individual is eating poorly, more specific inspection of the oral cavity may be indicated. If body odor is detected, more specific inspection of the skin may be indicated. If the nurse hears noisy breathing, more specific inspection of the lungs may be necessary. If gait is abnormal, more complete assessment of the joints, muscles, feet, and nervous system is indicated.

Inspection is used when assessing the overall level of function as well as when looking for specific areas of need within any particular area of function. When inspecting the aging individual, it is important that the nurse pay close attention to details. Adequate light (preferably natural light) should be used when trying to detect subtle changes in skin color. Size and mobility of body parts on one side of the body should be compared with that on the opposite side.

Palpation

Palpation employs the sense of touch in the fingers and hands to obtain data. Palpation is used for evaluation in many parts of a physical assessment, including pulses, temperature and texture of the skin, texture and condition of the hair, the presence and consistency of tumors or masses under the skin, distention of the urinary bladder, and the presence of pain or tenderness.

When palpating, the nurse should use the fingertips, which are the most sensitive part of the fingers. Warm hands and short fingernails promote comfort and reduce the risk of trauma to fragile elderly skin. Light touch should be used before deeper touch is attempted. When taking the pulse of an elderly person, deep palpation may occlude blood vessels. Deep pressure may also increase pain. Painful areas should be palpated last.

Auscultation

Auscultation uses the sense of hearing to detect sounds produced within the body. Heart, lung, and bowel sounds are typically assessed using auscultation. Auscultation involves the use of a stethoscope or other sound amplifier (such as a Doppler) to make the sounds louder and more easily heard. Sounds are described according to their quality, pitch, intensity, and duration. **Quality** describes the sound being heard using subjective terms such as crackling, whistling, or snapping. **Pitch** describes whether the sounds have a low or high tone. **Intensity** refers to the loudness or softness of the tone. **Duration** refers to the length of time a sound is heard. **Frequency** refers to how often a sound is heard. A sound can be continuous or intermittent. When sounds are intermittent, the number of times and the interval between occurrences should be determined.

Auscultation requires a quiet environment and spe-cial skills. Nurses who perform auscultation should have special training in the technique and should be knowledgeable regarding the significance of any findings.

Percussion

Percussion is a technique in which the size, position, and density of structures under the skin are assessed by tapping the area and listening to the resonance of the sound. Depending on the amount of vibration (sound) heard, the presence of masses, fluid, or air can be determined. This is the technique that is least often used by nurses. It requires special skill and training.

ASSESSING VITAL SIGNS IN THE ELDERLY

Assessment of vital signs involves all of the techniques previously discussed. When assessing vital signs, nurses should first complete a general inspection of the older adult to determine whether there are any subjective or objective observations that may affect the procedure or accuracy of the readings. Because activity level, medications, eating, stress, disease processes, and the environment can all affect vital signs, the possible contributions of these factors should be considered.

Baseline vital sign readings should be obtained during the initial contact with the elderly person. These readings are the basis for comparison with future readings, and they enable nurses to determine whether the person's health status is remaining constant or changing over time.

Temperature

The general inspection will help nurses select the most appropriate route for temperature assessment. The oral (sublingual) route is most commonly used for temperature assessment. Either glass or electronic thermometers can be used to take an oral temperature. Electronic thermometers are preferred because they can give an accurate temperature in less than a minute instead of the recommended 3 minutes for a glass thermometer. However, using the oral route is not always possible with the elderly. Edentulous (without teeth) older adults or those with poor muscle control may be unable to close the mouth tightly enough to obtain an accurate reading. Older adults who are unable to follow directions are also poor candidates for oral temperature checks.

Although acceptable, the rectal route should be used with caution. Use of the rectal route can be psychologically traumatic to the elderly, particularly if they are alert but unable to cooperate with an oral temperature. The rectal route should not be used in elderly persons who have undergone rectal surgery or have rectal bleeding. Rectal readings can be affected by the presence of stool in the rectum. Rectal temperature readings reflect changes in core body temperature more slowly than do oral readings.

Use of the axillary route is not common in the elderly. This route is time consuming, and the accuracy of temperature readings may be affected by environmental conditions.

Determination of body temperature using a sensor that measures the temperature of the tympanic membrane has received mixed reviews. This method has both advantages and disadvantages. Use of the tympanic sensor takes only seconds, is not invasive, and does not require patient cooperation; however, the readings obtained using this method are not as accurate as originally claimed, particularly when the device is not used precisely as directed. Individual agencies need to determine whether this method of assessment is adequate for their needs.

Healthy, active elderly individuals are generally able to maintain core body temperature within normal limits. The accepted norm for oral temperature is 98.6° F ±1° F or 37° C ±0.6° C. Studies have shown that older adults, particularly those over 75, have an average core body temperature of 97.2° F (36° C). This decrease may be due to inactivity, decreased subcutaneous fat, an inadequate diet, or environmental factors. Environmental temperature appears to play a greater role in the elderly because their thermoregulatory control systems are not as efficient as in younger individuals.

Pulse

Before assessing the pulse, the patient should be positioned so that he or she is comfortable and the nurse has access to the desired site. Position should be consistent (e.g., lying, sitting, or standing) each time the pulse is checked to provide meaningful readings for comparison.

Pulse can be assessed at various sites on the body, including the temporal, carotid, brachial, radial, femoral, popliteal, posterior tibial, and dorsalis pedis arteries as well as the apex of the heart (Fig. 8-2). Whenever possible the pulses on both sides of the body should be assessed and compared.

The radial artery is the site most commonly used for routine pulse assessment. The radial pulse is normally palpable at the medial aspect of the wrist. This pulse should be palpated gently in the elderly because excessive pressure may occlude the blood vessel. The pulse rate should be counted, and the rate, rhythm, and volume should be noted. Consistency of the blood

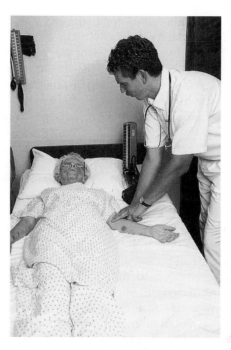

FIG. 8-2 Assessing vital signs. (From Elkin MK, Perry AG, Potter PA: *Nursing interventions and clinical skills*, St Louis, 1996, Mosby.)

vessel should also be assessed. The normal pulse rate in adults ranges from 60 to 90 beats per minute. Rates outside this range or significant changes from an individual's normal readings indicate the need for further assessment. Elderly persons, particularly those with a history of cardiovascular problems and those receiving digitalis, require prompt, thorough assessment if there is a significant change in the pulse rate.

The arteries of the elderly may feel stiff and knotty because of decreased elasticity. In aging individuals, it is common to observe irregularities in rhythm. These may be related to medical conditions, or they may have no identified cause. Detection of irregular pulse in an aging person whose pulse was previously regular is significant and requires further assessment. A change in pulse volume may indicate the need to assess fluid balance. Weak, thready pulses are often seen in individuals with fluid volume deficits or electrolyte imbalances; full or bounding pulses may indicate excessive fluid volume. Weakness of a radial pulse may make palpation impossible and necessitate use of the apical route.

When assessing the apical pulse, nurses should help their aging patients assume a comfortable position and should drape them to prevent chilling and to provide for modesty. The apical site is located on the left side of the chest. The apical heartbeat is best heard by placing the stethoscope over the fifth intercostal space even with the middle of the clavicle. The apical pulse should be counted for a full minute. Each *lub-dub* sound heard is counted as one heartbeat. The apical pulse should be assessed for regularity and the presence of any unusual sounds.

When assessing elderly women with sagging breasts, nurses should lift the tissue gently and place the stethoscope at the lower edge of the breast. Apical pulse may be difficult to assess in obese older adults or in those who have a change in the shape of the chest cavity.

Apical and radial readings, even when taken at the same time by two nurses, may be different. This is referred to as a **pulse deficit.** Inadequate force of the heart or disease of the blood vessels may prevent transmission from the heart to the peripheral vessels. Of the two, the apical pulse rate is considered more reliable.

The peripheral pulses of legs and feet should be palpated and assessed to determine whether they are present and to determine the quality of the pulse. Peripheral pulse rate is not normally counted. Altered peripheral circulation may be an early indicator of decreased cardiac functioning or vascular changes. Pulses on one side of the body should be compared with those on the other side to determine whether changes have affected one or both sides of the body.

Cardiovascular changes with aging, particularly arteriosclerotic changes, often result in a decrease or complete loss of palpable pulses in the lower extremities. Start with the pedal pulses. If these are not detectable, proceed upward toward the trunk and assess the popliteal and then the femoral pulses. If pulses cannot be palpated, it may be necessary to use a sound amplifier called a Doppler to evaluate circulation to the extremities.

If peripheral pulses are diminished or absent, the nurse should suspect circulatory impairment and assess the extremity for capillary refill time, temperature, color changes, and the absence of hair, all of which may indicate serious problems.

Respiration

After completing a general assessment of all of the factors that influence respiration, the aging person should be placed in a comfortable position to maximize ease of breathing. The rate, depth, and ease of breathing must be assessed. Each combination of inspiration and expiration is counted as one respiration. The normal respiratory rate for elderly individuals is similar to that of younger adults. A range of 12 to 20 breaths per minute is considered normal. A decrease in the resting respiratory rate is significant in the elderly person. It may be an indication of impending infection and may appear before an elevation in temperature is observed. Increased respiratory rate is common with anxiety, pain, elevated temperatures, and increased activity.

The depth of respiration tends to decrease with aging. Chest expansion is often decreased because of alterations in the shape of the thoracic cavity, muscle weakness, sedentary lifestyle, or disease processes.

Slightly irregular breathing rhythms are not unusual in the aging population. However, a highly irregular rhythm, dyspnea, or breathlessness with exertion are not normal and require further assessment to determine the cause.

Blood Pressure

Blood pressure readings are an important part of the physical assessment. It is essential that these readings be properly obtained. To obtain the most accurate readings, the person should be positioned so that the upper arm is at the level of the heart.

Equipment should be carefully chosen if meaningful results are to be obtained. Cuff selection should be based on the patient's upper arm size. It is a common mistake to use a one-size-fits-all blood pressure cuff. Many elderly persons, particularly those who are frail, have lost a great deal of upper arm mass. A cuff that is too wide for the size of the individual's arm will result in falsely low readings. A properly sized cuff is 20% wider than the diameter at the midpoint of the arm. Once the proper cuff has been obtained, it should be applied gently but snugly to the arm. Nurses should pay close attention not to pinch the skin in the cuff, which can easily lead to bruising.

The technique used when obtaining the measurement should follow the methods approved by the American Heart Association. This includes taking the blood pressure first by palpation, then by auscultation. The practice of pumping the cuff to excessively high pressures can result in inaccurate readings.

Blood pressure readings vary widely among the elderly. Some elderly have blood pressure readings in the low–normal range; others have significantly elevated readings. Hypertension is a common problem in the elderly population because of renal and cardiovascular changes of aging. Blood pressure elevations can also be caused by emotional upset, pain, exertion, eating, or smoking. This type of elevation disappears when the precipitating event is removed. To obtain accurate readings, nurses should attempt to reduce or minimize these factors before assessing blood pressure. Persistent elevations in blood pressure (i.e., systolic readings 160 mm Hg or higher; diastolic readings 90 mm Hg or higher; or elevations of both systolic and diastolic readings) indicate hypertension. Elevated blood pressure readings should be reported promptly, particularly if they are unusual for an individual.

Many aging individuals take medication for hypertension. Nurses should follow through with careful blood pressure monitoring when these medications are administered, and all precautions related to the specific medication should be followed rigorously.

Aging individuals are susceptible to posture-related changes in blood pressure. Older adults who have an inactive lifestyle and those who take drugs such as vasodilators, antihypertensives, or tricyclic antidepressants are particularly prone to orthostatic, or postural, hypotension. **Orthostatic hypotension** is a sudden drop in blood pressure that occurs when a person changes from a lying to a sitting or standing position. It may also occur when the person moves from sitting to standing. Those experiencing postural hypotension complain of lightheadedness or dizziness when changing positions. In severe cases, the person may even lose consciousness. Orthostatic hypotension is commonly observed in individuals who are on extended bedrest or are receiving medication for hypertension.

To determine the existence and severity of postural hypotension, it is necessary to obtain several blood pressure readings in succession. Performing this assessment requires the nurse to be somewhat skillful. The nurse should first take the blood pressure when the patient is at rest in bed. Then the person should sit at the edge of the bed, and the nurse should take the blood pressure again in 1 to 5 minutes. The patient should then stand for 1 to 5 minutes, and the nurse should take a third reading. All readings should be recorded along with any subjective information provided by the patient regarding dizziness, loss of balance, or other sensations. A drop of more than 20 mm Hg is always significant and should be reported promptly. A standing systolic blood pressure that is less than 100 mm Hg should also be reported. If the individual complains of symptoms such as dizziness, safety precautions should be taken.

SENSORY ASSESSMENT OF THE ELDERLY

Simple assessments of vision and hearing ability are based on empiric data (the way the individual responds to visual or auditory clues). Nurses should observe whether the person is able to read or do close work that requires good central vision or whether he or she participates in television viewing or other sight-related activities. If the elderly person uses eyeglasses, the ability to see with and without them should be assessed.

Talking with the elderly can reveal the presence or absence of hearing. Difficulty gaining attention, the frequent need to repeat information, or mistakes in understanding directions are good indicators of hearing problems. If applicable, hearing aid assessment should take place when the elderly person is wearing the aid, but only after it has been checked for proper functioning. Special assessment by a vision or audiometric specialist can reveal more precise information regarding vision and hearing.

PSYCHOSOCIAL ASSESSMENT OF THE ELDERLY

Psychologic assessment is performed to determine whether elderly people are alert and aware of their surroundings or suffer from some level of confusion, delirium, or dementia. More about the differences between these conditions is discussed in Chapter 15. Psychologic status is best assessed by direct observation and by means of standardized assessment tools. Many assessment tools are available to assist nurses in assessing mental status in the elderly. Probably the best known and most highly regarded is the Mini-Mental State Examination (MMSE), a sample of which is provided in Figure 8-3. Performing this assessment requires little time and only a pencil and blank sheet of paper. Scoring of this tool is simple and self-explanatory. Other assessment tools may also be used. Several of these are available in computerized form on the Internet (Box 8-1).

Assessment of social function is determined by observing the amount, frequency, and type of social interaction in which the elderly person participates. A wide variety of levels and degrees of social interaction can be classified as normal as long as the individual is happy or at least content with that level. Chapters 16, 17, and 18 deal more with socialization issues.

Special Assessments/The Minimum Data Set 2.0

In an attempt to improve the quality of care provided in extended-care facilities, the federal government instituted major reforms through the Omnibus Budget Reconciliation Act (OBRA) of 1987. An important focus of this law was the improvement and standardization of assessment procedures used in these facilities. The first reform produced by the U.S. Department of Health and Human Services was the Resident Assessment Instrument (RAI), introduced in 1990. This tool specified a comprehensive, standardized assessment that was to be completed on admission, with significant change in status, and thereafter on a yearly basis. The first version of the database used to conduct this assessment was a printed document called the **Minimum Data Set (MDS) 1.0**. This tool was designed not only to help assess residents but also to help caregivers identify problems, develop intervention plans, and monitor outcomes. It was hoped that use of this tool

Mini-Mental State Examination

Give one point for each correct response.		Score	Points
Orientation			
1. What is the	Year	____	1
	Season	____	1
	Date	____	1
	Day	____	1
	Month	____	1
2. Where are we?	State	____	1
	County	____	1
	Town or city	____	1
	Hospital/nursing home/other building	____	1
	Floor	____	1
Registration			
3. Name three objects, taking one second to say each. Then ask the patient to repeat all three. (Give one point for each correct answer. Repeat the answers until patient learns all three.)		____	3
Attention and calculation			
4. Serial sevens: Ask the patient to count backwards from 100 by sevens, as 93, 86, 79, etc. (Stop after five answers; give one point for each correct answer.) Alternative: Spell WORLD backwards.		____	5
Recall			
5. Ask for names of the three objects learned in question 3. (Give one point for each correct answer.)		____	3
Language			
6. Point to a pencil and a watch. Ask the patient to name each as you point.		____	2
7. Ask the patient to repeat "No ifs, ands, or buts."		____	1
8. Ask the patient to follow a three-stage command: "Take a paper in your right hand. Fold the paper in half. Put the paper on the floor."		____	3
9. Ask the patient to read and obey the following command: "CLOSE YOUR EYES." (Write in large letters.)		____	1
10. Ask the patient to write a sentence of his or her choice. (The sentence should contain a subject and an object and should make sense. Ignore spelling errors when scoring.)		____	1
11. Ask the patient to copy the design shown. (Give one point if all sides and angles are preserved and if the intersecting sides form a quadrangle.)	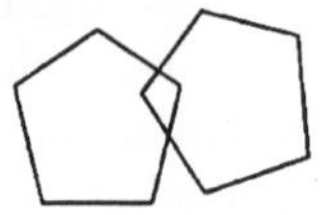	____	1
		____	30
		(Total)	(Total)

FIG. 8-3 Mini-Mental State Examination. (Adapted with permission from Folstein MF, Folstein SE, McHugh PR: *J Psychiatr Res* 12:189, 1975. Copyright 1975, Pergamon Press, Inc.)

BOX 8-1

Examples of Psychologic Assessment
Tools on the Internet

- Cornell Scale for Depression in Dementia
- Short Test for Dementia
- Functional Activities Questionnaire
- Clinical Dementia Rating Scale
- Informant Questionnaire on Cognitive Decline in
  the Elderly (IQCODE)
- Confusion Assessment Method

BOX 8-2

Core Data Set—Topics Assessed in
All Residents

- Cognitive patterns
- Vision patterns
- Physical functioning and structural problems
- Continence
- Psychosocial well-being
- Mood and behavior patterns
- Activity pursuit patterns
- Disease diagnoses
- Health conditions
- Oral nutritional status
- Oral/dental status
- Skin condition
- Medication use
- Special treatments and procedures

BOX 8-3

Resident Assessment Protocol Topics

- Delirium
- Cognitive loss/dementia
- Visual function
- Communication
- Activities of daily living function/rehabilitation
  potential
- Urinary incontinence/indwelling catheterization
- Psychosocial well-being
- Mood
- Behavior
- Activities
- Falls
- Nutrition
- Feeding tubes
- Dehydration/fluid maintenance
- Dental care
- Pressure ulcers
- Psychotropic drug use
- Physical restraints

---

would make the assessment process more consistent and reliable throughout the country. MDS 1.0 did help improve assessment and care in many cases, but information was often difficult to locate and interdepartmental monitoring of problems and outcomes was difficult because the assessment was paper based. A newer form called the **MDS 2.0** is an upgraded, computerized version of the older document (Fig. 8-4). By the end of 1997, all health care agencies that receive federal funding were mandated to use the computerized MDS and must be capable of transmitting the results to state and federal agencies.

The MDS 2.0 is a comprehensive assessment tool that assesses core areas of function (Box 8-2). Any unusual findings discovered with MDS 2.0 will initiate further evaluation using more detailed focus assessments such as Resident Assessment Protocols (RAPs). RAPs provide guidelines for more in-depth assessment of conditions that affect the functional well-being of residents of extended-care facilities (Fig. 8-5). The most common areas assessed using RAPs are identified in Box 8-3. Information revealed by more detailed RAP assessment can then be used to develop a specific plan of care for the resident.

Use of a computer-based system improves the process of assessment and planning. Use of a computer database helps to make the process more comprehensive, more complete, and (once the users become familiar with the program) easier for the nursing staff and other departments. Computerization of records in this database will enhance the flow of information between departments within a facility. For example, the pharmacy can verify that psychotropic and antidepressant medications are only administered when appropriate medical diagnoses exist, and the physicians and nurses can correlate dosage changes with observed behaviors. The dietary department can validate that appropriate diets are ordered based on medical diagnosis and can detect changes in weight that may indicate the need for further intervention. Nurses can

identify interventions that will be most beneficial at preventing pressure ulcers, constipation, or other common problems.

The computerized MDS 2.0 enhances the ability to access and correlate data from every long-term care facility in the United States and will provide an unprecedented database of information regarding the nursing home population. As the database grows,

Text continued on p. 141

Numeric Identifier_____

MINIMUM DATA SET (MDS) — *VERSION 2.0*
FOR NURSING HOME RESIDENT ASSESSMENT AND CARE SCREENING

BASIC ASSESSMENT TRACKING FORM

SECTION AA. IDENTIFICATION INFORMATION

1.	RESIDENT NAME©				
		a. (First)	b. (Middle Initial)	c. (Last)	d. (Jr/Sr)
2.	GENDER©	1. Male	2. Female		
3.	BIRTHDATE©	☐☐ — ☐☐ — ☐☐☐☐ Month Day Year			
4.	RACE/© ETHNICITY	1. American Indian/Alaskan Native 2. Asian/Pacific Islander 3. Black, not of Hispanic origin	4. Hispanic 5. White, not of Hispanic origin		
5.	SOCIAL SECURITY© AND MEDICARE NUMBERS© [C in 1st box if non med. no.]	a. Social Security Number ☐☐☐ — ☐☐ — ☐☐☐☐ b. Medicare number (or comparable railroad insurance number)			
6.	FACILITY PROVIDER NO.©	a. State No. b. Federal No.			
7.	MEDICAID NO. ["+" if pending, "N" if not a Medicaid recipient] ©				
8.	REASONS FOR ASSESS-MENT	[Note—Other codes do not apply to this form] a. Primary reason for assessment 1. Admission assessment (required by day 14) 2. Annual assessment 3. Significant change in status assessment 4. Significant correction of prior full assessment 5. Quarterly review assessment 10. Significant correction of prior quarterly assessment 0. *NONE OF ABOVE* b. *Codes for assessments required for Medicare PPS or the State* 1. Medicare 5 day assessment 2. Medicare 30 day assessment 3. Medicare 60 day assessment 4. Medicare 90 day assessment 5. Medicare readmission/return assessment 6. Other state required assessment 7. Medicare 14 day assessment 8. Other Medicare required assessment			
9.	SIGNATURES OF PERSONS COMPLETING THESE ITEMS:				
a.	Signatures	Title			Date
b.					Date

GENERAL INSTRUCTIONS

Complete this information for submission with all full and quarterly assessments (Admission, Annual, Significant Change, State or Medicare required assessments, or Quarterly Reviews, etc.)

© = Key items for computerized resident tracking

☐ = When box blank, must enter number or letter   a.☐ = When letter in box, check if condition applies

MDS 2.0 01/30/98

Fig. 8-4   Minimum Data Set (MDS)—Version 2.0. (Courtesy of the United States Department of Health and Human Services.)

Resident_____   Numeric Identifier_____

MINIMUM DATA SET (MDS) — *VERSION 2.0*
FOR NURSING HOME RESIDENT ASSESSMENT AND CARE SCREENING
BACKGROUND (FACE SHEET) INFORMATION AT ADMISSION

SECTION AB. DEMOGRAPHIC INFORMATION

1.	DATE OF ENTRY	*Date the stay began. Note — Does not include readmission if record was closed at time of temporary discharge to hospital, etc. In such cases, use prior admission date*

□□ — □□ — □□□□
Month — Day — Year

2.	ADMITTED FROM (AT ENTRY)	1. Private home/apt. with no home health services 2. Private home/apt. with home health services 3. Board and care/assisted living/group home 4. Nursing home 5. Acute care hospital 6. Psychiatric hospital, MR/DD facility 7. Rehabilitation hospital 8. Other	■
3.	LIVED ALONE (PRIOR TO ENTRY)	0. No 1. Yes 2. In other facility	■
4.	ZIP CODE OF PRIOR PRIMARY RESIDENCE	□□□□□	
5.	RESIDENTIAL HISTORY 5 YEARS PRIOR TO ENTRY	(*Check all settings* resident *lived in* during 5 years prior to date of entry given in item AB1 above)	
		Prior stay at this nursing home	a.
		Stay in other nursing home	b.
		Other residential facility—board and care home, assisted living, group home	c.
		MH/psychiatric setting	d.
		MR/DD setting	e.
		NONE OF ABOVE	f.
6.	LIFETIME OCCUPA-TION(S) [Put "/" between two occupations]	□□□□□□□□□□□□□□□□	
7.	EDUCATION (*Highest Level Completed*)	1. No schooling 5. Technical or trade school 2. 8th grade/less 6. Some college 3. 9-11 grades 7. Bachelor's degree 4. High school 8. Graduate degree	■
8.	LANGUAGE	(*Code for correct response*) **a. Primary Language** 0. English 1. Spanish 2. French 3. Other	■
		b. If other, specify □□□□□□	■
9.	MENTAL HEALTH HISTORY	Does resident's RECORD indicate any history of mental retardation, mental illness, or developmental disability problem? 0. No 1.Yes	■
10.	CONDITIONS RELATED TO MR/DD STATUS	(*Check all conditions* that are related to MR/DD status that were manifested before age 22, and are likely to continue indefinitely)	
		Not applicable—no MR/DD (Skip to AB11)	a. ■
		MR/DD with organic condition	
		Down's syndrome	b.
		Autism	c.
		Epilepsy	d.
		Other organic condition related to MR/DD	e.
		MR/DD with no organic condition	f.
11.	DATE BACK-GROUND INFORMA-TION COMPLETED	□□ — □□ — □□□□ Month — Day — Year	

SECTION AC. CUSTOMARY ROUTINE

1.	CUSTOMARY ROUTINE	(*Check all that apply.* If all information UNKNOWN, check last box only.)
	(*In year prior to DATE OF ENTRY to this nursing home, or year last in community if now being admitted from another nursing home*)	**CYCLE OF DAILY EVENTS**

Stays up late at night (e.g., after 9 pm)	a.
Naps regularly during day (at least 1 hour)	b.
Goes out 1+ days a week	c.
Stays busy with hobbies, reading, or fixed daily routine	d.
Spends most of time alone or watching TV	e.
Moves independently indoors (with appliances, if used)	f.
Use of tobacco products at least daily	g.
NONE OF ABOVE	h.
EATING PATTERNS	
Distinct food preferences	i.
Eats between meals all or most days	j.
Use of alcoholic beverage(s) at least weekly	k.
NONE OF ABOVE	l.
ADL PATTERNS	
In bedclothes much of day	m.
Wakens to toilet all or most nights	n.
Has irregular bowel movement pattern	o.
Showers for bathing	p.
Bathing in PM	q.
NONE OF ABOVE	r.
INVOLVEMENT PATTERNS	
Daily contact with relatives/close friends	s.
Usually attends church, temple, synagogue (etc.)	t.
Finds strength in faith	u.
Daily animal companion/presence	v.
Involved in group activities	w.
NONE OF ABOVE	x.
UNKNOWN—Resident/family unable to provide information	y.

SECTION AD. FACE SHEET SIGNATURES

SIGNATURES OF PERSONS COMPLETING FACE SHEET:

a. Signature of RN Assessment Coordinator				Date
b. Signatures		Title	Sections	Date
c.				Date
d.				Date
e.				Date
f.				Date
g.				Date

□ = When box blank, must enter number or letter |a.| = When letter in box, check if condition applies

MDS 2.0 01/30/98

FIG. 8-4, cont'd   For legend see opposite page.   *Continued*

Resident_____   Numeric Identifier_____

MINIMUM DATA SET (MDS) — *VERSION 2.0*
FOR NURSING HOME RESIDENT ASSESSMENT AND CARE SCREENING
FULL ASSESSMENT FORM
(Status in last 7 days, unless other time frame indicated)

SECTION A. IDENTIFICATION AND BACKGROUND INFORMATION

1.	RESIDENT NAME	
		a. (First) b. (Middle Initial) c. (Last) d. (Jr/Sr)
2.	ROOM NUMBER	
3.	ASSESS-MENT REFERENCE DATE	a. *Last day of MDS observation period* — Month / Day / Year
		b. Original (0) or corrected copy of form (enter number of correction)
4a.	DATE OF REENTRY	Date of reentry from most recent temporary discharge to a hospital in last 90 days (or since last assessment or admission if less than 90 days) — Month / Day / Year
5.	MARITAL STATUS	1. Never married 3. Widowed 5. Divorced 2. Married 4. Separated
6.	MEDICAL RECORD NO.	

7. CURRENT PAYMENT SOURCES FOR N.H. STAY — *(Billing Office to indicate; check all that apply in last 30 days)*

Medicaid per diem	a.	VA per diem		f.
Medicare per diem	b.	Self or family pays for full per diem		g.
Medicare ancillary part A	c.	Medicaid resident liability or Medicare co-payment		h.
Medicare ancillary part B	d.	Private insurance per diem (including co-payment)		i.
CHAMPUS per diem	e.	Other per diem		j.

8. REASONS FOR ASSESS-MENT

[Note—If this is a discharge or reentry assessment, only a limited subset of MDS items need be completed]

a. Primary reason for assessment
1. Admission assessment (required by day 14)
2. Annual assessment
3. Significant change in status assessment
4. Significant correction of prior full assessment
5. Quarterly review assessment
6. Discharged—return not anticipated
7. Discharged—return anticipated
8. Discharged prior to completing initial assessment
9. Reentry
10. Significant correction of prior quarterly assessment
0. *NONE OF ABOVE*

b. *Codes for assessments required for Medicare PPS or the State*
1. *Medicare 5 day assessment*
2. *Medicare 30 day assessment*
3. *Medicare 60 day assessment*
4. *Medicare 90 day assessment*
5. *Medicare readmission/return assessment*
6. *Other state required assessment*
7. *Medicare 14 day assessment*
8. *Other Medicare required assessment*

9. RESPONSI-BILITY/ LEGAL GUARDIAN — *(Check all that apply)*

Legal guardian	a.	Durable power attorney/financial	d.
Other legal oversight	b.	Family member responsible	e.
Durable power of attorney/health care	c.	Patient responsible for self	f.
		NONE OF ABOVE	g.

10. ADVANCED DIRECTIVES — *(For those items with supporting documentation in the medical record, check all that apply)*

Living will	a.	Feeding restrictions	f.
Do not resuscitate	b.	Medication restrictions	g.
Do not hospitalize	c.	Other treatment restrictions	h.
Organ donation	d.	*NONE OF ABOVE*	i.
Autopsy request	e.		

SECTION B. COGNITIVE PATTERNS

1.	COMATOSE	*(Persistent vegetative state/no discernible consciousness)* 0. No 1. Yes **(If yes, skip to Section G)**

2.	MEMORY	*(Recall of what was learned or known)*
		 a. Short-term memory OK—seems/appears to recall after 5 minutes
		    0. Memory OK 1. Memory problem
		 b. Long-term memory OK—seems/appears to recall long past
		    0. Memory OK 1. Memory problem

3.	MEMORY/ RECALL ABILITY	*(Check all that resident was **normally able to recall during** last 7 days)*
		Current season — a. Location of own room — b. That he/she is in a nursing home — d. Staff names/faces — c. *NONE OF ABOVE* are recalled — e.

4.	COGNITIVE SKILLS FOR DAILY DECISION-MAKING	*(Made decisions regarding tasks of daily life)* 0. *INDEPENDENT*—decisions consistent/reasonable 1. *MODIFIED INDEPENDENCE*—some difficulty in new situations only 2. *MODERATELY IMPAIRED*—decisions poor; cues/supervision required 3. *SEVERELY IMPAIRED*—never/rarely made decisions

5.	INDICATORS OF DELIRIUM— PERIODIC DISOR-DERED THINKING/ AWARENESS	*(Code for behavior in the last 7 days.)* **[Note: Accurate assessment requires conversations with staff and family who have direct knowledge of resident's behavior over this time].** 0. Behavior not present 1. Behavior present, not of recent onset 2. Behavior present, over last 7 days appears different from resident's usual functioning (e.g., new onset or worsening)

a. EASILY DISTRACTED—(e.g., difficulty paying attention; gets sidetracked)

b. PERIODS OF ALTERED PERCEPTION OR AWARENESS OF SURROUNDINGS—(e.g., moves lips or talks to someone not present; believes he/she is somewhere else; confuses night and day)

c. EPISODES OF DISORGANIZED SPEECH—(e.g., speech is incoherent, nonsensical, irrelevant, or rambling from subject to subject; loses train of thought)

d. PERIODS OF RESTLESSNESS—(e.g., fidgeting or picking at skin, clothing, napkins, etc; frequent position changes; repetitive physical movements or calling out)

e. PERIODS OF LETHARGY—(e.g., sluggishness; staring into space; difficult to arouse; little body movement)

f. MENTAL FUNCTION VARIES OVER THE COURSE OF THE DAY—(e.g., sometimes better, sometimes worse; behaviors sometimes present, sometimes not)

6.	CHANGE IN COGNITIVE STATUS	Resident's cognitive status, skills, or abilities have changed as compared to status of **90 days ago** (or since last assessment if less than 90 days) 0. No change 1. Improved 2. Deteriorated

SECTION C. COMMUNICATION/HEARING PATTERNS

1.	HEARING	*(With hearing appliance, if used)* 0. *HEARS ADEQUATELY*—normal talk, TV, phone 1. *MINIMAL DIFFICULTY* when not in quiet setting 2. *HEARS IN SPECIAL SITUATIONS ONLY*—speaker has to adjust tonal quality and speak distinctly 3. *HIGHLY IMPAIRED*/absence of useful hearing

2.	COMMUNI-CATION DEVICES/ TECH-NIQUES	*(Check all that apply during last 7 days)*	
		Hearing aid, present and used	a.
		Hearing aid, present and not used regularly	b.
		Other receptive comm. techniques used (e.g., lip reading)	c.
		NONE OF ABOVE	d.

3.	MODES OF EXPRESSION	*(Check all used by resident to make needs known)*
		Speech — a. Signs/gestures/sounds — d. Writing messages to express or clarify needs — b. Communication board — e. Other — f. American sign language or Braille — c. *NONE OF ABOVE* — g.

4.	MAKING SELF UNDER-STOOD	*(Expressing information content—however able)* 0. *UNDERSTOOD* 1. *USUALLY UNDERSTOOD*—difficulty finding words or finishing thoughts 2. *SOMETIMES UNDERSTOOD*—ability is limited to making concrete requests 3. *RARELY/NEVER UNDERSTOOD*

5.	SPEECH CLARITY	*(Code for speech in the last 7 days)* 0. *CLEAR SPEECH*—distinct, intelligible words 1. *UNCLEAR SPEECH*—slurred, mumbled words 2. *NO SPEECH*—absence of spoken words

6.	ABILITY TO UNDER-STAND OTHERS	*(Understanding verbal information content—however able)* 0. *UNDERSTANDS* 1. *USUALLY UNDERSTANDS*—may miss some part/intent of message 2. *SOMETIMES UNDERSTANDS*—responds adequately to simple, direct communication 3. *RARELY/NEVER UNDERSTANDS*

7.	CHANGE IN COMMUNI-CATION/ HEARING	Resident's ability to express, understand, or hear information has changed as compared to status of **90 days ago** (or since last assessment if less than 90 days) 0. No change 1. Improved 2. Deteriorated

☐ = When box blank, must enter number or letter   [a.☐] = When letter in box, check if condition applies

MDS 2.0 01/30/98

FIG. 8-4, cont'd   For legend see p. 132.

Resident _____   Numeric Identifier _____

SECTION D. VISION PATTERNS

1.	VISION	(Ability to see in adequate light and with glasses if used)
		0. *ADEQUATE*—sees fine detail, including regular print in newspapers/books
		1. *IMPAIRED*—sees large print, but not regular print in newspapers/books
		2. *MODERATELY IMPAIRED*—limited vision; not able to see newspaper headlines, but can identify objects
		3. *HIGHLY IMPAIRED*—object identification in question, but eyes appear to follow objects
		4. *SEVERELY IMPAIRED*—no vision or sees only light, colors, or shapes; eyes do not appear to follow objects

2.	VISUAL LIMITATIONS/ DIFFICULTIES	Side vision problems—decreased peripheral vision (e.g., leaves food on one side of tray, difficulty traveling, bumps into people and objects, misjudges placement of chair when seating self)	a.
		Experiences any of following: sees halos or rings around lights; sees flashes of light; sees "curtains" over eyes	b.
		NONE OF ABOVE	c.

| 3. | VISUAL APPLIANCES | Glasses; contact lenses; magnifying glass |
| | | 0. No   1. Yes |

SECTION E. MOOD AND BEHAVIOR PATTERNS

1.	INDICATORS OF DEPRESSION, ANXIETY, SAD MOOD	(Code for indicators observed in last 30 days, irrespective of the assumed cause)
		0. Indicator not exhibited in last 30 days
		1. Indicator of this type exhibited up to five days a week
		2. Indicator of this type exhibited daily or almost daily (6, 7 days a week)

VERBAL EXPRESSIONS OF DISTRESS

a. Resident made negative statements—e.g., "*Nothing matters; Would rather be dead; What's the use; Regrets having lived so long; Let me die*"

b. Repetitive questions—e.g., "*Where do I go; What do I do?*"

c. Repetitive verbalizations—e.g., calling out for help, ("*God help me*")

d. Persistent anger with self or others—e.g., easily annoyed, anger at placement in nursing home; anger at care received

e. Self deprecation—e.g., "*I am nothing; I am of no use to anyone*"

f. Expressions of what appear to be unrealistic fears—e.g., fear of being abandoned, left alone, being with others

g. Recurrent statements that something terrible is about to happen—e.g., believes he or she is about to die, have a heart attack

h. Repetitive health complaints—e.g., persistently seeks medical attention, obsessive concern with body functions

i. Repetitive anxious complaints/concerns (non-health related) e.g., persistently seeks attention/ reassurance regarding schedules, meals, laundry, clothing, relationship issues

SLEEP-CYCLE ISSUES

j. Unpleasant mood in morning

k. Insomnia/change in usual sleep pattern

SAD, APATHETIC, ANXIOUS APPEARANCE

l. Sad, pained, worried facial expressions—e.g., furrowed brows

m. Crying, tearfulness

n. Repetitive physical movements—e.g., pacing, hand wringing, restlessness, fidgeting, picking

LOSS OF INTEREST

o. Withdrawal from activities of interest—e.g., no interest in long standing activities or being with family/friends

p. Reduced social interaction

2.	MOOD PERSIS-TENCE	One or more indicators of depressed, sad or anxious mood **were not easily altered** by attempts to "cheer up", console, or reassure the resident over last 7 days
		0. No mood 1. Indicators present, 2. Indicators present, indicators easily altered not easily altered

3.	CHANGE IN MOOD	Resident's mood status has changed as compared to status of **90 days ago** (or since last assessment if less than 90 days)
		0. No change 1. Improved 2. Deteriorated

4.	BEHAVIORAL SYMPTOMS	**(A)** *Behavioral* symptom **frequency in last 7 days**
		0. Behavior not exhibited in last 7 days
		1. Behavior of this type occurred 1 to 3 days in last 7 days
		2. Behavior of this type occurred 4 to 6 days, but less than daily
		3. Behavior of this type occurred daily

(B) *Behavioral* symptom *alterability* in last 7 days
0. Behavior not present OR behavior was easily altered
1. Behavior was not easily altered   (A)   (B)

a. WANDERING (moved with no rational purpose, seemingly oblivious to needs or safety)

b. VERBALLY ABUSIVE BEHAVIORAL SYMPTOMS (others were threatened, screamed at, cursed at)

c. PHYSICALLY ABUSIVE BEHAVIORAL SYMPTOMS (others were hit, shoved, scratched, sexually abused)

d. SOCIALLY INAPPROPRIATE/DISRUPTIVE BEHAVIORAL SYMPTOMS (made disruptive sounds, noisiness, screaming, self-abusive acts, sexual behavior or disrobing in public, smeared/threw food/feces, hoarding, rummaged through others' belongings)

e. RESISTS CARE (resisted taking medications/ injections, ADL assistance, or eating)

5.	CHANGE IN BEHAVIORAL SYMPTOMS	Resident's behavior status has changed as compared to **status of 90 days ago** (or since last assessment if less than 90 days)
		0. No change 1. Improved 2. Deteriorated

SECTION F. PSYCHOSOCIAL WELL-BEING

1.	SENSE OF INITIATIVE/ INVOLVE-MENT	At ease interacting with others	a.
		At ease doing planned or structured activities	b.
		At ease doing self-initiated activities	c.
		Establishes own goals	d.
		Pursues involvement in life of facility (e.g., makes/keeps friends; involved in group activities; responds positively to new activities; assists at religious services)	e.
		Accepts invitations into most group activities	f.
		NONE OF ABOVE	g.

2.	UNSETTLED RELATION-SHIPS	Covert/open conflict with or repeated criticism of staff	a.
		Unhappy with roommate	b.
		Unhappy with residents other than roommate	c.
		Openly expresses conflict/anger with family/friends	d.
		Absence of personal contact with family/friends	e.
		Recent loss of close family member/friend	f.
		Does not adjust easily to change in routines	g.
		NONE OF ABOVE	h.

3.	PAST ROLES	Strong identification with past roles and life status	a.
		Expresses sadness/anger/empty feeling over lost roles/status	b.
		Resident perceives that daily routine (customary routine, activities) is very different from prior pattern in the community	c.
		NONE OF ABOVE	d.

SECTION G. PHYSICAL FUNCTIONING AND STRUCTURAL PROBLEMS

1. (A) ADL SELF-PERFORMANCE—(*Code for resident's PERFORMANCE OVER ALL SHIFTS during last 7 days—Not including setup*)

0. INDEPENDENT—No help or oversight —OR— Help/oversight provided only 1 or 2 times during last 7 days

1. SUPERVISION—Oversight, encouragement or cueing provided 3 or more times during last 7 days —OR— Supervision (3 or more times) plus physical assistance provided only 1 or 2 times during last 7 days

2. *LIMITED ASSISTANCE*—Resident highly involved in activity; received physical help in guided maneuvering of limbs or other nonweight bearing assistance 3 or more times — OR—More help provided only 1 or 2 times during last 7 days

3. *EXTENSIVE ASSISTANCE*—While resident performed part of activity, over last 7-day period, help of following type(s) provided 3 or more times:
—Weight-bearing support
— Full staff performance during part (but not all) of last 7 days

4. *TOTAL DEPENDENCE*—Full staff performance of activity during entire 7 days

8. *ACTIVITY DID NOT OCCUR* during entire 7 days

(B) ADL SUPPORT PROVIDED—(*Code for MOST SUPPORT PROVIDED OVER ALL SHIFTS during last 7 days; code regardless of resident's self-performance classification*)

0. No setup or physical help from staff
1. Setup help only
2. One person physical assist   8. ADL activity itself did not
3. Two+ persons physical assist   occur during entire 7 days

			(A) SELF-PERF	(B) SUPPORT
a.	BED MOBILITY	How resident moves to and from lying position, turns side to side, and positions body while in bed		
b.	TRANSFER	How resident moves between surfaces—to/from: bed, chair, wheelchair, standing position (EXCLUDE to/from bath/toilet)		
c.	WALK IN ROOM	How resident walks between locations in his/her room		
d.	WALK IN CORRIDOR	How resident walks in corridor on unit		
e.	LOCOMO-TION ON UNIT	How resident moves between locations in his/her room and adjacent corridor on same floor. If in wheelchair, self-sufficiency once in chair		
f.	LOCOMO-TION OFF UNIT	How resident moves to and returns from off unit locations (e.g., areas set aside for dining, activities, or treatments). **If facility has only one floor**, how resident moves to and from distant areas on the floor. If in wheelchair, self-sufficiency once in chair		
g.	DRESSING	How resident puts on, fastens, and takes off all items of **street clothing**, including donning/removing prosthesis		
h.	EATING	How resident eats and drinks (regardless of skill). Includes intake of nourishment by other means (e.g., tube feeding, total parenteral nutrition)		
i.	TOILET USE	How resident uses the toilet room (or commode, bedpan, urinal); transfer on/off toilet, cleanses, changes pad, manages ostomy or catheter, adjusts clothes		
j.	PERSONAL HYGIENE	How resident maintains personal hygiene, including combing hair, brushing teeth, shaving, applying makeup, washing/drying face, hands, and perineum (EXCLUDE baths and showers)		

MDS 2.0 01/30/98

FIG. 8-4, cont'd For legend see p. 132.

Continued

Resident_____   Numeric Identifier _____

2.	BATHING	How resident takes full-body bath/shower, sponge bath, and transfers in/out of tub/shower (EXCLUDE washing of back and hair.) *Code for most dependent in self-performance and support.* **(A) BATHING SELF-PERFORMANCE codes appear below**	(A)	(B)
		0. Independent—No help provided		
		1. Supervision—Oversight help only		
		2. Physical help limited to transfer only		
		3. Physical help in part of bathing activity		
		4. Total dependence		
		8. Activity itself did not occur during entire 7 days *(Bathing support codes are as defined in Item 1, code B above)*		

3.	TEST FOR BALANCE *(see training manual)*	*(Code for ability during test in the last 7 days)* 0. Maintained position as required in test 1. Unsteady, but able to rebalance self without physical support 2. Partial physical support during test; or stands (sits) but does not follow directions for test 3. Not able to attempt test without physical help	
		a. Balance while standing	
		b. Balance while sitting—position, trunk control	

4.	FUNCTIONAL LIMITATION IN RANGE OF MOTION *(see training manual)*	*(Code for limitations during last 7 days that interfered with daily functions or placed resident at risk of injury)* **(A)** *RANGE OF MOTION* **(B)** *VOLUNTARY MOVEMENT* 0. No limitation 0. No loss 1. Limitation on one side 1. Partial loss 2. Limitation on both sides 2. Full loss	(A)	(B)
		a. Neck		
		b. Arm—Including shoulder or elbow		
		c. Hand—Including wrist or fingers		
		d. Leg—Including hip or knee		
		e. Foot—Including ankle or toes		
		f. Other limitation or loss		

5.	MODES OF LOCOMO-TION	*(Check all that apply during last 7 days)*		
		Cane/walker/crutch	a.	Wheelchair primary mode of locomotion	d.
		Wheeled self	b.	
		Other person wheeled	c.	NONE OF ABOVE	e.

6.	MODES OF TRANSFER	*(Check all that apply during last 7 days)*		
		Bedfast all or most of time	a.	Lifted mechanically	d.
		Bed rails used for bed mobility or transfer	b.	Transfer aid (e.g., slide board, trapeze, cane, walker, brace)	e.
		Lifted manually	c.	NONE OF ABOVE	f.

7.	TASK SEGMENTA-TION	Some or all of ADL activities were broken into subtasks during **last 7 days** so that resident could perform them 0. No 1.Yes	

8.	ADL FUNCTIONAL REHABILITA-TION POTENTIAL	Resident believes he/she is capable of increased independence in at least some ADLs	a.
		Direct care staff believe resident is capable of increased independence in at least some ADLs	b.
		Resident able to perform tasks/activity but is very slow	c.
		Difference in ADL Self-Performance or ADL Support, comparing mornings to evenings	d.
		NONE OF ABOVE	e.

9.	CHANGE IN ADL FUNCTION	Resident's ADL self-performance status has changed as compared to status of **90 days ago** (or since last assessment if less than 90 days) 0. No change 1.Improved 2.Deteriorated	

SECTION H. CONTINENCE IN LAST 14 DAYS

1.	CONTINENCE SELF-CONTROL CATEGORIES *(Code for resident's PERFORMANCE OVER ALL SHIFTS)*
	0. *CONTINENT*—Complete control *[includes use of indwelling urinary catheter or ostomy device that does not leak urine or stool]*
	1. *USUALLY CONTINENT*—BLADDER, incontinent episodes once a week or less; BOWEL, less than weekly
	2. *OCCASIONALLY INCONTINENT*—BLADDER, 2 or more times a week but not daily; BOWEL, once a week
	3. *FREQUENTLY INCONTINENT*—BLADDER, tended to be incontinent daily, but some control present (e.g., on day shift); BOWEL, 2-3 times a week
	4. *INCONTINENT*—Had inadequate control BLADDER, multiple daily episodes; BOWEL, all (or almost all) of the time

a.	BOWEL CONTI-NENCE	Control of bowel movement, with appliance or bowel continence programs, if employed	
b.	BLADDER CONTI-NENCE	Control of urinary bladder function (if dribbles, volume insufficient to soak through underpants), with appliances (e.g., foley) or continence programs, if employed	

2.	BOWEL ELIMINATION PATTERN	Bowel elimination pattern regular—at least one movement every three days	a.	Diarrhea	c.
				Fecal impaction	d.
		Constipation	b.	NONE OF ABOVE	e.

MDS 2.0 01/30/98

3.	APPLIANCES AND PROGRAMS	Any scheduled toileting plan	a.	Did not use toilet room/commode/urinal	f.
		Bladder retraining program	b.	Pads/briefs used	g.
		External (condom) catheter	c.	Enemas/irrigation	h.
		Indwelling catheter	d.	Ostomy present	i.
		Intermittent catheter	e.	NONE OF ABOVE	j.

4.	CHANGE IN URINARY CONTI-NENCE	Resident's urinary continence has changed as compared to status of **90 days ago** (or since last assessment if less than 90 days) 0. No change 1. Improved 2. Deteriorated	

SECTION I. DISEASE DIAGNOSES

Check only those diseases that have a relationship to current ADL status, cognitive status, mood and behavior status, medical treatments, nursing monitoring, or risk of death. (Do not list inactive diagnoses)

1.	DISEASES	*(If none apply, CHECK the NONE OF ABOVE box)*			
		ENDOCRINE/METABOLIC/NUTRITIONAL		Hemiplegia/Hemiparesis	v.
				Multiple sclerosis	w.
		Diabetes mellitus	a.	Paraplegia	x.
		Hyperthyroidism	b.	Parkinson's disease	y.
		Hypothyroidism	c.	Quadriplegia	z.
		HEART/CIRCULATION		Seizure disorder	aa.
		Arteriosclerotic heart disease (ASHD)	d.	Transient ischemic attack (TIA)	bb.
		Cardiac dysrhythmias	e.	Traumatic brain injury	cc.
		Congestive heart failure	f.	**PSYCHIATRIC/MOOD**	
		Deep vein thrombosis	g.	Anxiety disorder	dd.
		Hypertension	h.	Depression	ee.
		Hypotension	i.	Manic depression (bipolar disease)	ff.
		Peripheral vascular disease	j.	Schizophrenia	gg.
		Other cardiovascular disease	k.	**PULMONARY**	
		MUSCULOSKELETAL		Asthma	hh.
		Arthritis	l.	Emphysema/COPD	ii.
		Hip fracture	m.	**SENSORY**	
		Missing limb (e.g., amputation)	n.	Cataracts	jj.
		Osteoporosis	o.	Diabetic retinopathy	kk.
		Pathological bone fracture	p.	Glaucoma	ll.
		NEUROLOGICAL		Macular degeneration	mm.
		Alzheimer's disease	q.	**OTHER**	
		Aphasia	r.	Allergies	nn.
		Cerebral palsy	s.	Anemia	oo.
		Cerebrovascular accident (stroke)	t.	Cancer	pp.
				Renal failure	qq.
		Dementia other than Alzheimer's disease	u.	NONE OF ABOVE	rr.

2.	INFECTIONS	*(If none apply, CHECK the NONE OF ABOVE box)*			
		Antibiotic resistant infection (e.g., Methicillin resistant staph)	a.	Septicemia	g.
				Sexually transmitted diseases	h.
		Clostridium difficile (c. diff.)	b.	Tuberculosis	i.
		Conjunctivitis	c.	Urinary tract infection **in last 30 days**	j.
		HIV infection	d.	Viral hepatitis	k.
		Pneumonia	e.	Wound infection	l.
		Respiratory infection	f.	NONE OF ABOVE	m.

3.	OTHER CURRENT OR MORE DETAILED DIAGNOSES AND ICD-9 CODES	a. _____	.
		b. _____	.
		c. _____	.
		d. _____	.
		e. _____	.

SECTION J. HEALTH CONDITIONS

1.	PROBLEM CONDITIONS	*(Check all problems present in last 7 days unless other time frame is indicated)*			
		INDICATORS OF FLUID STATUS		Dizziness/Vertigo	f.
				Edema	g.
		Weight gain or loss of 3 or more pounds within a 7 day period	a.	Fever	h.
				Hallucinations	i.
				Internal bleeding	j.
		Inability to lie flat due to shortness of breath	b.	Recurrent lung aspirations in **last 90 days**	k.
		Dehydrated; output exceeds input	c.	Shortness of breath	l.
				Syncope (fainting)	m.
		Insufficient fluid; did NOT consume all/almost all liquids provided during **last 3 days**	d.	Unsteady gait	n.
				Vomiting	o.
		OTHER		NONE OF ABOVE	p.
		Delusions	e.		

FIG. 8-4, cont'd   For legend see p. 132.

Resident _____ Numeric Identifier _____

2.	PAIN SYMPTOMS	*(Code the **highest level of pain** present in the **last 7 days**)*				
		a. FREQUENCY with which resident complains or shows evidence of pain		**b. INTENSITY** of pain		
		0. No pain *(skip to J4)*		1. Mild pain		
		1. Pain less than daily		2. Moderate pain		
		2. Pain daily		3. Times when pain is horrible or excruciating		

3.	PAIN SITE	*(If pain present, **check all sites** that apply in **last 7 days**)*				
		Back pain	a.	Incisional pain		f.
		Bone pain	b.	Joint pain (other than hip)		g.
		Chest pain while doing usual activities	c.	Soft tissue pain (e.g., lesion, muscle)		h.
		Headache	d.	Stomach pain		i.
		Hip pain	e.	Other		j.

4.	ACCIDENTS	*(**Check all that apply**)*			
		Fell in **past 30 days**	a.	Hip fracture in **last 180 days**	c.
		Fell in **past 31-180 days**	b.	Other fracture in **last 180 days**	d.
				NONE OF ABOVE	e.

5.	STABILITY OF CONDITIONS	Conditions/diseases make resident's cognitive, ADL, mood or behavior patterns unstable—(fluctuating, precarious, or deteriorating)	a.
		Resident experiencing an acute episode or a flare-up of a recurrent or chronic problem	b.
		End-stage disease, 6 or fewer months to live	c.
		NONE OF ABOVE	d.

SECTION K. ORAL/NUTRITIONAL STATUS

1.	ORAL PROBLEMS	Chewing problem	a.
		Swallowing problem	b.
		Mouth pain	c.
		NONE OF ABOVE	d.

2.	HEIGHT AND WEIGHT	Record **(a.)** height in inches and **(b.)** weight in pounds. Base weight on most recent measure in **last 30 days**; measure weight consistently in accord with standard facility practice—e.g., in a.m. after voiding, before meal, with shoes off, and in nightclothes
		a. HT (in.) [ ][ ] **b.** WT (lb.) [ ][ ][ ]

3.	WEIGHT CHANGE	a. Weight loss—5 % or more in **last 30 days**; or 10 % or more in **last 180 days**
		0. No 1. Yes
		b. Weight gain—5 % or more in **last 30 days**; or 10 % or more in **last 180 days**
		0. No 1. Yes

4.	NUTRI-TIONAL PROBLEMS	Complains about the taste of many foods	a.	Leaves 25% or more of food uneaten at most meals	c.
		Regular or repetitive complaints of hunger	b.	NONE OF ABOVE	d.

5.	NUTRI-TIONAL APPROACH-ES	*(**Check all that apply** in **last 7 days**)*			
		Parenteral/IV	a.	Dietary supplement between meals	f.
		Feeding tube	b.		
		Mechanically altered diet	c.	Plate guard, stabilized built-up utensil, etc.	g.
		Syringe (oral feeding)	d.	On a planned weight change program	h.
		Therapeutic diet	e.		
				NONE OF ABOVE	i.

6.	PARENTERAL OR ENTERAL INTAKE	*(Skip to Section L if neither 5a nor 5b is checked)*
		a. Code the proportion of **total calories** the resident received through parenteral or tube feedings in the **last 7 days**
		0. None 3. 51% to 75%
		1. 1% to 25% 4. 76% to 100%
		2. 26% to 50%
		b. Code the average **fluid intake** per day by IV or tube in **last 7 days**
		0. None 3. 1001 to 1500 cc/day
		1. 1 to 500 cc/day 4. 1501 to 2000 cc/day
		2. 501 to 1000 cc/day 5. 2001 or more cc/day

SECTION L. ORAL/DENTAL STATUS

1.	ORAL STATUS AND DISEASE PREVENTION	Debris (soft, easily movable substances) present in mouth prior to going to bed at night	a.
		Has dentures or removable bridge	b.
		Some/all natural teeth lost—does not have or does not use dentures (or partial plates)	c.
		Broken, loose, or carious teeth	d.
		Inflamed gums (gingiva); swollen or bleeding gums; oral abcesses; ulcers or rashes	e.
		Daily cleaning of teeth/dentures or daily mouth care—by resident or staff	f.
		NONE OF ABOVE	g.

SECTION M. SKIN CONDITION

1.	ULCERS (Due to any cause)	*(Record the number of ulcers at each ulcer stage—regardless of cause. If none present at a stage, record "0" (zero). Code all that apply during **last 7 days**. Code 9 = 9 or more.) **[Requires full body exam.]***	Number at Stage
		a. Stage 1. A persistent area of skin redness (without a break in the skin) that does not disappear when pressure is relieved.	
		b. Stage 2. A partial thickness loss of skin layers that presents clinically as an abrasion, blister, or shallow crater.	
		c. Stage 3. A full thickness of skin is lost, exposing the subcutaneous tissues - presents as a deep crater with or without undermining adjacent tissue.	
		d. Stage 4. A full thickness of skin and subcutaneous tissue is lost, exposing muscle or bone.	

2.	TYPE OF ULCER	*(For each type of ulcer, **code for the highest stage** in the **last 7 days** using scale in item M1—i.e., 0=none; stages 1, 2, 3, 4)*
		a. Pressure ulcer—any lesion caused by pressure resulting in damage of underlying tissue
		b. Stasis ulcer—open lesion caused by poor circulation in the lower extremities

3.	HISTORY OF RESOLVED ULCERS	Resident had an ulcer that was resolved or cured **in LAST 90 DAYS**
		0. No 1. Yes

4.	OTHER SKIN PROBLEMS OR LESIONS PRESENT	*(**Check all that apply** during **last 7 days**)*	
		Abrasions, bruises	a.
		Burns (second or third degree)	b.
		Open lesions other than ulcers, rashes, cuts (e.g., cancer lesions)	c.
		Rashes—e.g., intertrigo, eczema, drug rash, heat rash, herpes zoster	d.
		Skin desensitized to pain or pressure	e.
		Skin tears or cuts (other than surgery)	f.
		Surgical wounds	g.
		NONE OF ABOVE	h.

5.	SKIN TREAT-MENTS	*(**Check all that** apply during **last 7 days**)*	
		Pressure relieving device(s) for chair	a.
		Pressure relieving device(s) for bed	b.
		Turning/repositioning program	c.
		Nutrition or hydration intervention to manage skin problems	d.
		Ulcer care	e.
		Surgical wound care	f.
		Application of dressings (with or without topical medications) other than to feet	g.
		Application of ointments/medications (other than to feet)	h.
		Other preventative or protective skin care (other than to feet)	i.
		NONE OF ABOVE	j.

6.	FOOT PROBLEMS AND CARE	*(**Check all that apply** during **last 7 days**)*	
		Resident has one or more foot problems—e.g., corns, callouses, bunions, hammer toes, overlapping toes, pain, structural problems	a.
		Infection of the foot—e.g., cellulitis, purulent drainage	b.
		Open lesions on the foot	c.
		Nails/calluses trimmed during **last 90 days**	d.
		Received preventative or protective foot care (e.g., used special shoes, inserts, pads, toe separators)	e.
		Application of dressings (with or without topical medications)	f.
		NONE OF ABOVE	g.

SECTION N. ACTIVITY PURSUIT PATTERNS

1.	TIME AWAKE	*(**Check appropriate time periods** over **last 7 days**)* Resident awake all or most of time (i.e., naps no more than one hour per time period) in the:			
		Morning	a.	Evening	c.
		Afternoon	b.	NONE OF ABOVE	d.

(If resident is comatose, skip to Section O)

2.	AVERAGE TIME INVOLVED IN ACTIVITIES	*(When awake and not receiving treatments or ADL care)*
		0. Most—more than 2/3 of time 2. Little—less than 1/3 of time
		1. Some—from 1/3 to 2/3 of time 3. None

3.	PREFERRED ACTIVITY SETTINGS	*(**Check all settings** in which activities are **preferred**)*			
		Own room	a.		
		Day/activity room	b.	Outside facility	d.
		Inside NH/off unit	c.	NONE OF ABOVE	e.

4.	GENERAL ACTIVITY PREFER-ENCES (adapted to resident's current abilities)	*(**Check all PREFERENCES** whether or not activity is currently available to resident)*			
		Cards/other games	a.	Trips/shopping	g.
		Crafts/arts	b.	Walking/wheeling outdoors	h.
		Exercise/sports	c.	Watching TV	i.
		Music	d.	Gardening or plants	j.
		Reading/writing	e.	Talking or conversing	k.
		Spiritual/religious activities	f.	Helping others	l.
				NONE OF ABOVE	m.

MDS 2.0 01/30/98

FIG. 8-4, cont'd   For legend see p. 132.

Continued

Resident _____   Numeric Identifier _____

| 5. | PREFERS CHANGE IN DAILY ROUTINE | Code for resident preferences in daily routines
0. No change 1. Slight change 2. Major change
a. Type of activities in which resident is currently involved | |
| | | b. Extent of resident involvement in activities | |

SECTION O. MEDICATIONS

1.	NUMBER OF MEDICA-TIONS	(Record the number of different medications used in the last 7 days; enter "0" if none used)	
2.	NEW MEDICA-TIONS	(Resident currently receiving medications that were initiated during the last 90 days) 0. No 1. Yes	
3.	INJECTIONS	(Record the number of DAYS injections of any type received during the last 7 days; enter "0" if none used)	
4.	DAYS RECEIVED THE FOLLOWING MEDICATION	(Record the number of DAYS during last 7 days; enter "0" if not used. Note—enter "1" for long-acting meds used less than weekly)	

a. Antipsychotic		d. Hypnotic	
b. Antianxiety		e. Diuretic	
c. Antidepressant			

SECTION P. SPECIAL TREATMENTS AND PROCEDURES

| 1. | SPECIAL TREAT-MENTS, PROCE-DURES, AND PROGRAMS | a. SPECIAL CARE—Check treatments or programs received during the last 14 days | |

TREATMENTS		PROGRAMS	
		Ventilator or respirator	l.
Chemotherapy	a.	PROGRAMS	
Dialysis	b.	Alcohol/drug treatment program	m.
IV medication	c.	Alzheimer's/dementia special care unit	n.
Intake/output	d.	Hospice care	o.
Monitoring acute medical condition	e.	Pediatric unit	p.
Ostomy care	f.	Respite care	q.
Oxygen therapy	g.	Training in skills required to return to the community (e.g., taking medications, house work, shopping, transportation, ADLs)	r.
Radiation	h.		
Suctioning	i.		
Tracheostomy care	j.		
Transfusions	k.	NONE OF ABOVE	s.

b. THERAPIES - Record the number of days and total minutes each of the following therapies was administered (for at least 15 minutes a day) in the last 7 calendar days (Enter 0 if none or less than 15 min. daily) [Note—count only post admission therapies]
(A) = # of days administered for 15 minutes or more
(B) = total # of minutes provided in last 7 days

	DAYS (A)	MIN (B)
a. Speech - language pathology and audiology services		
b. Occupational therapy		
c. Physical therapy		
d. Respiratory therapy		
e. Psychological therapy (by any licensed mental health professional)		

2.	INTERVEN-TION PROGRAMS FOR MOOD, BEHAVIOR, COGNITIVE LOSS	(Check all interventions or strategies used in last 7 days—no matter where received)	
		Special behavior symptom evaluation program	a.
		Evaluation by a licensed mental health specialist in last 90 days	b.
		Group therapy	c.
		Resident-specific deliberate changes in the environment to address mood/behavior patterns—e.g., providing bureau in which to rummage	d.
		Reorientation—e.g., cueing	e.
		NONE OF ABOVE	f.

| 3. | NURSING REHABILITA-TION/ RESTOR-ATIVE CARE | Record the NUMBER OF DAYS each of the following rehabilitation or restorative techniques or practices was provided to the resident for more than or equal to 15 minutes per day in the last 7 days (Enter 0 if none or less than 15 min. daily) | |

a. Range of motion (passive)		f. Walking	
b. Range of motion (active)		g. Dressing or grooming	
c. Splint or brace assistance		h. Eating or swallowing	
TRAINING AND SKILL PRACTICE IN:		i. Amputation/prosthesis care	
d. Bed mobility		j. Communication	
e. Transfer		k. Other	

4.	DEVICES AND RESTRAINTS	(Use the following codes for last 7 days:) 0. Not used 1. Used less than daily 2. Used daily	
		Bed rails	
		a. — Full bed rails on all open sides of bed	
		b. — Other types of side rails used (e.g., half rail, one side)	
		c. Trunk restraint	
		d. Limb restraint	
		e. Chair prevents rising	
5.	HOSPITAL STAY(S)	Record number of times resident was admitted to hospital with an overnight stay in last 90 days (or since last assessment if less than 90 days). (Enter 0 if no hospital admissions)	
6.	EMERGENCY ROOM (ER) VISIT(S)	Record number of times resident visited ER without an overnight stay in last 90 days (or since last assessment if less than 90 days). (Enter 0 if no ER visits)	
7.	PHYSICIAN VISITS	In the LAST 14 DAYS (or since admission if less than 14 days in facility) how many days has the physician (or authorized assistant or practitioner) examined the resident? (Enter 0 if none)	
8.	PHYSICIAN ORDERS	In the LAST 14 DAYS (or since admission if less than 14 days in facility) how many days has the physician (or authorized assistant or practitioner) changed the resident's orders? Do not include order renewals without change. (Enter 0 if none)	
9.	ABNORMAL LAB VALUES	Has the resident had any abnormal lab values during the last 90 days (or since admission)? 0. No 1. Yes	

SECTION Q. DISCHARGE POTENTIAL AND OVERALL STATUS

1.	DISCHARGE POTENTIAL	a. Resident expresses/indicates preference to return to the community 0. No 1. Yes	
		b. Resident has a support person who is positive towards discharge 0. No 1. Yes	
		c. Stay projected to be of a short duration— discharge projected within 90 days (do not include expected discharge due to death) 0. No 2. Within 31-90 days 1. Within 30 days 3. Discharge status uncertain	
2.	OVERALL CHANGE IN CARE NEEDS	Resident's overall self sufficiency has changed significantly as compared to status of 90 days ago (or since last assessment if less than 90 days) 0. No change 1. Improved—receives fewer 2. Deteriorated—receives supports, needs less more support restrictive level of care	

SECTION R. ASSESSMENT INFORMATION

1.	PARTICIPA-TION IN ASSESS-MENT	a. Resident: 0. No 1. Yes	
		b. Family: 0. No 1. Yes 2. No family	
		c. Significant other: 0. No 1. Yes 2. None	

2. SIGNATURES OF PERSONS COMPLETING THE ASSESSMENT:

a. Signature of RN Assessment Coordinator (sign on above line)

b. Date RN Assessment Coordinator signed as complete

Month	Day	Year
☐ ☐	☐ ☐	☐ ☐ ☐ ☐

c. Other Signatures	Title	Sections	Date
d.			Date
e.			Date
f.			Date
g.			Date
h.			Date

MDS 2.0 01/30/98

FIG. 8-4, cont'd   For legend see p. 132.

Resident _____   Numeric Identifier _____

SECTION T. THERAPY SUPPLEMENT FOR MEDICARE PPS

1.	SPECIAL TREAT-MENTS AND PROCE-DURES	**a. RECREATION THERAPY**—*Enter number of days and total minutes of recreation therapy administered (**for at least 15 minutes a day**) in the **last 7 days** (Enter 0 if none)*		

			DAYS (A)	MIN (B)
		(A) = # of days administered for 15 minutes or more		
		(B) = total # of minutes provided in last 7 days		

Skip unless this is a Medicare 5 day or Medicare readmission/return assessment.

b. ORDERED THERAPIES—*Has physician ordered any of following therapies to begin in FIRST 14 days of stay—physical therapy, occupational therapy, or speech pathology service?*
    0. No   1. Yes

If not ordered, skip to item 2

c. Through day 15, provide an estimate of the number of days when at least 1 therapy service can be expected to have been delivered.

d. Through day 15, provide an estimate of the number of therapy minutes (across the therapies) that can be expected to be delivered?

2.	WALKING WHEN MOST SELF SUFFICIENT	*Complete item 2 if ADL self-performance score for TRANSFER (G.1.b.A) is 0,1,2, or 3 AND at least one of the following are present:*

  • Resident received physical therapy involving gait training (P.1.b.c)
  • Physical therapy was ordered for the resident involving gait training (T.1.b)
  • Resident received nursing rehabilitation for walking (P.3.f)
  • Physical therapy involving walking has been discontinued within the past 180 days

Skip to item 3 if resident did not walk in last 7 days

(FOR FOLLOWING FIVE ITEMS, BASE CODING ON THE EPISODE WHEN THE RESIDENT WALKED THE FARTHEST WITHOUT SITTING DOWN. INCLUDE WALKING DURING REHABILITATION SESSIONS.)

a. Furthest distance walked without sitting down during this episode.

  0. 150+ feet   3. 10-25 feet
  1. 51-149 feet   4. Less than 10 feet
  2. 26-50 feet

b. Time walked without sitting down during this episode.

  0. 1-2 minutes   3. 11-15 minutes
  1. 3-4 minutes   4. 16-30 minutes
  2. 5-10 minutes   5. 31+ minutes

c. Self-Performance in walking during this episode.

  0. *INDEPENDENT*—No help or oversight
  1. *SUPERVISION*—Oversight, encouragement or cueing provided
  2. *LIMITED ASSISTANCE*—Resident highly involved in walking; received physical help in guided maneuvering of limbs or other nonweight bearing assistance
  3. *EXTENSIVE ASSISTANCE*—Resident received weight bearing assistance while walking

d. Walking support provided associated with this episode (code regardless of resident's self-performance classification).

  0. No setup or physical help from staff
  1. Setup help only
  2. One person physical assist
  3. Two+ persons physical assist

e. Parallel bars used by resident in association with this episode.

  0. No   1. Yes

3.	CASE MIX GROUP	Medicare [ ][ ][ ][ ][ ] State [ ][ ][ ][ ][ ]

MDS 2.0 01/30/98

FIG. 8-4, cont'd   For legend see p. 132.

SECTION V. RESIDENT ASSESSMENT PROTOCOL SUMMARY   Numeric Identifier _____

Resident's Name:	Medical Record No.:

1. Check if RAP is triggered.

2. For each triggered RAP, use the RAP guidelines to identify areas needing further assessment. Document relevant assessment information regarding the resident's status.

- Describe:
  — Nature of the condition (may include presence or lack of objective data and subjective complaints).
  — Complications and risk factors that affect your decision to proceed to care planning.
  — Factors that must be considered in developing individualized care plan interventions.
  — Need for referrals/further evaluation by appropriate health professionals.

- Documentation should support your decision-making regarding whether to proceed with a care plan for a triggered RAP and the type(s) of care plan interventions that are appropriate for a particular resident.

- Documentation may appear anywhere in the clinical record (e.g., progress notes, consults, flowsheets, etc.).

3. Indicate under the Location of RAP Assessment Documentation column where information related to the RAP assessment can be found.

4. For each triggered RAP, indicate whether a new care plan, care plan revision, or continuation of current care plan is necessary to address the problem(s) identified in your assessment. The Care Planning Decision column must be completed within 7 days of completing the RAI (MDS and RAPs).

A. RAP PROBLEM AREA	(a) Check if triggered	Location and Date of RAP Assessment Documentation	(b) Care Planning Decision—check if addressed in care plan
1. DELIRIUM			
2. COGNITIVE LOSS			
3. VISUAL FUNCTION			
4. COMMUNICATION			
5. ADL FUNCTIONAL/ REHABILITATION POTENTIAL			
6. URINARY INCONTINENCE AND INDWELLING CATHETER			
7. PSYCHOSOCIAL WELL-BEING			
8. MOOD STATE			
9. BEHAVIORAL SYMPTOMS			
10. ACTIVITIES			
11. FALLS			
12. NUTRITIONAL STATUS			
13. FEEDING TUBES			
14. DEHYDRATION/FLUID MAINTENANCE			
15. DENTAL CARE			
16. PRESSURE ULCERS			
17. PSYCHOTROPIC DRUG USE			
18. PHYSICAL RESTRAINTS			

B.
1. Signature of RN Coordinator for RAP Assessment Process   2. Month — Day — Year

3. Signature of Person Completing Care Planning Decision   4. Month — Day — Year

MDS 2.0 01/30/98

FIG. 8-5 Resident Assessment Protocol Summary. (Courtesy of the United States Department of Health and Human Services.)

caregivers will learn more about the infirm elderly population, their most common medical problems, and the most- or least-effective treatments and interventions.

The new MDS enables state and federal agencies to evaluate the performance of an individual institution in any number of categories and facilitates a level of comparison between treatment methods that has not previously been available. For example, the frequency, location, and extent of pressure ulcers can be determined and correlated to age, disease, diet, and other factors. It also enables the supervising government agency to compare various long-term care providers with each other.

The ability to assemble these data on a regional or national basis excites the better health care providers because this correlative data will enable them to identify critical parameters in resident status and develop more effective models for care. Other providers, particularly those who may not meet the expected standards of care, view this oversight capability less favorably.

Because the MDS plays such an important role in determining resident status and planning and evaluating care, it must be completed in a timely manner and updated regularly. Licensed nursing staff must pay close attention to the times specified in the statutes and complete all records in a timely manner.

SUMMARY

Although the initial health assessment of the elderly is important, it is only a starting point. It is important to remember that assessment is a continuous and ongoing process. As each aging person's condition changes, objective and subjective data will also change. OBRA mandates that the total assessment be revised and updated whenever a significant change occurs in a resident's mental or physical condition. Because nurses spend the greatest amount of time with the elderly, they have the greatest opportunity to assess and recognize significant changes. It is the responsibility of nurses to assess continually and to institute changes in care based on those observations.

READINGS AND REFERENCES

Arguelles T, Loewnstein DA: Cognitive tests and test translations: research says si to development of culturally appropriate cognitive assessment tools, *Generations* 21:30, 1997.

Beck JC, Freedman ML, Warshaw GA: Geriatric assessment: focus on function, *Patient Care* 28:10, 1994.

Cognitive performance scale developed from MDS items, *Brown University Long-Term Care Quality Letter* 6:7, 1994.

Comprehensiveness and accuracy improve with the MDS, *Brown University Long-Term Care Quality Letter* 6:5, 1994.

Cefalu CA: The cognitive assessment screening tests (CAST), *Am Fam Physician* 54: 1877, 1996.

Cohen G: Comprehensive assessment: capturing strengths, not just weaknesses, *Generations* 17:47, 1993.

Drachman DA, Swearer JM: Screening for dementia: cognitive assessment screening test, *Am Fam Physician* 54:1957, 1996.

Dubin S: Geriatric assessment: a holistic multidisciplinary approach goes beyond the admitting diagnosis, *Am J Nurs* 96:49, 1996.

Elders functional status may not be best predictor of nursing home placement, *Brown University Long-Term Care Quality Letter* 7:8, 1995.

Fries BE: Changing technology of assessing the elderly: the example of the R.A.I., *Generations* 21:59, 1997.

Functional decline is reversible, *Brown University Long-Term Care Quality Letter* 7:S1, 1995.

Genevay B: See me! Hear me! I am! An experience in being assessed, *Generations* 21:16, 1997.

George LK: Choosing among established assessment tools, scientific demands and practical constraints, *Generations* 21:32, 1997.

Geron SM: Multidimensional assessment measures, *Generations* 21:52, 1997.

Greganti MA, Hanson LC: Comprehensive geriatric assessment: where do we go from here? *Arch Intern Med*, 156:15, 1996.

Ikegami N: Functional assessment and its place in health care, *N Engl J Med* 332:598, 1995.

Impaired vision contributes most to functional disability, *Brown University Long-Term Care Quality Letter* 6:7, 1994.

Inpatients who get comprehensive geriatric assessment found no better off at 12-month follow-up, *Brown University Long-Term Care Quality Letter* 7:9, 1995.

Jagger C, Spiers NA, Clarke M: Factors associated with decline in function, institutionalization and mortality of elderly people, *Age Aging*, 22:190, 1993.

Judge KM: Geriatric need assessment, *Independent Living Provider* 11:28, 1996.

Kane RA, Degenholtz H: Assessing values and preferences: should we, can we? *Generations* 21:19, 1997.

Kinney ED, et al: Automating assessment for community based long-term care: Indiana's experience, *Generations* 21:62, 1997.

King C: Guidelines for improving assessment skills, *Generations* 21:73, 1997.

Koch M, et al: An impairment and disability assessment and treatment protocol for community living elderly persons, *Phys Ther* 74:286, 1994.

Level of cognitive dysfunction should indicate the need for long-term care, *Brown University Long-Term Care Quality Letter* 6:1, 1994.

McGrew KB, Quinn CA: Examining the effectiveness of telephone assessment and care planning for home care services, *Generations* 21:66, 1997.

Paist SS, Jafri A: Functional assessment in older patients: key to improving quality of life, *Postgrad Med* 99:101, 1996.

Rabins PV: Nursing aides can use brief behavioral symptom rating scale for cognitively impaired, *Brown University Long-Term Care Quality Letter* 6:7, 1994.

Rogers H, Curless R, James OFW: Standardized functional assessment scales for elderly patients, *Age Aging* 22:161, 1993.

Schneider B, Amerman E, Ratajczak E: Clinical protocols: guiding case management assessment and care planning, *Generations* 21:69, 1997

Siu AL, et al: Measuring functioning and health in the very old, *J Gerontol* 48:M10, 1993.

Yee DL: Can long term care assessments be culturally responsive? *Generations* 21:25, 1997.

Zarit SH: Brief measures of depression and cognitive function, *Generations* 21:41, 1997.

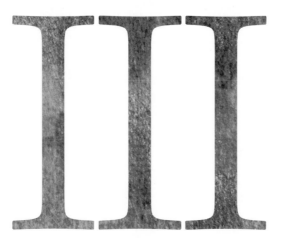

PHYSICAL CARE
OF THE
ELDERLY

MEETING SAFETY NEEDS OF THE ELDERLY

LEARNING OBJECTIVES

1. Discuss the types and extent of safety problems experienced by the aging population.
2. Describe internal and external factors that increase safety risks for the elderly.
3. Discuss interventions that will promote safety for the elderly.
4. Discuss factors that place the elderly at risk for altered thermoregulation.
5. Describe those older adults who are most at risk for developing problems related to altered thermoregulation.
6. Identify signs and symptoms of thermoregulatory problems.
7. Identify interventions that will assist the elderly in maintaining normal body temperature.

Safety is a major concern when working with or providing care to the elderly. Although the elderly comprise about 11% of the population, they account for approximately 23% of accidental deaths. A report from the National Safety Council reveals that about 24,000 people over 65 years of age die from accidental injuries each year, and at least 800,000 sustain injuries serious enough to disable them for at least 1 day.

Falls, burns, poisoning, and automobile accidents are the most common safety problems among the elderly. Exposure to temperature extremes also places the elderly at risk for injury or death. Older adults are more susceptible to accidents and injuries than are younger adults because of both internal and external factors. Internal factors include: the normal physiologic changes with aging, increased incidence of chronic disease, increased use of medications, and cognitive or emotional changes. External factors include a variety of environmental factors that present hazards to the elderly.

INTERNAL RISK FACTORS

Vision and hearing are protective senses. When the acuteness of the senses diminishes with aging, the risk for injury increases. Vision and hearing changes are common with aging. Diminished range of peripheral vision and changes in depth perception are common and can interfere with the ability of the elderly to judge the distance and height of stairs and curbs or to determine the position and speed of motor vehicles. Night vision diminishes. In dim light or glare, the elderly may be unable to see that a curb, step, or other hazard is present. They may be unable to see or read stationary road signs that provide directions or warnings. Falls or motor vehicle accidents often result from altered vision.

Changes in visual acuity make it more difficult to read labels with small print. This can make it difficult for the elderly to read the directions on prescriptions. Many elderly have taken incorrect medications or wrong doses or have even consumed poisonous substances because they could not see adequately to read the labels.

Decreased auditory acuity reduces an elderly person's ability to detect and respond appropriately to warning calls, whistles, or alarms. For example, the elderly may not hear a warning call of impending danger, may not hear a motor vehicle or siren in time to avoid an accident, or may not respond to a fire alarm in time to leave a building safely.

The elderly frequently experience one or more of the following problems: altered balance, decreased mobility, decreased flexibility, decreased muscle strength, slowed reaction time, gait changes, difficulty lifting the feet, altered sense of balance, or postural changes. Any of these changes alone or in combination can reduce the elderly person's ability to respond quickly enough to prevent an accident or injury. When these problems are combined with chronic diseases or health problems, the risk for falls increases dramatically.

Conditions affecting the cardiovascular, nervous, and musculoskeletal systems are most likely to contribute to safety problems. Any cardiovascular condition that results in decreased cardiac output and decreased oxygen supply to the brain can cause the elderly to experience vertigo (dizziness) or syncope (fainting). Common disorders with this result include anemia, heart block, and orthostatic hypotension. Studies have shown that approximately 52% of long-term nursing home residents older than 60 years of age experience four or more episodes of orthostatic hypotension a day.

Elderly persons with neurologic disorders such as Parkinson's disease or stroke experience weakness and alterations in gait and balance that increase the risk of falls. Neurologic and circulatory changes can also decrease the ability to sense painful stimuli or temperature changes, increasing the risk of tissue injuries, burns, and frostbite.

Musculoskeletal conditions such as arthritis further reduce joint mobility and flexibility, decreasing the ability of the elderly person to move and respond to hazards and intensifying the likelihood of accidents or injury. See Box 9-1 for a list of injury risks for older adults.

Medications frequently contribute to falls, and because the elderly often take one or more medications their risk of untoward effects is increased. Any medication that alters sensation or perception, slows reaction time, or causes orthostatic hypotension is potentially dangerous for the elderly. Common types of hazardous medications include sedatives, hypnotics, tranquilizers, diuretics, antihypertensives, and antihistamines. Alcohol, although not a prescription medication, acts as a drug in the body. Alcoholic beverages, particularly in combination with prescription drugs, increase the risk of falls and other injuries. More information regarding safe use of medications is included in Chapter 7.

BOX 9-1
Injury Risks for Older Adults
• Impaired physical mobility • Sensory deficits • Lack of knowledge of health practices or safety precautions • A hazardous environment • A history of accidents or injuries

Cognitive changes or emotional disturbance and depression may be overlooked as risk factors for falls or injury. These disturbances reduce the elderly person's ability to recognize and process information. Distracted or preoccupied elderly people are less likely to pay full attention to what is happening or what they are doing. This lack of attention and caution increases the risk for accidents and injury.

Falls are the most common safety problems in the elderly. Consider the following statistical facts revealed in the literature: (1) One third to one half of people over age 65 are prone to falling. (2) Two thirds of those who have experienced one fall will fall again within 6 months. (3) The older a person becomes, the more likely he or she is to suffer serious consequences, such as a hip fracture, from a fall. (4) Falls are the fifth leading cause of death in people over age 65. (5) Approximately one fourth of elderly people who experience falls will die within a year. (6) The incidence of falls is higher among those elderly residing in long-term care facilities than among those who live independently in the community.

Elderly people need to be aware of things they can do to reduce their risk of falls. Some helpful approaches are summarized in Box 9-2.

BOX 9-2

Reducing the Risk of Falls

- *Allow adequate time to complete an activity or task.* Haste increases the risk of falls or other injuries.
- *Wear good-fitting footwear.* Shoes with nonslip soles and low heels are recommended because high-heeled shoes contribute to balance problems. Shoes should have closures that are easy to manipulate. Check that laces do not come loose and cause tripping. Loose-fitting slippers or shoes can drop off the foot and lead to a fall.
- *Use assistive devices if needed.* A cane or walker provides security by enlarging the base of support. These devices should be kept close at hand to avoid leaning or reaching. The tips should have solid rubber grips to prevent slipping and may need to be modified on icy surfaces to promote gripping.
- *Ask for help when necessary.* The Bible saying, "Pride goeth before destruction, and a haughty spirit before a fall," provides good advice. Failure to seek help can lead to serious injury. The elderly should be encouraged to recognize that good judgement is a sign of healthy aging and not a sign of weakness.

EXTERNAL RISK FACTORS

Environmental hazards include everything that surrounds the elderly. Potential hazards are presented by the people and wide variety of objects a person comes in contact with on a daily basis. Even the climate in which a person lives can present an environmental hazard. Environmental hazards are everywhere: in the home, on the street, in public buildings, and in health care settings. Although injuries can and do occur frequently in the home, changes in environment such as hospitalization, travel, or any other move from a familiar environment increases the likelihood of injury for the elderly (Box 9-3).

People, particularly strangers, present a risk to the elderly. The elderly are more vulnerable than younger persons to attack and injury from that segment of the population who preys on weaker or more defenseless people such as the infirm or elderly. The elderly need to be aware of the risks presented by strangers and learn to institute measures to reduce the likelihood of injury (Box 9-4).

Things like motor vehicles, sharp or pointed objects, ladders, and electric and mechanical devices all present threats to safety. Probably the most dangerous hazards, because of their size and speed, are motor vehicles. Motor vehicle accidents are more likely to occur with aging whether the elderly person is a pedestrian or a driver.

Studies reveal facts that demonstrate the magnitude of the problem. One study revealed that only 1% of independent persons over 72 years of age were able to cross a street before the traffic signal changed. Elderly drivers who are unable to respond quickly enough are involved in a disproportionate number of accidents for the amount of miles driven. The National Institute on Aging reports that motor vehicle accidents are the most common cause of accidental death in the 65- to 74-year-old age group and are the second most common cause among the elderly in general.

Driving ability is affected by all of the internal factors previously discussed. The elderly are often unwilling to stop driving even though they are a serious risk to themselves and others. This is a major concern in communities in which large numbers of senior citizens reside. Currently there are few legal measures that are effective in terminating driving privileges.

While people are usually aware of the need to modify their homes and activity levels as they age, the elderly may not be equally aware of the need to make adjustments in driving. Initiating safe driving modifications can enable the elderly to enjoy the freedom of movement provided by automobiles while protecting themselves and others (Box 9-5).

Extremes in environmental climate are an external factor that presents risks to the elderly. Elderly persons in extreme conditions (temperatures below 60° F

BOX 9-3

Preventing Injuries in the Home

- *Ensure that all rugs are firmly fixed to the floor.* Tack down loose edges, ensure that rubber skid proofing is secure, and remove decorative "scatter rugs."
- *Maintain electric safety.* Check regularly to ensure that there are no broken or frayed electric cords or plugs. Any defective electric plug or cord should be repaired by an approved repair person. Discard all electric appliances that cannot be repaired. Install ground fault interrupt electric sockets near water sources to prevent accidental shocks when using appliances.
- *Decrease clutter and other hazards.* Throw out unnecessary items such as old newspapers. Keep shoes, wastebaskets, and electric or telephone cords out of traffic areas. Never place or store anything on stairs. Ice should be cleared promptly from sidewalks and outside staircases. "Kitty litter" can help provide traction on icy surfaces.
- *Provide adequate lighting.* This is particularly important in stairwells. Switches should be located at both the top and bottom of stairs. Use night lights in the bedroom, bathroom, and hallways. The kitchen should have adequate lighting in food preparation areas to facilitate label reading and reduce the risk of injury when using sharp objects.
- *Provide grip assistance wherever appropriate.* Handrails should be installed in all stairwells to provide support when climbing stairs. Grab bars alongside the toilet and in the bathtub and shower also help provide support. Lightweight cooking utensils with large handles and enlarged stove knobs make cooking easier and safer for the elderly.
- *Place frequently used items at shoulder height or lower where they can be reached easily.* Keeping frequently used items available decreases the need to use climbing devices. Use only approved devices such as step stools when reaching for items that cannot be reached easily. Ladders are not recommended for use by the elderly, but if they are used ensure that they are fully open and locked. Excessive reaching should be avoided and another person should stand by to steady the ladder, reducing the risk of tipping.
- *Take measures to prevent burns.* Avoid smoking or the use of open flames whenever possible. Do not wear loose, long sleeves when cooking on a gas stove. Check that the hot water tank setting does not exceed 120° F. Use a mixer valve to prevent sudden bursts of hot water. Have a plan for leaving the residence in case of fire.

---

or above 90° F) are at increased risk of developing problems related to thermoregulation (Box 9-6). It is estimated that 10% of all persons over age 65 have some thermal regulating defect that puts them at risk. Elderly persons who are sick, frail, inactive, or taking medications such as sedatives, tranquilizers, antidepressants, and cardiovascular drugs that prevent the body from regulating body temperature normally are at serious risk when exposed to even minor climate changes. Even active, healthy elderly persons are at increased risk when exposed to extremely hot or cold temperatures.

Thermoregulation, which is the ability to maintain body temperature in a safe range, is controlled by the hypothalamus. The normal core body temperature is maintained between 97° F and 99° F. Body temperature can be affected by a wide range of internal and external factors. Internal factors include muscle activity, peripheral circulation, amount of subcutaneous fat, metabolic rate, amount and type of foods and fluids ingested, medications, and disease processes. External factors include humidity, environmental temperature, air movement, and amount and type of clothing or covering.

Normal changes that occur with aging affect the

body's ability to regulate temperature. Decreased muscle tissue, decreased muscle activity, diminished peripheral circulation, reduced subcutaneous fat, and decreased metabolic rate affect the amount of heat produced and retained by the body. Changes in the skin reduce the elderly person's ability to perceive dangerously hot or cold environments. The normal processes used by the body to produce and lose heat are affected by aging.

Heat is produced by metabolic processes and by muscular activity such as shivering. As a person ages, metabolism slows, activity decreases, and shivering diminishes. Thus the elderly person becomes increasingly susceptible to hypothermia. **Hypothermia** is defined as a core body temperature of 95° F or lower. When the elderly person is exposed to low environmental temperatures, body temperature drops further. These changes further decrease activity and heat production and allow the body temperature to decrease even further. If this cycle is not stopped, the person may die. The National Institute on Aging estimates that over 2.5 million elderly are at risk for hypothermia, and a Harvard study estimates that 25,000 adults may die every year from hypothermia.

In addition to decreased body temperature, the el-

BOX 9-4

Home Security Guidelines

- *Think and plan ahead to reduce risks to personal safety.* Unfortunately, we live in a society that is less safe than it was when the elderly grew up. Precautions that may not have been necessary in the past now should be part of each person's daily planning.
- *Identify ways an intruder could enter the home.* Defective locks on windows or doors should be replaced. Locks should be secured and checked each time the person enters and leaves. Lost or stolen keys may necessitate lock changes.
- *Maintain regular contact with friends and family.* Daily phone calls or some sort of signal should be used to indicate that everything is all right.
- *Use the telephone safely.* Keep a phone at the bedside and near the favorite sitting area. This will eliminate the need to hurry to another room. If possible, obtain a phone with large numbers, which will enable accurate dialing in a stressful situation. An auto-dial function with emergency numbers is also helpful. An answering machine is useful in screening nuisance or late-night calls. Women living alone should never broadcast this fact to strangers. Using a male voice on the answering machine is a wise precaution.
- *Answer the door safely.* Ensure that doors are secure with a peephole at eye level for viewing visitors before opening the door. Make sure that outside lighting is available and working so nighttime visitors can be observed. Ask for proper identification before opening the door for a stranger. *Do not* open the door if there is any doubt about who is there; any authentic sales agent or service employee will wait and not take exception to having the identification checked with their company.
- *Bank safely.* Withdraw cash in small-denomination bills. *Do not* carry or display large amounts of cash. Secure money immediately in a wallet, money belt, or handbag. It is wise not to put large sums of money in a shoulder or strap handbag that can be pulled away easily. It is better to keep wallets in an internal pocket or body pouch. Keep large amounts of cash and valuables in a bank or other financial institution. Vary the day and time that banking is done. When using an automated teller machine, avoid nighttime visits and whenever possible have another person along for safety.
- *Prepare for emergencies.* Have emergency numbers posted in large, clear lettering near each telephone. If entry door locks have dead bolts, they should be left unlocked with the key in place while the elderly person is inside. This will reduce the risk of the elderly person being trapped in the building in case of fire and will enable emergency care providers to enter the housing unit if services are needed.

BOX 9-5

Safe Driving Practices for the Elderly

Do:
- Plan ahead to know where you are going.
- Wear appropriate eyeglasses and hearing aids.
- Pace trips to allow for frequent rest breaks.
- Use extra caution when approaching intersections.
- Drive at a safe distance behind other cars.

Avoid driving:
- If taking medications that affect driving skills.
- During rush hour.
- At night when lighting is limited or during inclement weather.
- On busy streets and in congested traffic areas.
- On limited-access roads with high speed limits and complex intersections such as freeways.

BOX 9-6

Thermoregulation Risks for Older Adults

- Exposure to excessively cold or hot environments
- Limited financial resources to pay for heat or clothing that is suitable for environmental temperature
- Neurologic, endocrine, or cardiovascular disease
- Hypometabolic or hypermetabolic disorders (diabetes, cancer, hypothyroidism, hyperthyroidism, malnutrition, obesity)
- Infection or other febrile illness
- Dehydration or electrolyte imbalances
- Inactivity or excessive activity
- Temperature-altering medications (alcohol, antidepressants, barbiturates, reserpine, benzodiazepines, phenothiazines, anticholinergics)

BOX 9-7

Signs of Hypothermia

- Mental confusion
- Decreased pulse and respiratory rate
- Decreased body temperature
- Cool/cold skin
- Pallor or cyanosis
- Swollen or puffy face
- Muscle stiffness
- Fine tremors
- Altered coordination
- Changes in gait and balance
- Lethargy, apathy, irritability, hostility, or aggression

---

derly person experiencing hypothermia may manifest other signs or symptoms (Box 9-7). One of the first signs of hypothermia in the elderly is growing mental confusion that can progress from simple memory loss or changes in logical thinking to total disorientation. Pulse and respiratory rate slow with hypothermia and may be difficult to detect in severe cases. The skin becomes cool or cold to the touch, and pallor or cyanosis is often present (particularly on the extremities). The face may appear swollen or puffy. Muscles appear to be stiff, and fine tremors may occur. Changes in coordination, including poor balance or gait changes are common. Behavior changes such as lethargy or apathy may occur, but irritability, hostility, and aggression are also possible responses. Shivering, an indication that the body is having difficulty maintaining adequate body temperature, may or may not be evident in the elderly because this response often diminishes or disappears with aging. Because many of the signs and symptoms of hypothermia are similar to those of other disorders in the elderly, they can easily be missed or mistaken for something else.

The body needs time to adjust to hot weather. Sudden increases in temperature can place a significant strain on the heart and blood vessels of the elderly. Heat is normally lost through vasodilation and through the evaporation of perspiration. It takes longer for older adults to begin sweating, and they produce less perspiration when they do sweat. Medications can compromise the body's normal adaptation to heat. Diuretics prevent the body from storing fluids and can diminish superficial vasodilation, and some antiparkinsonian agents (benztropine, trihexyphenidyl) interfere with perspiration. These factors render older adults more likely to develop heat exhaustion and heatstroke.

Mild, early signs of heat stress include feeling hot, listless, or uncomfortable. Serious indications of heat-related problems include hot, dry skin without perspiration, tachycardia, chest pain, breathing problems, throbbing headache, dizziness, profound weakness, changes in mentation, vomiting, abdominal cramps, nausea, and diarrhea.

Heat exhaustion occurs gradually and is caused by water or sodium depletion. Both active and inactive elderly people can develop heat exhaustion if they do not consume adequate fluids and electrolytes when exposed to hot environments. If heat exhaustion is not recognized and treated, it can progress to a more severe condition called **heatstroke.**

Heatstroke, which is life-threatening, results from a decreased ability to regulate body temperature, high environmental temperatures, and excessive activity. Heatstroke is a very real concern for active elderly persons, particularly those living in hot climates.

Psychologic trauma caused by falls, assaults, motor vehicle accidents, thermal events, or other injuries can be more serious than the physical trauma itself. Fear of injury often confines the elderly to their homes and can cause them to lose confidence in their ability to perform even simple actions. They may restrict their activity, thereby contributing to further loss of strength, decreased mobility, social isolation, and increased dependence. If too much function is lost, institutionalization may be necessary.

NURSING PROCESS

RISK FOR INJURY

Risk Assessment

- Does the person have a history of falls or other injuries?
- If yes, what types of injuries are most common?
- How often does the person suffer injuries?
- What is the person's level of vision? Hearing? Temperature perception?
- Does the person suffer from any memory impairment?
- Is the person forgetful?
- Does the person live alone?
- What medications does the person take?
- Does the person suffer from dizziness or fainting?
- Is the person able to follow directions?
- Does the person drive? Does he or she wear seat belts when riding in a car?
- If living at home, where does the person store his or her medications?
- Where does the person store chemicals and cleaning supplies?

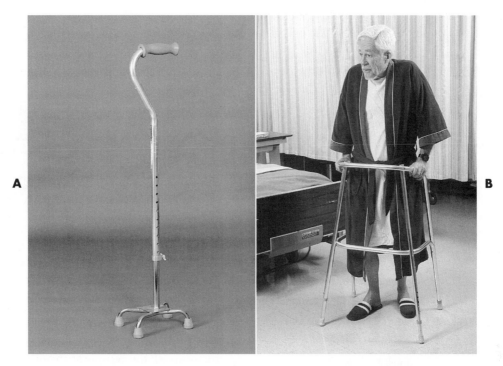

FIG. 9-1 Assistive devices promote support and safety. **A,** Quad cane. **B,** Walker. (From Sorrentino SA: *Mosby's textbook for nursing assistants,* ed 4, St. Louis, 1996, Mosby.)

Nursing Diagnoses

Risk for injury, trauma, poisoning

Nursing Goals/Outcomes

The nursing goals for an elderly person at risk for injury, trauma, or poisoning are to experience a decrease in the frequency and severity of injuries and to identify unsafe conditions and behaviors.

Nursing Interventions

The following nursing interventions are for those at risk for injury, trauma, or poisoning should take place in hospitals or extended-care facilities:

1. **Evaluate the person for the risk of falls.** Elderly individuals who experience dizziness or fainting with position changes are at increased risk for falls. These symptoms are often caused by a sudden drop in blood pressure (orthostatic hypotension). These individuals should be instructed to move slowly and to remain seated until the dizziness passes. Episodes of orthostatic hypotension are more likely to occur early in the morning, particularly before breakfast, and may be aggravated by dehydration or medications. Episodes of dizziness may have other causes and should be reported to the physician so that their cause can be determined.

   Elderly individuals should be encouraged to move at a comfortable pace and not to hurry. Hurrying increases the risk of falling. They should be encouraged to wear comfortable footwear that helps with support and balance. Assistive devices that improve stability by providing a wider base of support (e.g., canes and walkers) may be needed (Fig. 9-1).

   The call signal should be readily available whether the person is in bed or in a chair. Lounges and bathrooms should be equipped with call signals. Calls from the elderly should be answered promptly. If the elderly have to wait too long for assistance, they may attempt to stand or walk even if they know it is unsafe.

2. **Modify the environment to reduce risks.** To prevent falls resulting from visual changes, stairwells should be well illuminated. The edges of stairs, shower lips, and any other elevations should be marked using a dark or contrasting color stripe to help the aging individual recognize the edge. Hallways should have strong grip rails to provide support during ambulation (Fig. 9-2). Beds should be kept in the low position unless the caregiver is at the bedside. If the caregiver has to leave the person, even briefly, the bed should be lowered. Whenever the bed is elevated, the opposite side rail should be up to reduce the chance of falls.

   Medication carts should be locked and properly stored when not in use. Medications should never

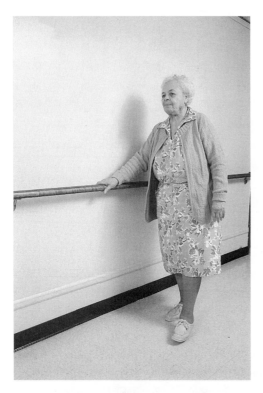

FIG. 9-2   An elderly woman using the handrails for support while walking. (From Sorrentino SA: *Mosby's textbook for nursing assistants*, ed 4, St Louis, 1996, Mosby.)

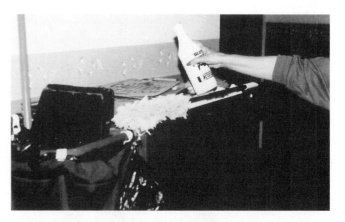

FIG. 9-3   Poisons must be kept out of reach of all residents. (From Castillo HM: *The nurse assistant in long-term care: a rehabilitative approach*, St Louis, 1992, Mosby.)

be left at the bedside unless this is permitted by the physician. Medications intended for one individual can easily be taken by a confused person who wanders into the room. Cleaning carts and supplies should also be locked in cabinet or closet when not in use (Fig. 9-3).

Use restraints with caution only when there is a documented reason for them and only after the person or his or her guardian agrees to their use. This includes use of foot pedals, vest and waist restraints, and even chair tables and safety belts. Omnibus Budget Reconciliation Act (OBRA) regulations are very specific about when and what types of restraints are permitted. Most facilities require a physician's order to use restraints.

The following interventions should take place in the home:

1. **Assess the environment for hazards and modify it to reduce the likelihood of injury.** The home environment can be dangerous for the elderly. To reduce the likelihood of poisoning, all cleaning supplies should be stored well away from food or medications. If the elderly person has impaired judgment, it may be necessary to keep all poisonous substances in a locked cabinet or closet. All medications should be labeled clearly in large letters so individuals can distinguish their names and directions.

Individuals with circulatory changes should be taught the importance of checking the temperature of bath water with a thermometer. They should not add hot water when sitting in a tub, nor should they adjust the temperature of the water while in the shower.

Aging individuals should be discouraged from climbing because falls from higher places are more likely to cause serious injury. Chairs, footstools, and other pieces of furniture are generally unsafe. If the person needs to reach a high area, a good step stool with a broad base of support should be used.

The floor should be checked for hazards such as clutter, scatter rugs, or loose carpet edges that when rolled up may trip a person. All hazardous items should be removed or fixed to reduce the risk of falls.

2. **Recruit the assistance of a family member or friend to check on the elderly person at regular intervals.** Regular visits to the home permit a quick check of the most obvious hazards. Any unsafe conditions can be corrected before an injury occurs. The nurse should review the most common concerns with the visitors so that they are more alert and aware. Although frequent checks will not always prevent injury, they can reduce the chance of an injured elderly person lying helpless for extended periods of time. Some elderly persons invest in special call signal devices that can be worn on their bodies. These call signals can be activated in case of emergency to summon help. They should only be purchased after the reputation of the company who sells and services the device has been carefully checked with an agency such as the Better Business Bureau. Many of these so-called safety systems are worthless and provide a false sense of security to the elderly.

3. **Use any appropriate interventions that are used in the institutional setting.**

Hypothermia / Hyperthermia
Assessment of thermoregulation

- What is the person's body temperature?
- How does it change throughout the day?
- Is the person inactive or excessively active?
- Does the person show any signs of infection, including behavioral changes?
- Does the person complain of feeling hot or cold?
- Does the person have any disease conditions that increase the risk of altered thermoregulation?
- Does the person suffer from electrolyte imbalance?
- Does the person consume alcohol or other temperature-altering medications?
- Does the person suffer from dementia, depression, or other conditions that decrease awareness?
- Does the individual have adequate financial resources to pay for housing that has adequate heat and ventilation?
- Does the individual have clothing suitable for the environmental conditions?

See Box 9-6 for a list of thermoregulation risks for older adults.

Nursing Diagnoses

Hypothermia, hyperthermia, risk for altered body temperature, ineffective thermoregulation

Nursing Goals/Outcomes

The nursing goals for an elderly person with hypothermia, hyperthermia, altered body temperature, or ineffective thermoregulation are to maintain core body temperature within the normal range and to state the appropriate modifications in dress, activity, and environment needed to maintain body temperature within normal limits.

Nursing Interventions

The following nursing interventions should take place in hospitals or extended-care facilities:

1. **Monitor the environmental temperature, humidity, and air movement.** Room temperature should be maintained at a comfortable level between 70° F and 75° F. Relative humidity between 40% and 60% is comfortable for most people. Ventilation should provide an exchange of air without drafts that may cause chilling.
2. **Monitor body temperature at regular intervals.** The temperature of any person at risk for hyperthermia or hypothermia should be monitored regularly. In many cases, a thermometer that registers temperatures below 95° F is needed for accurate measurement. Electronic thermometers or thermal ear sensors provide accurate temperatures when used correctly.
3. **Provide clothing and bed covers that are suitable for the environment.** Extra clothing and blankets may be necessary for inactive persons. Knit undergarments, layered clothing, bed socks, nightcaps, and flannel sheets or blankets are particularly effective at retaining body heat. In the summer, clothing should be lightweight, loose, and nonconstricting to allow adequate movement of air over the body.
4. **Promote adequate fluid and food intake.** In hot weather, the elderly person should have fresh fluids at the bedside at all times. Pitchers of a cool sugar-free beverage should be available in day rooms, activity centers, and lounges. Because the elderly may have a diminished sense of thirst, frequent reminders to drink may be necessary.
5. **Monitor activity level in accordance with environmental temperature.** Increased physical activity will help the elderly person keep warm in cool weather. Excessive activity should be avoided during hot weather, particularly during daytime hours when heat is greatest.

The following interventions should take place in the home:

1. **Verify that the residence has adequate heat in cold weather and adequate ventilation in hot weather.** Many elderly, particularly those who live alone and those with limited financial resources, live in marginal or substandard housing. Frequently there is inadequate heat to provide warmth in winter or inadequate ventilation to keep cool in the summer. If the home is poorly heated, the person should be encouraged to stay active and dress warmly. If the house is too hot or is poorly ventilated, the person could be encouraged to reduce activity and dress in cool clothing. If air-conditioned public buildings such as shopping plazas, libraries, or senior citizen centers are available, the elderly should be encouraged to spend the hottest times of day in these facilities.
2. **Identify community resources that can help the elderly maintain a safe environment.** Many public utility companies have special programs designed to ensure that the elderly have adequate heat in winter. Some also provide fans or air conditioners in the summer. Often these are available to the elderly at reduced prices. Special payment plans that spread the cost of heating or air conditioning over the year are also available in most areas of the country. Such plans can enable the elderly to budget their limited resources while maintaining a safe thermal environment.
3. **Teach good health habits.**

To prevent hyperthermia: Decrease physical activity during the daytime. Do heavy chores such as laundry early in the morning or in the evening. Perform outdoor activities after sunset. (1) Dress in light-colored, loose-fitting cotton clothing. (2) Keep out of direct sunlight—use hats, umbrellas, awnings, or other types of sunscreens to reduce sun exposure. (3) In excessive heat, take cool baths or showers several times a day, or apply cool, wet towels or ice packs to the axilla and groin. (4) Drink a minimum of 8 to 10 glasses of water or cool beverages each day *regardless of thirst*. When there are medical restrictions on fluid intake, the physician should be consulted regarding the recommended amount of intake. (5) Avoid drinking hot beverages and alcohol. (6) Eat several small meals instead of a few large ones.

To prevent hypothermia: (1) Keep the heat within the safe temperature range of 70° F to 75° F. (2) Stay active. (3) Wear several layers of clothing rather than one heavy layer. Wool, knits, and flannel are particularly warm. (4) Drink 8 to 10 glasses of fluid daily, including warm beverages. (5) Avoid consuming alcohol. (6) Eat several small, warm meals throughout the day.

4. **Use any appropriate interventions that are used in the institutional setting.**

SUMMARY

The normal physiologic changes of aging, increased incidence of chronic illness, increased use of medications, and sensory or cognitive changes place the aging population at increased risk for injury. This is particularly true when the elderly are exposed to multiple environmental hazards. The most common injuries experienced by the elderly include falls, burns, poisoning, and automobile accidents. Nurses can play an important role by helping the elderly person recognize their risk factors, by planning coping strategies to promote safety, and by modifying their environment to minimize the likelihood of injury.

READINGS AND REFERENCES

Belkin L: Nursing homes without restraints, *New York Times* 142:A1, 24 March 1993.

Brocklehurst J, Dickinson E: Autonomy for elderly people in long term care, *Age Aging* 25:329, 1996.

Brody JE: For the elderly, lights change too fast, *New York Times* 143:B7, 23 March 1994.

Campbell AJ: Drug treatment as a cause of falls in old age, *Drugs Aging* 1:289, 1991.

Carr DB: Assessing older drivers for physical and cognitive impairment, *Geriatrics* 48:46, 1993.

Carter SE, et al: Environmental hazards in the homes of older people, *Age Aging* 26:195, 1997.

Clemson L, Cumming RG, Roland M: Case control study of hazards in the home and risk of falls and hip fractures, *Age Aging* 25:97, 1996.

Crane M: How to tell patients they're too old to drive, *Med Ec* 73:115, 1996.

Cutson TM: Falls in the elderly, *Am Fam Physician* 49:149, 1994.

Driving: how safe are you behind the wheel? Mayo Clinic Health Letter 14:7, 1996.

Fleck J Web site: *Prevention of falls in the elderly: an occupational therapist's perspective,* http://hippocrates.family.med.ualb ...letter.autumn_1995/prevention.html, 1995.

Hornbrook MC, et al: Preventing falls among community dwelling older persons: results of a randomized trial, *Gerontologist* 34:16, 1994.

Horowitz A: Vision impairment and functional disability among nursing home residents, *Gerontologist* 34:316, 1994.

Loew F: The elderly can avoid falls, *World Health* p 10, Jan–Feb 1993.

National Institute on Aging Web site: Age Page: accident prevention, http://www.mfaaa.org/center/agepage/accident_pre.html, 1991.

Safety assessment reliable tool for frail elderly in nursing homes, *Brown University Long-Term Care Quality Letter,* 6:5, 1994.

Tibbitts GM: Patients who fall: how to predict and prevent injuries, *Geriatrics* 51:24, 1996.

Tideiksaar R: Preventing falls: how to identify risk factors, reduce complications, *Geriatrics* 51:43, 1996.

Tinetti ME, et al: Fear of falling and fall related efficacy in relationship to functioning among community-living elders, *J Gerontol* 49:M140, 1994.

Wiseman EJ, Souder E: The older driver: a handy tool to assess competence behind the wheel, *Geriatrics* 51:36, 1996.

MEETING NUTRITIONAL AND FLUID NEEDS

LEARNING OBJECTIVES

1. Describe methods of assessing the nutritional status and practices of older adults.
2. Identify the older adults who are most at risk for problems related to nutrition and hydration.
3. Identify selected nursing diagnoses related to nutritional or metabolic problems.
4. Identify interventions that will help elderly persons meet their nutrition and hydration needs.

Nutrition plays an important role in health maintenance, in rehabilitation, and in the prevention and control of disease (Fig. 10-1). When dealing with nutritional issues, nurses who work with older adults must consider the following: (1) How the normal physiologic changes of aging will change nutritional needs; (2) how the physiologic changes of aging may interfere with the purchase, preparation, and consumption of nutrients; (3) how the disease processes commonly seen in aging will impact nutritional needs; and (4) how psychosocial changes associated with aging may affect nutritional practices.

Good nutrition has been shown to be one of the most significant factors in the prevention of skin breakdown. Indicators of nutritional and metabolic alterations are most commonly observed in the skin, mucous membranes, hair, and nails. Assessment of these structures can indicate a great deal about an aging person's nutritional status and fluid balance.

NUTRITION AND AGING

Nutritional needs do not remain static throughout life. As with other needs, the nutritional needs of the elderly are not exactly the same as those of younger individuals. An understanding of the nutritional needs of the elderly is essential to providing good nursing care. In order to assess nutritional adequacy and select interventions that promote good nutrition, nurses must be knowledgeable about basic nutrition and diet therapy. Basic concepts related to nutrition are presented in Chapter 6. For more information, explore texts that focus on geriatric nutrition.

Good nutrition practices play a vital role in health maintenance and health promotion. Good eating habits throughout life promote physical wellness and mental well-being. Inadequate nutrition and fluid intake can result in serious problems such as malnutrition and dehydration. Poor nutrition practices can contribute to the development of osteoporosis and skin ulcers or can complicate existing conditions such as cardiovascular disease and diabetes mellitus.

Information derived from the Elderly Nutrition Program of the Older Americans Act reveals that 67% to 88% of the participants were at moderate to high nutritional risk. The greatest problems were found among frail, homebound elderly. Other studies show that 8% to 16% of older adults do not have ready access at all times to nutritionally adequate and culturally acceptable meals.

There are many reasons for inadequate nutritional intake. As with safety problems the causes can be internal or external. Internal problems include sensory changes in vision, taste, and smell; cognitive changes;

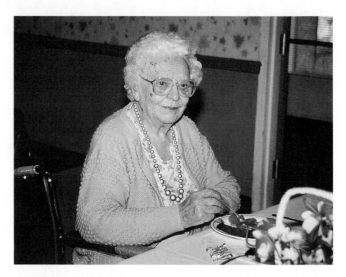

FIG. 10-1   Good nutrition plays an important role in health maintenance. (Courtesy of Michael S. Clement, MD, Mesa, Ariz.)

weakness or activity intolerance; loss of interest in food; and depression. External causes include medications and problems related to the procurement of food.

Changes in vision can make shopping and food preparation more difficult for the elderly. Even reading a simple recipe can become so difficult that it becomes too much trouble to cook. The appearance of food also has an affect on appetite. Expensive restaurants know this and serve meals that appeal to the eye as well as the taste buds. The senses of taste and smell begin to decline at approximately 60 years of age and become more pronounced with advanced age. The elderly have two to three times more difficulty detecting flavors than do young adults. These changes make foods less appealing and fats more difficult for the elderly to detect. The elderly may consume excessive amounts of relatively non-nutritious salty, sweet, or fatty foods in an attempt to detect flavors. Use of monosodium glutamate (MSG) to enhance flavors in food served to the elderly has been suggested as a way of improving appetite. MSG should be used cautiously because a percentage of the population is allergic to it.

Cognitive changes such as confusion or dementia can affect nutrition. Severely affected elderly require total assistance in meal preparation and often require feeding assistance. Without help and support they face almost certain malnutrition if not starvation. Appetite changes are common and unpredictable. Some seriously confused elderly will maintain a good appetite as long as food is provided, whereas others demonstrate little or no interest in food.

Weakness or activity intolerance increases the risk of malnourishment. Shopping, transporting food, and preparing meals require more physical endurance than many elderly persons possess. Elderly individuals suffering from cardiovascular disease, obstructive pulmonary disease, or severe arthritis are at high risk due to their physical limitations. Some compensate by using shopping services, prepared meals, or a meal service such as Meals on Wheels. Those who fail to compensate suffer serious nutritional consequences.

Depression or other emotional stress can cause anyone to lose their appetite. This is particularly true for an elderly person who is already dealing with other factors that diminish appetite. Eating alone or dining in a community setting with strangers is often not conducive to a good appetite. Pleasant surroundings and company can help lift an older person's mood and improve his or her appetite.

Medications can significantly affect appetite. Many medications cause food to have a "strange" or "metallic" taste. Some medications suppress the appetite, and others decrease saliva production so mastication is more difficult than normal. Good oral hygiene and the use of artificial saliva can help reduce these problems.

Food procurement problems include both cost and accessibility. Cost is a real factor for elderly people who live on a fixed income. As money is spent on costly medications or other more "necessary" items, less is left to purchase food. Although food stamps and meal delivery services are available to the elderly, many are unaware of these programs or are unwilling to accept such assistance. This problem is discussed more fully in Chapter 6.

Symptoms of nutritional problems include unintentional weight loss, lightheadedness, disorientation, lethargy, and loss of appetite. The same or similar symptoms often occur with a variety of illnesses, making it difficult to determine whether the primary problem is medical or nutritional in origin.

NURSING PROCESS

ALTERED NUTRITION

Changes in weight may be an early indication of actual or potential nutritional problems in the elderly. Current weight should be compared with standard height-and-weight charts that list the desirable weight for various heights (see Table 6-1). The height used should reflect the person's current height, not the height from a younger age that is commonly reported by aging individuals and recorded on their charts. If the individual appears well proportioned and if his or her weight falls within recommended norms, then the individual is probably receiving adequate calories. A slow increase or decrease in weight indicates an im-

balance between caloric intake and energy expenditure. A decrease in activity with static caloric intake normally results in gradual weight gain, whereas an increase in activity with consistent caloric intake normally results in weight loss. Nurses should investigate changes in intake or activity that could account for changes in weight (see Chapter 6).

Adequate caloric intake is not enough. It is also essential that the elderly obtain adequate amounts of essential nutrients. To determine whether these nutritional needs are being met, it is necessary to gather additional information.

Laboratory values may help support other observations. Hemoglobin level, hematocrit level, red blood cell (RBC) count, blood urea nitrogen (BUN) level, creatinine level, albumin levels, and other nutritional indices should be reviewed to determine whether specific nutritional deficiencies exist. These laboratory values can be evaluated in the same way for younger and older persons because they do not routinely change with aging (see Chapter 6).

Hemoglobin is a complex protein–iron molecule that is responsible for the transport of oxygen and carbon dioxide within the bloodstream. If inadequate iron is available, the hemoglobin level and RBC count will fall below the normal levels. Low hemoglobin levels may result from anemia or blood loss. Common forms of anemia, as discussed in Chapter 3, include iron-deficiency anemia and pernicious anemia. Iron-deficiency anemia may result from blood loss. In the elderly, this rarely takes the form of a massive hemorrhage, although a significant amount of blood may be lost from frequent nosebleeds or recent surgery. More common in the elderly is subtle blood loss from bleeding gastric or duodenal ulcers, diverticulitis, tumors, or pathology of the lower gastrointestinal tract.

The blood glucose level of a healthy person changes throughout the day. It is low during periods of fasting, but it rises after a meal and then peaks approximately 30 to 60 minutes after eating. Within 3 hours, it returns to its normal range of 80 to 120 mg/dl. Those who have diabetes, are receiving steroid therapy or total parenteral nutrition, or are experiencing high levels of stress are likely to experience problems with control of blood sugar levels.

Electrolyte imbalances may be a result of inadequate electrolyte intake or excessive loss. Abnormal levels of calcium, sodium, and potassium are most commonly observed. The diet should be assessed to see whether there is adequate intake of the necessary electrolytes. Medications that may cause electrolyte depletion should be considered. Vomiting, diarrhea, and gastric suction are likely to contribute to electrolyte imbalances.

Assessment of Nutritional Status
Weight changes

- Does the person appear noticeably overweight or underweight?
- Does the person's clothing appear abnormally loose or tight?
- What are the person's current height and weight? (Check the chart or weigh the patient if current information is not available.)
- Is the person's weight within normal limits (see Table 6-2)?
- Has the person's weight significantly increased or decreased in the past 3 to 6 months? How much has it changed?
- How long has this weight change been occurring?

Appetite changes

- What does the person say about his or her appetite?
- Does the person feel that his or her appetite has changed?
- Why does the person think this is happening?
- How does food taste to the person?
- What does the person like or dislike about the meals he or she eats (or is served)?
- What would the person prefer to eat?
- Does the person have any cultural food preferences that are not being recognized?
- Does the person have any dietary restrictions? Are they understood?
- Does the person complain of nausea or hyperacidity before, during, or after meals?
- Does the person complain of a strange taste in the mouth?
- Does the person have any feeling of chest pain after meals?
- Does the person show an unusual reaction to any foods (e.g., dairy products)?
- Does the person experience increased eructation or flatulence related to particular foods?
- Is the person depressed?

Nutritional intake

- Are the person's hemoglobin, hematocrit, and RBC parameters within normal limits?
- Has the person's blood sugar level been taken? Was this a fasting blood sugar? If taken at a non-fasting time, was it before or after a meal? How long before or after?
- Are the person's electrolyte levels (e.g., sodium, potassium, calcium) within normal limits?
- Does the person have a history of diabetes mellitus, anemia, or electrolyte imbalances?

- Are there any other observations such as pallor, dizziness, or easy fatigue that may indicate anemia?
- Does the person show any signs of hyperglycemia or hypoglycemia?
- Does the person show any signs of electrolyte imbalance?
- How are the electrolyte levels (especially potassium and sodium)?
- Is the person on a prescribed diet that restricts sodium, calorie, sugar, or fluid intake? Are there any other dietary restrictions?
- Does the person receive calcium supplements?
- Does the person drink milk and eat dairy products? (Is the person lactose intolerant?)
- Does the person receive iron supplements?
- Does the person receive any drugs that can alter electrolyte levels (e.g., diuretics or cardiotonics)?
- Has the person had any recent episodes of vomiting?
- Are there certain foods that the person never consumes? (Look particularly at meats or vegetables that may require more chewing, and compare this information to the dental status.)
- What types of foods does the person consume most? First? Not at all?
- What percentage of food in general and of each type does the person actually consume?
- What fluids does the person consume during and between meals?
- Is the person consuming snacks or supplements between meals?
- Are these snacks prescribed?
- Is the person sneaking snacks that are not allowed on a therapeutic diet?
- Does the person receive any medications that could alter the taste of food?
- When are these medications given?
- Is the person receiving any drugs that require a restricted diet (e.g., monoamine oxidase inhibitors)?

Social and cultural factors

- Does the person eat alone in his or her room, or in the dining room?
- Does the person socialize with others during meals?
- Does the person's family ever bring favorite foods from home?
- How do these favorite foods meet the individual's nutritional needs?
- Do the favorite foods violate any dietary restrictions (e.g., sodium or calorie restrictions)?

Risk Factors Related to Nutritional Intake in the Elderly

- Metabolic disorders (diabetes, thyroid disturbances)
- Neurologic or musculoskeletal problems that interfere with food preparation, eating, or swallowing
- Disturbances of the gastrointestinal tract
- Inadequate resources to obtain food
- Loss of nutrients as a result of medications, hemorrhage, vomiting, or diarrhea
- Inadequate or excessive energy because of exercise patterns or disease processes
- Living alone
- Selective eating habits related to culture or habit
- Grief or other emotional difficulties

Home care or discharge planning

- Does the person live alone or with others?
- What are the person's health management and health maintenance abilities?
- If the person lives at home, does he or she have adequate food in the house?
- Does the person have adequate financial resources to buy food?
- Can the person get to a store to purchase food?
- Does the person have family or friends who will assist with going to the grocery store?
- Can the person prepare the food, or do problems with vision, stamina, or coordination interfere?
- Does the person tire too easily, so that by the time the food is prepared he or she is too tired to eat?
- Does the person have adequate equipment for refrigeration and cooking?
- Is the person aware of community resources for nutrition (e.g., Meals on Wheels, senior citizen center meal programs)?

See Box 10-1 for a list of risk factors for problems related to nutritional intake.

Nursing Diagnoses

Altered nutrition: less than body requirements
Altered nutrition: risk for more than body requirements
Altered nutrition: more than body requirements

Nursing Goals/Outcomes

The nursing goals for elderly individuals diagnosed with some form of altered nutrition are (1) to maintain body weight within normal limits for height; (2) to obtain adequate nutrients to maintain healthy tissue; (3) to identify internal and external cues that influence eating patterns; and (4) to adhere to a prescribed therapeutic diet.

Nursing Interventions

The following nursing interventions should take place in hospitals or extended-care facilities:

1. **Assess the individual carefully to determine the causes of a problem (e.g., dental problems, depression, cultural factors, activity level).** The types of approaches used by nurses will vary with the type and extent of the problem.
2. **Schedule weekly weight checks.** Weight changes related to nutritional intake do not occur rapidly as they do with fluid imbalance. Often there are daily weight fluctuations. Weighing an elderly person too often can cause frustration. Weekly weight checks are more reliable indicators of success.
3. **Keep a dietary record of the amount, type, and frequency of food intake.** A careful dietary record will help nurses and the elderly to determine problem areas, which will help nurses and dietitians develop a dietary plan that is most likely to have the desired outcome. When possible, older adults should be actively involved in this record keeping.
4. **Explain the importance of nutrition to overall health or disease control.** Many elderly individuals are already aware of normal nutritional needs. If the changes related to aging or disease require dietary modifications, it is important that the modifications and the reasons behind them be explained carefully to the individual. If older adults understand the rationale of dietary changes, they are more likely to cooperate with the new plan.
5. **Determine food likes and dislikes.** People tend to seek the things they like and avoid what they do not like. Knowledge of food preferences can be used when selecting nutritious yet acceptable foods for the elderly. Many elderly individuals are set in their likes and dislikes and are unwilling to change late in life.
6. **Monitor laboratory values.** RBC parameters, hematocrit, and hemoglobin values will help determine whether iron intake is adequate. Electrolyte levels should be monitored to verify that they are within normal limits.
7. **Assess the condition of the skin, hair, nails, and mucous membranes.** Signs of nutritional inadequacy can be detected by observation of external surfaces. Cracks at the corner of the mouth, changes in the appearance of the tongue, loss or change in consistency of the hair, and slow tissue healing provide clues to nutritional status.

8. **Consult with the dietitian.** Dietitians are specially trained to assess nutritional needs and have in-depth knowledge of the nutritional value of foods. If an aging individual has serious nutritional problems or medical conditions with nutritional implications, it is essential that the dietitian be actively involved in the nutritional plan of care.

9. **Institute measures to increase or decrease nutritional intake.**

To increase intake

Provide a selection of nutritious foods. Nurses should attempt to provide choices for those who are most in need of nutrients. Many institutions, particularly long-term care facilities, have limited menus for each meal. If the meal served does not appeal to aging individuals, they may eat very little if at all. Most institutions have alternatives that do not appear on the menu, usually including simple foods such as eggs, cheese sandwiches, or soup. The elderly individual may not be aware of these choices or may not wish to cause additional work for the staff. It is the nurse's responsibility to explore these options with the individual.

Supplement food intake with nutritious snacks. It is often difficult for the elderly to consume adequate calories and nutrients within the three routine daily meals. If allowed within the prescribed diet, nutritious snacks that are high in calories and nutrients (e.g., bananas, graham crackers, dried fruits, or milkshakes) can be offered between meals. These snacks should be scheduled so that they do not interfere with the person's appetite for regular meals. Many elderly individuals like to "stash" snacks in the bedside stand or closet. Nurses can ensure that snacks are not stored where they can spoil or attract insects. Any snacks that are not consumed promptly should be discarded.

Ask the person's family to bring his or her favorite dishes from home. Family favorites are rarely on the menu in an institutional setting. Special favorites and foods connected with fond memories are most likely to be consumed by the elderly. Before the family brings food, however, nurses should be sure to discuss the care plan with them to ensure that these foods are permitted. It is very frustrating for the family to make a special effort, only to have the meal rejected at the institution.

Serve meals in an attractive manner. Foods that are well prepared and served in an attractive manner are more appealing. Taking plates and cups off of the tray or setting a table with placemats and flowers can improve the appearance of a meal. Serving food on fancier dishes, using a special teacup, or making an effort to reduce the institutional character of the food can help improve appetite (Fig. 10-2). Foods should always be served fresh and at the appropriate temperature.

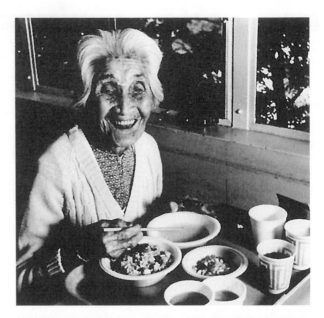

FIG. 10-2 Chopsticks and oriental food make the meal enjoyable for this elderly Japanese woman. (Courtesy of Ken Yamaguchi. In Castillo HM: *The nurse assistant in long-term care: a rehabilitative approach,* St Louis, 1992, Mosby.)

Provide a social environment for meals by encouraging the elderly to eat in the dining room. The nature of meals tends to be social. Aging individuals often have better appetites when eating in groups than when isolated in individual rooms. Alert individuals should be grouped with other alert people. Noise and distraction from confused patients can be disturbing and can decrease appetite. Separate seatings or rooms can provide the best environment, depending on the needs of the individual. Many elderly individuals living in institutional settings make friends with whom they prefer to sit. Aging individuals should have the opportunity to seek mutually agreeable seating arrangements in dining rooms without staff interference. If significant others are present at mealtime, they may want to eat with the elderly individual. Some institutions will provide special trays or bag lunches for guests at a nominal charge.

Prepare food by opening cartons, buttering toast, or performing other activities that may be difficult for the elderly person. Problems setting up food and opening cartons may lead the elderly to skip or avoid certain foods. Many containers are difficult to open—even healthy young adults can have difficulty. These should be opened with minimum fuss so that the aging person does not feel helpless. Assistance in getting the individual ready to eat by cutting meats or buttering bread should be done unobtrusively.

Avoid hurrying the individual during meals. If an elderly person eats too rapidly, indigestion, heartburn, or regurgitation may result. If rushed, many elderly individuals will stop eating before they are truly satisfied. Avoid a rushed environment, and allow adequate time for the elderly to eat at their own pace.

Request a modification in the form of food served if the individual has difficulty chewing. It may be difficult for older adults to chew some foods, particularly meats and undercooked vegetables. Chopped or ground meat is easier to eat for people with dentures or missing teeth. The dietary department should be notified about these modifications, and the physician should be contacted if an order is required. If the person is alert, pureed foods should be avoided because of their similarity to baby food (unless the individual has *severe* trouble chewing). If vegetables are routinely a problem, dicing or additional cooking may help. The dietary department should be contacted if problems are detected.

Provide assistive devices such as plate sides, gripper spoons, adaptive cups. Most elderly prefer to feed themselves whenever possible. An occupational therapist should be consulted regarding utensils that enable aging individuals to eat without undue difficulty.

Provide oral hygiene before meals. There are normal decreases in taste and saliva production with aging. The decrease in saliva production reduces the normal cleansing mechanism within the mouth, leading to a buildup of debris and microorganisms that alter the taste of food and decrease the appetite. Good oral hygiene will freshen the mouth and make food taste better.

Assist the individual to the toilet before meals. Many elderly have less awareness of the need to eliminate. If the need to eliminate occurs during mealtime, the person may become distracted and lose interest in the meal.

Provide supplemental tube feedings, if ordered. Supplemental gastric or nasogastric tube feedings are ordered for individuals who cannot consume adequate nutrients by eating. These supplemental feedings should be given only after the individual has had adequate opportunity for oral intake. All attempts at oral feeding should be made *before* the supplement is given. If nasogastric feeding is required, all safety precautions (including checks for tube placement and positioning) should be taken.

Time the administration of medications so that they do not interfere with meals. Some medications leave a bad taste in the mouth or otherwise upset the individual. If possible, these medications should be scheduled away from normal mealtimes.

Refer individuals for special counseling if emotional difficulties are interfering with appetite. Individuals with extreme grief and emotional disturbances may require special nutritional approaches. Therapists trained to deal with eating disorders should be consulted to determine the most effective interventions.

To decrease intake

Assist in the selection of low-calorie foods. Decreasing caloric intake will help the person lose weight. Foods high in bulk and low in calories such as fresh fruits and vegetables provide a sense of fullness without a sense of deprivation.

Plan low-calorie snacks into the daily routine. Snacks such as diet beverages and unbuttered popcorn are appropriate for elderly individuals unless they have a medical condition that contraindicates their inclusion. The sodium content of "diet" beverages should be checked if the person is on a sodium-restricted diet. Individuals with diverticulitis should avoid corn with husks. Planned snacks can actually prevent mealtime overeating and consumption of high-calorie snacks if they are part of the aging person's dietary habits.

Increase diversional activities to decrease snacking. Some older and younger people snack when they are bored. Activities that occupy the hands and mind may reduce the urge to eat.

Encourage increased activity levels. Increased activity helps burn calories. Walking is an exercise tolerated well by most elderly individuals, and it is effective as a means of weight reduction.

10. **Complete a thorough documentation of nutritional status, including assessment, interventions, referrals, and patient response.**

The following interventions should take place in the home:

1. **Assist the individual in obtaining resources such as Meals on Wheels, food stamps, a housekeeper, or shopping services.** Many community agencies and programs have been developed to help the elderly meet their nutritional needs. Each community has different services available. Social workers often maintain directories of these agencies and can help the elderly establish contact with them. Nurses can clarify and explain the available programs and provide the means for the elderly or their families to contact the agencies.

2. **Involve the family in shopping and meal planning.** If the elderly person is unable to meet his or her nutritional needs without assistance, the family can often provide help. Elderly individuals are often too proud to ask for help, even from their own families. With help from a nurse, the elderly person may be willing to accept this assistance. Family members can provide transportation to the store, can read labels, and can assist with food preparation. Variety can be provided through meals prepared and then frozen in family members' homes for the elderly person's use. Family members should be taught about their loved one's relevant dietary restrictions so that meals do not endanger his or her well-being.

3. **Identify senior citizen meal programs available in**

the community. Many communities offer meals at churches or senior citizen centers. These meals are prepared by dietitians who are well versed in the nutritional needs of the aging population. These inexpensive meals provide the opportunity for social interaction.

4. **Use any appropriate interventions that are used in the institutional setting.**

NURSING PROCESS

ALTERATIONS IN FLUID VOLUME

Fluid balance is not a problem in healthy older adults. However, if there is a sudden change in fluid volume, an elderly person is more likely to experience significant problems than is a younger person. A seemingly minor problem with fluid balance can quickly become a serious concern in an aging individual. If not detected and treated, dehydration can easily become a significant problem, possibly resulting in death. The very old, blacks, and men are most likely to experience dehydration.

The elderly have a lower percentage of body fluid (approximately 45% lower), than younger persons, even when they are well hydrated. Anything that restricts adequate intake of fluids or causes the body to lose water excessively can contribute to the risk of dehydration.

Common risk factors include (1) a decreased thirst sensation; (2) decreased effectiveness of the kidney at concentrating urine; (3) hormonal changes including decreased aldosterone secretion and renin activity; (4) side effects of medications; (5) altered level of mentation; (6) altered levels of functional ability; and (7) fear of incontinence or pain leading to inappropriate fluid restriction.

As at younger ages, elderly men have a higher percentage of body fluid than do elderly women. The decrease in the kidneys' concentrating ability reduces the body's ability to adapt to changes in fluid volume. The aging body is less able to respond rapidly to fluid volume changes. When the many diseases that affect fluid balance are added to the normal changes of aging, maintaining fluid balance becomes a challenge.

Body fluids are distributed into two major compartments: the intracellular and the extracellular compartments. **Intracellular fluid** is found within the cells and comprises about two thirds of the total body fluid. Extracellular fluid (ECF) comprises about one third of the total body fluid. ECFs are further classified as **intravascular** (plasma) and **interstitial fluids.** ECF is in constant motion throughout the body, carrying nutrients to the cells and removing waste products. The movement of body fluids is affected by the levels of various electrolytes and proteins in the various compartments. Albumin, an important plasma protein responsible for maintaining adequate intravascular fluid levels, is frequently deficient, contributing to tissue edema and orthostatic hypotension.

Although the intracellular fluid is affected when the body experiences fluid imbalance, the ECF changes most rapidly and significantly. ECF deficit, or fluid volume deficit, can result in hypovolemia or dehydration. ECF excess, or fluid volume excess, can result in hypervolemia (circulatory overload) or edema (excessive fluid in the interstitial spaces).

Assessment of Fluid Volume

- What are the vital signs (i.e., blood pressure, pulse, respiration, temperature)?
- What is the appearance of the skin? Is it moist? Dry?
- What is the skin turgor? Skin temperature?
- Does the individual complain of thirst? Weakness?
- Does the individual manifest any mood changes, such as restlessness or confusion?
- What is the fluid intake per nursing shift? Per day?
- Is the person receiving fluids through non-oral routes such as nasogastric feeding or intravenous fluid therapy?
- How does this individual's fluid intake compare with the recommended intake?
- Is the person's weight changing rapidly? Is it increasing? Decreasing?
- Is the urine output within normal limits?
- What is the color and consistency of the urine? What is its specific gravity?
- Is there excessive fluid loss through hemorrhage, wound drains, gastric suction, diaphoresis, or mouth breathing?
- Does the person complain about the fit of rings, shoes, or other clothing? Are they too loose or too tight?
- Is the person receiving medication that is likely to cause fluid retention or loss?
- Are laboratory values within normal limits (hemoglobin, hematocrit, electrolytes, BUN, creatinine)?

See Boxes 10-2 and 10-3 for lists of risks for fluid volume deficit or excess in the elderly.

Fluid volume deficit

Fluid volume deficit occurs when an individual has inadequate intake or excessive loss of fluids. A wide variety of conditions can contribute to fluid volume deficit in the elderly.

BOX 10-2

Risk Factors for Fluid Volume Deficit in the Elderly

- Altered swallow reflex (stroke victims)
- Nausea and an unwillingness to eat or drink
- Acute emotional distress and decreased interest in personal needs
- Inability to obtain adequate fluids without assistance (bedridden patients)
- Altered cognition (Alzheimer's disease or dementia) and lack of awareness of the need for fluids
- Draining wounds, open sores, or ulcers
- Diuretic medications
- Kidney disease
- Tube feedings of low-sodium preparations

BOX 10-3

Risk Factors for Fluid Volume Excess in the Elderly

- Increased fluid intake secondary to excess sodium intake, hyperglycemia, or medications
- Compulsive water-drinking
- Decreased urine output secondary to kidney dysfunction
- Heart failure
- Insufficient protein intake or excessive protein loss
- Steroid therapy
- A history of alcoholism or liver disease
- Kidney disease
- Diaphoresis
- Intermittent or persistent vomiting
- Intermittent or persistent diarrhea

Individuals experiencing fluid volume deficit are likely to manifest dry mucous membranes, thirst, decreased skin turgor, rapid weight loss, weakness, and decreased volume or increased concentration of urine. Vital signs are likely to be affected. An increase in heart rate and decrease in pulse pressure can indicate a decrease in fluid volume. Hypotension, and particularly orthostatic hypotension, are common. An increase in body temperature may indicate dehydration. Blood studies are likely to change with fluid volume deficit. Hematocrit normally increases as the blood plasma level decreases. Electrolyte levels, creatinine, and BUN are likely to be altered.

Fluid volume excess

Fluid volume excess can result from excessive intake or inadequate elimination of fluids.

A primary indication of fluid volume excess is **edema,** which may manifest as swelling of dependent extremities and increased abdominal girth. Pulmonary edema may result in shortness of breath, dyspnea, cough, gurgling sounds on respiration, and frothy sputum. Because fluid intake exceeds fluid output, weight gain can be sudden and dramatic. The amount of weight gained reflects the amount of fluid being retained. One liter of fluid results in a 1-kg weight gain. Skin over edematous areas may appear shiny and taut. The amount of and the concentration of urine produced are likely to change with fluid volume excess. Hematocrit normally decreases as the blood plasma level increases. Electrolyte levels, creatinine, and BUN are also likely to be altered. The individual may experience behavioral changes, including restlessness and anxiety.

Nursing Diagnoses

Fluid volume deficit
Risk for fluid volume deficit
Fluid volume excess

Nursing Goals/Outcomes

The nursing goals for elderly individuals with or at risk for fluid volume deficit or excess are (1) to manifest vital signs within normal limits or limits specified by the physician; (2) to evidence moist oral mucous membranes and good skin turgor without evidence of edema; (3) to maintain a stable weight within normal limits; (4) to exhibit balanced fluid intake and output; (5) to report no problems related to thirst or weakness; (6) to exhibit blood studies within normal limits (hemoglobin, hematocrit, serum electrolytes, BUN, and creatinine); (7) to verbalize an understanding of the recommended dietary and fluid intake; (8) to demonstrate behaviors necessary to maintain appropriate fluid intake; (9) to demonstrate selection of appropriate foods and fluids; (10) to verbalize an understanding of prescribed medication(s), including the frequency and any precautions; and (11) to verbalize signs and symptoms that should be reported to the physician.

Nursing Interventions

The following nursing interventions should take place in hospitals or extended-care facilities:

1. **Complete a thorough assessment.** A thorough assessment is necessary to determine the presence and severity of any problems related to fluid intake.

2. **Monitor vital signs.** Vital signs can change in response to changes in fluid volume. Orthostatic hypotension is more common in individuals who have inadequate fluid intake.
3. **Monitor intake and output.** Any individual with an actual or potential fluid imbalance should be placed on "I&O" (intake and output measurement). Shift and daily totals should be calculated and compared with previous totals. It is essential that all individuals who provide care know how to measure intake and output correctly. All caregivers should be aware that the individual is on intake and output so that all fluids are recorded. If family members assist with feeding, they should be taught how to record fluid intake. Keeping intake and output sheets in a convenient place will help ensure prompt recording. Too often, intake and output are monitored in a careless manner and the data collected are meaningless.
4. **Monitor laboratory values.** Shifts in hemoglobin, hematocrit, BUN, creatinine, albumin, or electrolytes may precede or may be a result of fluid imbalance. These changes should be reported promptly.
5. **Weigh the patient daily before breakfast.** Weights measured at a consistent time of day are the most accurate for comparison. The individual should be weighed each day wearing the same clothing. The same scale should be used consistently, and it should be checked for accuracy at regular intervals. Consistency is essential to eliminate errors in readings. Daily weight checks should be recorded promptly on the appropriate record.
6. **Measure changes in girth of body parts such as legs and abdomen.** Measurements should be taken at a consistent spot each day. A small ink mark can be made on the skin so that all staff will measure consistently. Retained fluid (edema) will increase girth; fluid loss will result in decreased girth.
7. **Maintain adequate fluid intake.**

To increase intake

Offer smaller amounts of fluid at more frequent intervals. Small amounts of fluids taken frequently add up to significant fluid intake. Fluids should be offered, or the individual should be reminded to take a drink every 30 to 60 minutes throughout the day.

Keep preferred beverages at the bedside. Many elderly have distinct preferences regarding the type and temperature of beverages they like. Because people are most likely to consume foods and fluids that they like, nurses should find out what is preferred.

Use smaller containers such as medication cups or small juice glasses when offering beverages. Small beverage containers are less intimidating than large containers.

An elderly person can often be coaxed into drinking four or five medicine cups of liquid (120 to 150 ml) far more easily than they can be persuaded to drink a glassful.

Keep beverages easily available for individuals who are not in their rooms (e.g., in day rooms, activity rooms, lounges, or other common areas). Low-sodium, low-sugar beverages are ideal because individuals on restricted diets can consume them. Making beverages easily accessible will remind and encourage individuals to drink. Passing a tray of assorted beverages around an area where several elderly are congregated can encourage social interchange and provide mutual encouragement for many to participate even when they might otherwise have refused.

Encourage the intake of foods with a high fluid content such as fruits, vegetables, soups, and cream cereals. Significant amounts of fluid are contained in these foods. Individuals who have difficulty drinking liquids can obtain significant amounts of fluid through these alternative sources.

Administer nasogastric, gastric, or parenteral fluids as ordered by the physician.

Individuals who cannot drink adequate fluids may need supplemental fluids administered by other routes. All fluid given by gastric or parenteral route must be counted as fluid intake.

To decrease intake

Avoid keeping fluids at the bedside. If fluids are easily available, the elderly are likely to consume them too freely.

Offer frequent oral hygiene. When fluids are restricted, saliva production will decrease and the mucous membranes will feel dry and uncomfortable. Thick, tenacious secretions can build up in the mouth if not removed regularly. Frequent oral hygiene is needed to compensate for the lack of oral fluids and diminished saliva production.

Provide lozenges or hard candy. Sucking on a hard lozenge stimulates the release of saliva. Candy and lozenges should only be given to those who are alert enough not to swallow or choke on them. Verify that there is no dietary prohibition to additional sugar intake.

Plan a schedule that distributes limited fluids throughout the day. The total fluid volume intake for the day should be planned within the prescribed limitations. The total can then be divided into appropriate amounts spaced throughout the day. For example, a 600-ml restriction could be divided into 12 servings of 50 ml offered at hourly intervals between 8:00 AM and 8:00 PM. This prevents the person from consuming all of their allowance too early in the day and then having to withstand long periods of thirst or to exceed pre-scribed limits.

Limit the quantity of foods that are high in fluid content. Fluids contained in solid foods can contribute to fluid volume excess and edema. Foods such as fresh fruits and vegetables have a high fluid content, whereas foods such as breads, dried fruits, and cooked meats have a lower fluid content.

8. **Administer medications as ordered by the physician.** Many individuals with fluid imbalances receive medication to prevent or correct this problem. Nurses must ensure that these medications are given on time and that the patient's response to the medications is assessed.

9. **Refer to the dietitian, if appropriate.** Individuals with medical conditions that are likely to cause excessive fluid loss or fluid retention will need detailed and specific diet modifications and instructions, which are best provided by a specialist. Nurses should reinforce this teaching.

10. **Provide appropriate skin care.** Persons with fluid volume excess or deficit require careful hygiene. Both dry, fragile skin and edematous tissue are highly susceptible to breakdown. The person's physical position should be changed frequently. Care should be taken when moving or handling the skin.

11. **Report and document significant findings promptly.** The signs and symptoms of fluid volume problems rarely occur suddenly. Rather, these problems tend to develop over time. Nurses must be sure that all changes are documented and reported promptly to the nurse in charge and/or to the physician.

The following interventions should take place in the home:

1. **Complete a thorough assessment.** A thorough assessment is necessary to determine the presence and severity of any problems. It may be necessary to bring a scale, measuring tape, and sphygmomanometer to the home in order to complete a good assessment.

2. **Teach the individual and his or her family members how to monitor fluid intake.** The individual and the family must be aware of methods used to keep track of fluid intake and loss. The family should learn to measure fluid intake using common household containers, and they should be taught to read cartons for fluid content. It is easier for laypersons to learn to keep track of fluid intake in terms of ounces than in terms of milliliters. A specimen pan or urinal should be provided to measure output.

3. **Promote wellness by reviewing the prescribed dietary and fluid intake with the individual.** It is im-portant that the individual understand the reason for consuming or avoiding certain foods and fluids. The importance of adequate fluid intake, particularly during hot weather, should be stressed. Individuals with no acute problems should be advised to consume a minimum of 64 ounces (2000 ml) of fluid each day. Those who live alone may need reminders to consume this amount. Fluid intake reminders are particularly important during hot weather when increased amounts of fluid are lost through perspiration.

4. **Explain methods of increasing or decreasing fluid intake.**

To increase intake

Develop a schedule for fluid intake. A planned schedule using a time list or clock will help to remind elderly persons, as well as their spouse or caregiver, to consume fluids at regular times. It will also help them keep track of how much fluid is being consumed. They should be encouraged to check off or write amounts next to the times so they are aware of making progress.

Post signs in the kitchen and other rooms reminding the individual to drink. Reminders will help the elderly remember the importance of drinking adequate amounts of fluid.

Encourage friends and family to visit and share a beverage with the individual. Social contact and sharing are natural over a cup of coffee, soda, juice, or other beverage. This is a pleasant way to promote social interaction and encourage fluid intake at the same time.

Encourage the use of fruit or other foods with high fluid content.

To decrease intake

Develop a schedule that spreads the limited amount of fluid throughout the day.

Encourage the use of hard candy or lozenges to keep the mouth moist.

Recommend frequent oral hygiene.

Discuss the importance of avoiding foods with high fluid content.

5. **Discuss signs and symptoms that should be reported promptly to the physician.** Fluid imbalance may result in hospitalization and serious complications. This is particularly important for elderly individuals who are receiving medications that influence fluid balance. The individual should know what signs and symptoms are important. A written list of symptoms should be given to the individual and to his or her significant others.

6. **Use any appropriate interventions that are used in the institutional setting.**

NURSING PROCESS

ALTERATIONS IN SWALLOWING

Chewing and swallowing are complex processes that involve coordinated movements of the oral cavity, pharynx, larynx, and esophagus. An individual who is unable to coordinate these movements will experience difficulty swallowing, or **dysphagia**. Dysphagia is often a result of abnormal muscle contraction, infection, scar tissue, cancer, or dental conditions. Problems related to eating, and particularly problems related to swallowing, are serious because they can lead to dehydration, malnutrition, or aspiration.

Neurologic damage due to disease or trauma that affects the cranial nerves or facial muscles places older adults at risk of swallowing difficulties. Elderly individuals with altered consciousness or severe fatigue are also at risk. Some individuals who are capable of swallowing may be hesitant to do so because of a lack of desire to eat or because of fear after an episode of choking.

Assessment of Swallowing Ability

- Is there any history of stroke or other neurologic disease that could interfere with chewing or swallowing?
- Is the individual alert and able to follow directions?
- Do you observe any facial drooping or difficulty chewing?
- Do you observe or does the person report difficulty swallowing?
- Does the person complain of something sticking in the throat?
- Does the person cough, choke, or drool when eating?
- Does the person complain of hoarseness or dry throat?
- Does the person store food in the cheek pockets?
- Is the person's gag reflex weak or absent?
- Can the person close his or her lips?
- Does the person experience problems with any particular foods or fluids?

See Box 10-4 for a list of risk factors associated with problems with swallowing in the elderly.

Nursing Diagnosis

Impaired swallowing

BOX 10-4

Risk Factors for Problems with Swallowing in the Elderly

- Neurologic problems that result in paralysis or weakness of the face, mouth, or throat
- Altered level of consciousness, awareness, or sensation
- Mechanical devices such as a tracheostomy tube or nasogastric tube
- A narrowing or obstruction of the pharynx or esophagus
- Excessive fatigue

Nursing Goals/Outcomes

The nursing goals for an elderly individual diagnosed with impaired swallowing are to (1) pass food from mouth to stomach without aspiration; (2) maintain adequate nutrition and hydration; and (3) maintain or achieve appropriate body weight.

Nursing Interventions

The following nursing interventions should take place in hospitals or extended-care facilities:

1. **Assess the individual to determine his or her unique problems and needs.** All swallowing disorders are not the same. Different approaches must be developed based on the individual's specific problems and needs.
2. **Consult with the speech therapist, occupational therapist, and dietitian to develop a dysphagia program.** These specialists have unique knowledge of the best techniques and methods for dealing with swallowing disorders. It is important for nurses to use their expertise when developing a feeding plan. Special adaptive equipment (e.g., special spoons) is often used to deliver food to the back of the throat where it is more easily swallowed. Special cups that allow the elderly individual to drink without tipping the head back are frequently used.
3. **Verify that dentures fit properly and maintain good oral hygiene.** Improperly fitted dentures can slip in the mouth, causing increased problems with swallowing. A dentist should be consulted if this is the problem. Good oral hygiene enhances the appetite and removes any old food or foreign materials that may interfere with swallowing.
4. **Position the person with head upright and the chin flexed slightly forward to facilitate swallowing. Help with head control if necessary.** Whenever possible, the elderly should be seated

in a chair for meals. If they must remain in bed, the head of the bed should be raised as high as possible. Malpositioning of the head can interfere with the ability to swallow. Excessive flexion or hyperextension of the neck can interfere with passage of food through the pharynx and into the esophagus. If a pillow is used for positioning, it should be placed behind the shoulder, not behind the head, which would interfere with swallowing. Individuals with swallowing problems should remain seated upright for at least 30 minutes after a meal to reduce the likelihood of aspiration.

5. **Encourage rest periods before meals.** Eating requires a great deal of effort from individuals with swallowing disorders. Providing rest before meals helps to increase the amount of energy and strength available.

6. **Allow adequate time for meals.** Hurrying a meal increases the risk of aspiration. Elderly persons with swallowing difficulties are even more likely to have problems if they try to swallow too quickly.

7. **Start with small amounts of food and thickened fluids.** Individuals with swallowing difficulties should be given a moderate amount of food (about 15 to 20 ml at a time). This amount is enough for the individual to detect the presence of food, but it is not so much that it is difficult to swallow. Individuals with swallowing disorders have a great deal of difficulty controlling and swallowing liquids. Therefore foods that have a high fluid content are necessary to ensure adequate fluid intake. Many facilities add a thickening agent to flavored beverages to turn them into a gelatinous form that is more easily managed by persons with impaired swallowing. Water is not usually given to individuals with swallowing disorders. Because water has no texture or taste, the individual may not be aware of its presence in the mouth and may aspirate it.

8. **Place foods into the unaffected or stronger side of the mouth.** The individual will be able to detect food more easily on this side.

9. **Present foods in an appealing manner.** The appearance of food affects the appetite. Even if its consistency is altered (ground or pureed), it should be served as pleasantly as possible. Foods should not be stirred together in an unappealing mixture. Each food should remain identifiable and served to the individual in the preferred order.

10. **Select foods based on taste, texture, temperature, and fluid content.** Individuals with swallowing disorders may have altered senses of taste, texture, and temperature. Foods that have distinct flavors and textures such as apple sauce are accepted more readily than are nondescript, pureed foods.

Seasonings and spices can be used to enhance the flavor of many foods. The food should have some consistency; however, foods that require chewing are not advised. Food should be served at a temperature that will not burn the mucous membranes of the mouth. Many individuals with swallowing disorders cannot sense temperature adequately. A variety of temperatures will make the person more aware of the presence of food.

11. **Ensure that the lips are closed by applying slight pressure or stroking.** It is almost impossible to swallow when the lips are open. To prevent aspiration it may be necessary to close the lips mechanically.

12. **Stimulate swallowing by stroking the side of the neck, and support the weakened side if appropriate.** Stroking the neck stimulates the urge to swallow. Supporting the muscles of the affected side of the throat can enhance swallowing.

13. **Give frequent verbal cues.** Individuals with swallowing difficulties may not remember to swallow when food is in the mouth. Some are able to swallow if they are reminded to do so.

14. **Reduce distractions.** The process of eating requires the full attention of the affected individual and the caregiver. Distractions such as television or visitors may interfere with concentration and lead to increased problems.

15. **Keep suction equipment available in case of problems.** When giving oral feedings to an individual with a swallowing disorder, it is wise to keep a suction apparatus nearby. Most of these people also have problems with other protective reflexes such as the gag and cough reflexes. They may be unable to clear an airway obstruction. The suction machine should be readily available because delay may lead to aspiration or more serious consequences.

16. **Provide oral hygiene before and after feedings.** Individuals with swallowing disorders are likely to retain food particles in the mouth, leading to altered taste. Good oral hygiene before and after meals will remove debris and tenacious saliva and might improve the person's appetite.

17. **Administer tube feedings as ordered by the physician to individuals who are unable to achieve adequate oral intake.** Some individuals with swallowing disorders may not be able to eat enough to meet their nutritional needs. These individuals will require feeding through either a nasogastric or gastric feeding tube. Tube feedings may be used to meet the total nutritional needs of the elderly or they may be given as a supplement for those who need additional fluid or calories. If the feeding is supplemental, it should be given

after the individual has had the opportunity to take as much oral nutrition as possible. These feedings are not meant as a time-saving method to replace oral feedings.

The following interventions should take place in the home:

1. **Use any appropriate interventions that are used in the institutional setting.**

NURSING PROCESS

RISK FOR ASPIRATION

Aspiration, the inhalation of solids or liquids into the upper respiratory tract, is a serious problem for many infirm elderly. Risk for aspiration is increased with gastroesophageal reflux problems. Symptoms are discussed in Chapter 3.

Assessment of Risk for Aspiration

- Does the person have cough and gag reflexes?
- Does the person have a reduced level of consciousness?
- Does the person have a tracheostomy?
- Is the person in the supine position during feedings?
- Is the person receiving feedings or medications through gastric tubes?
- Does the person have signs of abdominal distention?
- Are the person's stomach contents more than 150 ml before a scheduled feeding?
- Is there any noise with respiration?
- Is there a productive cough? What is the consistency of the sputum?
- Are the pulse and respiratory rates elevated?

See Box 10-5 for a list of risk factors for aspiration in the elderly.

Nursing Diagnosis

Risk for aspiration

BOX 10-5

Risk Factors for Aspiration in the Elderly

- Neurologic problems, particularly those that affect the cough and/or gag reflexes
- A reduced level of consciousness
- Continuous supine positioning
- Tracheostomy tubes
- Gastric tubes
- Decreased gastric motility, excessive amounts of residual gastric contents, or gas

---

Nursing Goals/Outcomes

The nursing goals for an elderly individual at risk for aspiration are to remain remain free from episodes of aspiration and maintain clear, noiseless breath sounds.

Nursing Interventions

The following nursing interventions should take place in hospitals or extended-care facilities:

1. **Position the person appropriately.** The person should be positioned in a Fowler's or semi-Fowler's position before both oral and gastric tube feedings. This position should be maintained for at least 30 to 45 minutes after each feeding. Elevating the head allows solutions to flow into the stomach and reduces the chance of regurgitation. If the person must remain flat in bed, a side-lying position is better than a supine position.

2. **Assess for stomach distention.** Stomach distention can be an indication of slow gastric emptying, which can lead to regurgitation and aspiration. Continued complaints of gastric fullness or excessive stomach gas should be monitored carefully and reported. If these problems persist, the amount or type of feeding may need to be changed.

3. **Avoid feeding too rapidly.** Rapid ingestion of food increases the likelihood of regurgitation and aspiration. Oral nourishment should be offered slowly, and adequate time should be allowed for chewing and swallowing.

4. **Avoid liquids and pureed foods.** Semisolid foods are less likely to be aspirated than are liquids or pureed foods. The consistency of liquids can be modified with commercial preparations that are available in most dietary departments.

5. **Monitor respiratory sounds and respiratory rate, and observe the amount and type of sputum produced.** Aspiration of food or fluids may result in coughing, choking, dyspnea, and respiratory distress. Increased amounts of frothy sputum are often noted. If the person has a tracheostomy, feeding solutions should be tinted with blue food coloring. If secretions removed during respiratory suctioning reveal a blue color, aspiration has occurred.

6. **Keep suction equipment available.** Aspiration can result in respiratory distress. Suction equipment should be kept on hand whenever feeding an individual at risk for aspiration.

7. **Consult with specialists such as speech therapists and dietitians.** A team approach to swallowing disorders and potential aspiration can help reduce the likelihood of problems. Speech therapists often have special training in swallowing disorders and can suggest modifications in feeding practices. Dietitians are specially trained to meet the needs of

---

NURSING CARE PLAN

NUTRITIONAL-METABOLIC

Mr. Thomas is a 74-year-old man who recently suffered a stroke. His level of consciousness is decreased, he has no gag reflex, and the left side of his face shows some paralysis. His physician has ordered intermittent feedings (every 4 hours) of a commercial nutrient solution through a nasogastric tube.

NURSING DIAGNOSIS

Risk for aspiration

DEFINING CHARACTERISTICS

- Decreased level of consciousness
- Facial paralysis
- Absence of gag reflex

GOAL/OUTCOME

Mr. Thomas will remain free from episodes of aspiration.

NURSING INTERVENTIONS

1. Assess for signs of stomach distention, cough, or excessive respiratory secretions.
2. Position Mr. Thomas in Fowler's position before feeding.
3. Verify placement of the nasogastric tube using approved methods.
4. Measure the stomach contents. Withhold feeding and notify the physician if the volume of stomach contents is greater than 50 to 100 ml.
5. Return the stomach contents via nasogastric tube.
6. Allow adequate time (approximately 30 minutes) for instillation of 250 ml.
7. Keep the head elevated for 30 to 45 minutes after feeding.
8. Keep suction equipment at the bedside. Check at regular intervals to verify that this equipment is functioning properly.

EVALUATION

Physical assessment reveals no signs of stomach distention. The residual stomach contents before feedings range from 25 to 70 ml. No episodes of coughing or silent tearing are noted with feedings. His lungs are clear on auscultation. You will continue the plan of care.

---

these individuals and can provide a nutritionally sound diet in a form modified to meet the needs of the person at risk for aspiration.

For persons receiving tube feedings

8. **Check placement of the nasogastric tube using the approved method.** Nasogastric tubes can become displaced into the lungs, resulting in aspiration. Tube placement should be verified before any solution is instilled. This should be done routinely according to institutional policy.
9. **Measure stomach contents before starting inter-**

mittent feeding, then reinstill stomach contents. Stomach distention, which is related to decreased gastric emptying time, increases the risk of regurgitation and aspiration. If possible, the volume of stomach contents should be measured before intermittent tube feedings. This may not be possible if a small-bore tube is used. If the volume of stomach contents exceeds 50 to 100 ml, the physician should be notified and the feeding withheld. Stomach contents should be replaced through the tube to maintain electrolyte balance.

The following interventions should take place in the home:

1. **Explain safety precautions to the individual and to the family or caregiver.** Explain the importance of proper positioning, proper rate of feeding, and modifications to food consistency that reduce the likelihood of aspiration.

2. **Encourage enrollment in a home safety course that includes the Heimlich maneuver and cardiopulmonary resuscitation (CPR).** Aspiration of solids can sometimes be relieved by use of the Heimlich maneuver. Respiratory distress related to aspiration may require other emergency interventions until medical assistance arrives. The family should be prepared to provide these lifesaving measures if they plan to provide care in the home.

3. **Use any appropriate interventions that are used in the institutional setting.** A nursing care plan for the risk for aspiration appears on p. 169.

SUMMARY

Nutritional and fluid problems are common in the aging population. Sensory or cognitive changes, weakness, activity intolerance, and loss of interest in food due to depression or other emotional disturbances all contribute to these problems. Nurses plays an important role in the recognition of nutritional and fluid balance problems, identification of contributing factors, and development of an appropriate plan of care. Nurses should recognize the importance of consultation with the dietitian and referral to community agencies that can provide nutritional support.

READINGS AND REFERENCES

Campbell SM: Maintaining hydration status in elderly persons: problems and solutions, *Support Line* 14:7

Chernoff R: Meeting the nutritional needs of the elderly in the institutional setting, *Nutr Rev* 52:132, 1994.

Chidester JC, Spangler AA: Fluid intake in the institutionalized elderly, *J Am Diet Assoc* 97:23, 1997.

Coulston AM, Craig L, Voss AC: Meals-on-Wheels applicants are a population at risk for poor nutritional status, *J Am Diet Assoc* 96:570, 1996.

Dietitians in Nutrition Support: *Suggested guidelines for nutrition and metabolic management of adult patients receiving nu-*trition support, ed 2, Chicago, 1993, American Dietetic Association.

Evans WJ, Cyr-Campbell D: Nutrition, exercise and healthy aging, *J Am Diet Assoc* 97:632, 1997.

Fiatarone MA, et al: Exercise training and nutritional supplementation for physical frailty in very elderly people, *N Engl J Med* 330:1769, 1994.

Fishman P: Healthy people 2000: what progress toward better nutrition, *Geriatrics* 51:38, 1996.

Frisone GB, et al: Food intake and mortality in the frail elderly, *J Gerontol* 50:M203, 1995.

Gerwick CL: *Nutrition care in nursing facilities*, ed 2, Chicago, 1992, American Dietetic Association.

Gilmore SA, et al: Clinical indicators associated with unintentional weight loss and pressure ulcers in elderly residents of nursing facilities, *J Am Diet Assoc* 95:984, 1995.

High-protein diets can promote healing of pressure ulcers, *Brown University Long-Term Quality Letter* 5:4, 1993.

Hoffman NB: Dehydration in the elderly: insidious and manageable, *Geriatrics* 46:35, 1991.

Houston DK, et al: Individual foods and food group patterns of the oldest old, *J Nutr Elderly* 13:5, 1994.

Kurtzweil P: Growing older, eating better, *FDA Consumer* 30:12, 1996.

Neyman M, Zidenberg-Cherr S, McDonald R: Effect of participation in congregate-site meal programs on nutritional status of the healthy elderly, *J Am Diet Assoc* 96:475, 1996.

O'Mahony D, McIntyre AS: Artificial feeding for elderly patients after stroke, *Age Aging* 24:533, 1995.

Phillips PA, Johnson CI, Gray L: Disturbed fluid and electrolyte homeostasis following dehydration in elderly people, *Age Aging* 22:S26, 1993.

Poor nutrient intakes in the frail elderly, *Nutrition Research Newsletter* 15:84, 1996.

Position of the American Dietetic Association: nutrition, aging, and the continuum of care, *J Am Diet Assoc* 96:1048, 1996.

Preventing frailty in the very elderly, *Nutrition Research Newsletter* 8:84, 1994.

Protein requirements of the elderly, *Nutrition Research Newsletter* 15:123, 1996.

Relationship between dietary protein and pressure ulcers, *Am Fam Physician* 48:663, 1993.

Sahyoun NR, et al: Nutrition screening initiative checklist may be a better awareness/educational tool than a screening one, *J Am Diet Assoc* 97:760, 1997.

CARE OF AGING SKIN AND MUCOUS MEMBRANES

The skin undergoes several changes with aging that make it more susceptible to damage. Over time, the epidermal layer becomes thinner and subcutaneous padding diminishes, increasing the risk of traumatic injuries such as skin tears or pressure ulcers. Decreased sebaceous secretions and circulatory changes contribute to the dry skin and scaliness of the lower extremities that are common with aging. Aging skin is more susceptible to inflammation, infection, and rashes. Pruritus, which is a common complaint in the elderly, may be due to dryness, irritation, or infection but can be related to diseases such as diabetes mellitus, kidney disease, malignancy, or anemia. Although skin problems are usually not life-threatening, they are significant because they can distress the elderly person and lead to decreased quality-of-life. Skin problems should be prevented whenever possible; in situations in which the problems are not preventable, they should be recognized, treated, and resolved in a timely manner.

NURSING PROCESS
ALTERATION IN SKIN INTEGRITY

Changes in the skin, hair, and nails may indicate a variety of problems related to nutritional and circulatory adequacy. Because these structures are the ones most easily observed, they can provide a great deal of information about the metabolic health of the entire body (Table 11-1).

Complete assessment of skin, hair, and nails is best done when the person is undressed so all skin surfaces can be inspected. Skin assessment can be performed during a bath, during daily personal hygiene, at bedtime, or at any other convenient time for the elderly person. Independent elderly persons should be aware of what is normal for themselves, and should bring any changes to the attention of the physician. In a hospital or extended-care setting, privacy must be maintained and modesty protected during the skin inspection. Assessment of the skin and ancillary structures is an important responsibility of nurses. Nursing assistants and attendant health care workers who assist with bathing or other care should be instructed to report any unusual or questionable observations promptly to a nurse for further investigation. Inspection should follow a logical order so that no pertinent observations are missed. Most nurses find that a head-to-toe progression is the most helpful, as is a body diagram on which observations are indicated (Fig. 11-1).

Skin color changes can indicate a variety of disorders. When assessing skin for color, it is important to be aware of the differences in skin pigments among ethnic groups. Examination of the skin should take place in good, preferably natural light; one side of the body should be compared with the other; and touch should be used to determine skin temperature or the presence of rashes or irritation. Stretching the skin slightly may also help in determining the underlying tones. Color changes, including pallor, cyanosis, jaundice, or erythema, can indicate a variety of problems. The extent and location of any color changes should be recorded and reported promptly.

Dry skin is one of the most common problems of aging. Various studies have shown that 75% to 85% of people over 65 years of age experience some degree of problem with dry skin. Physiologic changes as well as excessive bathing, the use of harsh soaps, and a dry environment contribute to problems with dry skin.

Dry skin can result in itching (pruritus), burning, and cracking of the skin (Fig. 11-2). Many elderly people develop a habit of scratching or picking at dry or cracked skin, increasing their risk for further tissue damage and infection. Skin irritation can be severe and cause intense discomfort to the elderly. In fact, it may be so distracting that affected individuals cease to participate in social activities.

Rashes and skin irritation can be caused by factors other than dryness. Medications, communicable diseases, and contact with chemical substances are common causes of skin rashes and pruritus (Fig. 11-3).

Allergic response to medications can manifest as diffuse rashes over the body. Whenever a rash develops soon after administration of new medication, an allergy should be suspected. It is appropriate to withhold that particular medication and contact the physician to report the symptom.

One communicable source of skin irritation and severe pruritus is **scabies.** Scabies is a superficial infection caused by a parasitic mite (*Sarcoptes scabiei* var *hominis*) that burrows under the skin (Fig. 11-4). The elderly, especially those who suffer from chronic illness, dementia, or a depressed immune system, are particularly vulnerable to scabies infections. Signs of scabies include intense itching and fine, dark, wavy lines at the flexor surface of the wrist or elbow, the webbed area of the fingers, the axilla, and the genitals. Recognition of scabies may be difficult in the elderly because there is an asymptomatic incubation period of 4 to 6 weeks and because atypical presentations are common. When infestation is suspected, skin scrapings should be examined to determine the presence of ova or mites.

Scabies is spread from person to person by direct contact. Because recognition is difficult, treatment may be delayed—allowing the parasite to infect other people. In order to reduce outbreaks of scabies infection within an institution, all new residents in extended-care settings should be assessed carefully on admission. All cases must be identified and treated

TABLE 11-1		
Changes Related to Aging in Skin, Hair, and Nails		
Parameters	**Observable changes**	**Cause**
SKIN		
Color	Paleness in white skin	Decreased vascularity of dermis; loss of melanocytes
	Brown spots (senile lentigines)	Hyperpigmentation
	Purple patches (senile purpura)	Blood leaking from poorly supported fragile capillaries
Moisture	Dry skin, decreased perspiration	Decreased sebaceous and sweat gland activity
Elasticity, turgor	Decreased elasticity	Loss of collagen and elastic fibers
	Loose folds and wrinkles	
	Decreased turgor	
Texture	Some rough areas	Environmental effects over time; less moisture
	Thin, more transparent skin	Thinning of epidermis from decreased vascularity of dermis; loss of underlying tissue
HAIR		
Color	Grayness	Decreased number of melanocytes in hair
Consistency	Thinner on head and body	Decreased density and rate of hair growth
	Coarser in noses of men	Increased density of nasal hair
Distribution	Loss of hair on head and body	Decreased rate of hair growth; decreased hormones; decreased peripheral circulation
	Increased hair on faces of women	Higher androgen:estrogen ratio
NAILS		
	More brittle	Slowing of nail growth; decreased peripheral circulation
	Longitudinal ridges	
	Thickening and yellowing of toenails	

From Phipps WJ, et al: *Medical-surgical nursing: concepts and clinical practice*, ed 4, St Louis, 1991, Mosby.

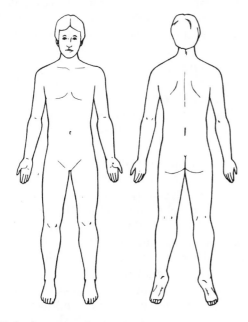

FIG. 11-1 Example of a body diagram that can be used in assessing elderly patients for skin alterations. (From Sorrention SA: *Mosby's textbook for nursing assistants*, ed 3, St Louis, 1992, Mosby.)

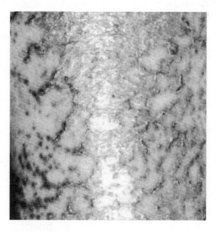

FIG. 11-2 Dry, scaly skin commonly seen in the elderly.

promptly to prevent spread or reinfestation with the parasite.

Changes in skin pigmentation are common with aging. These changes are discussed in Chapter 3. Many of the changes are cosmetic in nature and do not cause problems unless they are located on the face or

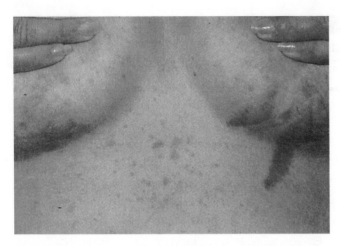

FIG. 11-3 Drug-induced skin reactions are seen more often among older patients. Use of a potent topical corticosteroid has resulted in severe striae under this woman's breasts—an occasional complication. (From Eaglstein WH, McKay M, Pariser DM: *Patient Care* 28:89, 1994.)

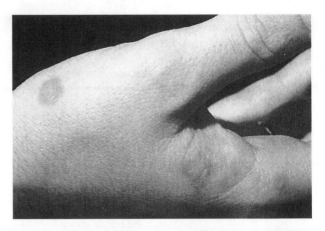

FIG. 11-4 Scabies lesions at three different stages are evident on this patient's hand. The lesion at the far left features a well-demarcated round border surrounding a blister, whereas the sore nearest the thumb fold has already erupted and appears to be healing. (From Eaglstein WH, McKay M, Pariser DM: *Patient Care* 28:89, 1994.)

arms, where they may be distressing to the affected person. Common conditions such as acne rosacea can be treated with topical medications, which help heal the skin and reduce redness, whereas others can be concealed by appropriate use of cosmetics. Changes in the size or pigmentation of moles are of greater significance because these changes may indicate the presence of a precancerous or cancerous condition that needs immediate medical attention.

Breaks in tissue integrity increase the elderly person's risk for infection and often result in the need for costly, time-consuming treatments. These breaks can cause disfigurement and are frightening to the elderly. Skin tears, abrasions, lacerations, and ulcers most often result from friction, shearing force, moisture, and pressure. Even simple incidents such as contact with furniture, sliding across bed linens, a grip during a transfer, or the removal of tape may result in significant skin trauma to the elderly person.

Pressure ulcers are a particular risk to older adults who suffer from compromised circulation, restricted mobility, altered level of consciousness, fecal or urinary incontinence, or nutritional problems (Table 11-2). It has been estimated that as many as 3 million pressure ulcers occur each year in the United States. Of these, 60% or more develop in hospitals, 18% in extended-care facilities, and 18% in the home.

Excessive pressure on tissues, particularly over bony prominences, can quickly lead to skin breakdown (Fig. 11-5). Ulcer development depends on the amount of pressure, the length of time pressure is exerted, and the underlying status of the tissues involved. Tissue that is subjected to excessive pressure does not receive adequate oxygen or nutrients. This can result in ischemia and increased susceptibility to breakdown.

When tissue is deprived of necessary nutrients for a longer period of time, necrosis and tissue destruction will result. Tissue that is fragile because of poor nutrition or circulation is most susceptible to breakdown. Early danger signs indicating a risk for breakdown include pale or reddened tissue. Pressure ulcers are categorized or "staged" based on their appearance and the depth of tissue penetration (Fig. 11-6).

Rather than wait for skin breakdown to occur, most health care agencies perform a formal risk assessment at the time of admission and then at regular intervals. The most common tools used for this assessment are the Braden and Norton Scales (Tables 11-3 and 11-4). Nurses use the information from this assessment to develop a plan of care that minimizes risk factors and promotes skin integrity.

The amount, distribution, appearance, and consistency of the hair changes with aging. The hair of both men and women will typically become thinner and have a finer consistency with advanced age. Heredity and gender play a role in hair loss patterns. Men tend to lose more hair than do women, although some men will retain a full head of hair throughout life. Male pattern baldness typically results in progressive loss of hair at the temples and back of the head. Sudden and excessive hair loss **(alopecia)** or breakage is likely to indicate a systemic problem. Abnormal hair loss can be related to high fevers, medications, nutrition problems, fungal or bacterial infections, endocrine disorders, or stress. Sudden or unusual hair loss should be reported so that the physician can determine the cause.

The amount and distribution of body hair also change with aging. Diminished or absent hair on the lower legs or feet—particularly when combined with

TABLE 11-2

A Quick Guide to Prevention of Pressure Ulcers

Risk factor	Nursing interventions
Immobility	Establish individualized turning schedule; reduce shear and friction; provide pressure-relief surface.
Inactivity	Provide assistive devices to increase activity.
Incontinence	Assess the need for incontinence management; clean and dry skin after soiling.
Malnutrition	Provide adequate nutritional and fluid intake; consult the dietitian for nutritional evaluation.
Diminished sensation, decreased mental status	Assess the client's and family's ability to provide care; educate caregivers regarding pressure ulcer prevention.
Impaired skin integrity	Avoid pressure; do not use donut-shaped cushions; lubricate skin; do not massage red areas; do not use heat lamps.

Modified from Maklebust J, Sieggreen M: *Pressure ulcers: guidelines for prevention and nursing management*, West Dundee, Ill, 1991, S-N Publications.

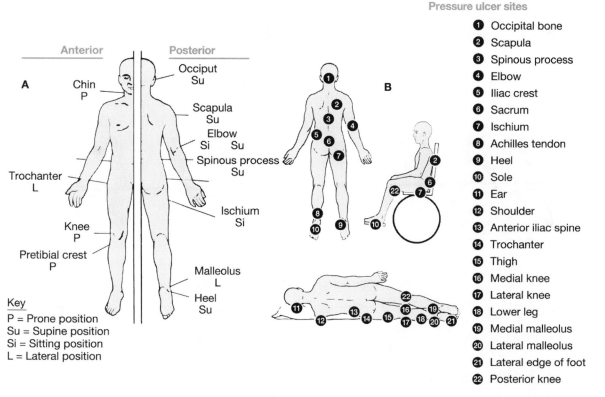

FIG. 11-5 **A,** Bony prominences most frequently underlying pressure ulcers. **B,** Pressure ulcer sites. (From Trelease CC: *Ostomty/Wound Manage* 20:46, 1988.)

excessively dry, scaly, or flaky skin and weak or absent pedal pulses—indicates decreased blood supply to the lower extremities.

Inspection of the tissue on the feet warrants special attention in the elderly. Because many aging individuals are unable to bend adequately to view the feet, a family member or friend can perform this inspection for independent elderly (Fig. 11-7). In an institutional setting, foot inspection should be done by the nursing staff. Many older adults neglect their feet simply because they cannot see or reach them. Unless foot inspection is done on a regular schedule, severe problems can occur before anyone is aware of them.

Aging results in hyperkeratosis of the nails, particularly those of the feet. Thick, hard nails are difficult to cut using normal foot care equipment. The strength

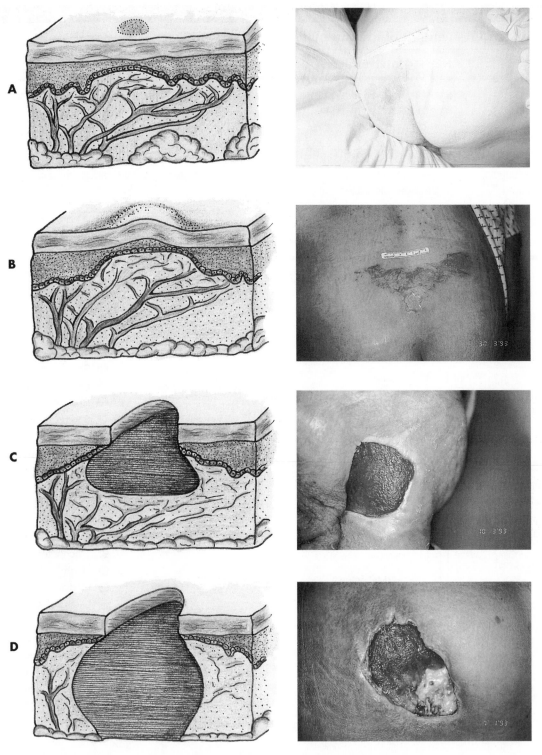

Fig. 11-6   Pressure ulcers. **A,** Stage I. **B,** Stage II. **C,** Stage III. **D,** Stage IV. (Courtesy of Laurel Wiersema, RN, MSN, Clinical Nurse Specialist, Barnes Hospital, St Louis.)

and effort required to cut these nails may exceed the elderly person's abilities, resulting in overgrowth. Soaking the feet in warm water before attempting to cut them may help soften the nails and make them easier to cut. Assistance from a family member or

health care provider is appropriate when there is no history of circulatory problem or diabetes. When diabetes or circulatory problems are present, care should be provided by a foot care specialist. Special heavy-duty equipment may be needed to accomplish proper

TABLE 11-3

Braden Scale for Predicting Pressure Sore Risk

Assessment tool	1 point	2 points	3 points	4 points
SENSORY PERCEPTION				
Ability to respond meaningfully to pressure-related discomfort	**Completely limited:** Unresponsive (does not moan, flinch, or grasp) to painful stimuli because of diminished level of consciousness or sedation **or** Limited ability to feel pain over most of body surface	**Very limited:** Responds only to painful stimuli; cannot communicate discomfort except by moaning or restlessness **or** Has a sensory impairment that limits the ability to feel pain or discomfort over half of body	**Slightly limited:** Responds to verbal commands but cannot always communicate discomfort or the need to be turned **or** Has some sensory impairment, which limits ability to feel pain or discomfort in one or two extremities	**No impairment:** Responds to verbal commands; has no sensory deficit that would limit ability to feel or voice pain or discomfort
MOISTURE				
Degree to which skin is exposed to moisture	**Constantly moist:** Skin is kept moist almost constantly by perspiration, urine, etc., dampness is detected every time patient is moved or turned	**Very moist:** Skin is often, but not always, moist; linens must be changed at least once a shift	**Occasionally moist:** Skin is occasionally moist, requiring an extra linen change approximately once a day	**Rarely moist:** Skin is usually dry; linen requires changing only at routine intervals
ACTIVITY				
Degree of physical activity	**Bedfast:** Confined to bed	**Chairfast:** Ability to walk severely limited or nonexistent; cannot bear own weight and/or must be assisted into chair or wheelchair	**Walks occasionally:** Walks occasionally during day, but for very short distances, with or without assistance; spends majority of each shift in bed or chair	**Walks frequently:** Walks outside room at least twice a day and inside room at least once every 2 hours during waking hours
MOBILITY				
Ability to change and control body position	**Completely immobile:** Does not make even slight changes in body or extremity position without assistance	**Very limited:** Makes occasional slight changes in body or extremity position but is unable to make frequent or significant changes independently	**Slightly limited:** Makes frequent although slight changes in body or extremity position independently	**No limitations:** Makes major and frequent body position changes without assistance

Continued

TABLE 11-3

Braden Scale for Predicting Pressure Sore Risk—cont'd

Assessment tool	1 point	2 points	3 points	4 points
NUTRITION Usual food intake pattern	**Very poor:** Never eats a complete meal; Rarely eats more than one third of any food offered; eats two servings or less of protein (meat or dairy products) per day; takes fluids poorly; does not take a liquid dietary supplement **or** Receives nothing by mouth and/or is maintained on clear liquids or intravenous solutions for more than 5 days	**Probably inadequate:** Rarely eats a complete meal and generally eats only about half of any food offered; protein intake includes only three servings of meat or dairy products per day; occasionally will take a dietary supplement **or** Receives less than optimal amount of liquid diet or tube feeding	**Adequate:** Eats over half of most meals; eats a total of four servings of protein (meat, dairy products) each day; occasionally will refuse a meal, but will usually take a supplement if offered **or** Is on a tube-feeding or total parenteral nutrition regimen that probably meets most of nutritional needs	**Excellent:** eats most of every meal; never refuses a meal; usually eats a total of four or more servings of meat and dairy products per day; occasionally eats between meals, does not require supplements
FRICTION AND SHEAR	**Problem:** Requires moderate to maximal assistance in moving; complete lifting without sliding against sheets is impossible; frequently slides down in bed or chair, requiring frequent repositioning with maximal assistance; spasticity, contractions, or agitation leads to almost constant friction	**Potential problem:** Moves feebly or requires minimal assistance; during a move skin probably slides to some extent against sheets, chair, restraints, or other devices; maintains relatively good position in chair or bed most of the time but occasionally slides down	**No apparent problem:** Moves in bed and in chair independently and has sufficient muscle strength to sit up completely during move; maintains good position in bed or chair at all times	

Instructions: Score client in each of the six subscales. Maximum score is 23, indicating little or no risk. A score of ≤ 16 indicates "at risk"; ≤ 9 indicates high risk.

TABLE 11-4

Norton Risk Assessment Scale

		Physical condition	**Mental condition**	**Activity**	**Mobility**	**Incontinent**	
							TOTAL SCORE
		Good 4 Fair 3 Poor 2 Very Bad 1	Alert 4 Apathetic 3 Confused 2 Stupor 1	Ambulant 4 Walk/help 3 Chairbound 2 Bad 1	Full 4 Sl. limited 3 V. limited 2 Immobile 1	Not 4 Occasional 3 Usually/Urine 2 Doubly 1	
Name	Date						

From the Centre for Policy on Ageing, London, England.

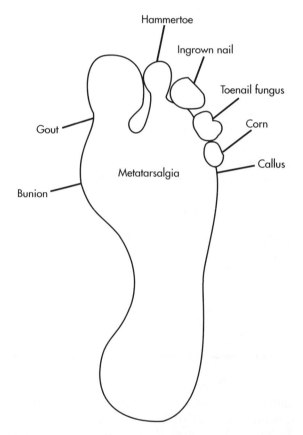

FIG. 11-7 Common foot problems in the elderly. (from Eber-sole P, Hess P: *Toward healthy aging: human needs and nursing response*, ed 5, St Louis, 1998, Mosby.)

nail care. Use of safety glasses is recommended during nail care to prevent eye injuries from flying nail particles.

If proper care is neglected, uncut nails confined in shoes will often begin to curl under the toes, resulting in a condition called **ram's horn nails.** In this condition, the nail curls over the top of the toe into the flesh on the bottom causing pain. When the discomfort becomes severe the elderly person may stop wearing shoes and decrease ambulation in an attempt to reduce the discomfort. In such severe cases, care from a podiatrist is advisable.

Other common foot problems include corns, calluses, blisters, and bunions, which usually result from years of wearing poorly fitted footwear. These conditions often cause discomfort for the elderly and lead to some degree of activity restriction. Many independent elderly use commercially available foot remedies or attempt to remove corns or calluses with a knife or scissors. This practice is dangerous and significantly increases the risk for serious foot infections, which may necessitate amputation of a toe, toes, or entire foot. Diabetics and elderly persons with impaired peripheral circulation are particularly prone to develop foot ulcers or infections and are at greatest risk for amputation.

Assessment of the Skin

- What is the general appearance of the person's skin?
- Are any sores evident on the scalp?
- What is the color of the skin? Are there any signs of pallor, jaundice, cyanosis, or erythema?
- Where?
- Are there any areas of dry skin? Where?
- Does the person complain of itching?
- Is there any evidence of scratching?
- Are there any signs of scabies (fine, wavy, dark lines or spots at the webs of the fingers or folds of the skin)?
- Are there any rashes? Where are they located? What is their appearance (e.g., macular, papular, vesicular)?

BOX 11-1

Risk Factors for Alterations in Skin, Hair, or Nails in the Elderly

- Circulatory problems
- Restricted mobility
- Nutritional or fluid imbalances
- Cognitive impairments
- Exposure to irritating chemicals, including body secretions or waste products
- Exposure to communicable diseases
- Lack of adequate hygiene facilities or assistance in the home

BOX 11-2

Products that Help Moisturize the Skin

All of these products are available without a prescription. You may find other moisturizers in stores. Ask your doctor or pharmacist whether they would work well for you.

CREAMS AND LOTIONS
Cetaphil Cream and Lotion
Complex 15 Hand and Body Cream and Lotion
Curel Moisturizing Cream and Lotion
Eucerin Cream and Lotion
EverSoft
Keri Lotion
Lubriderm Cream and Lotion
Moisturel Lotion
Nivea Moisturizing Lotion
Nivea Ultramoisturizing Cream
Nutraderm Cream and Lotion
Purpose Dry Skin Cream
Shepard's Cream Lotion
Shepard's Skin Cream

OINTMENTS
Aquaphor Natural Healing Ointment
Crisco vegetable shortening
Dermasil
Neutrogena Norwegian Formula Emulsion
Unibase
Vaseline Pure Petroleum Jelly

UREA OR LACTIC ACID–CONTAINING CREAMS AND LOTIONS
Aqua Care Cream
Carmol 10
Lac-Hydrin Five
LactiCare
Nutraplus

- Is there any sign of pallor or erythema over bony prominences?
- Are there any breaks in the skin integrity? Where? What do they look like?
- Are any abrasions (friction burns) or skin tears evident?
- What is the appearance of the toenails?
- Are any sores or lesions evident on the feet or ankles?
- Are there pedal pulses? Are these pulses easy or difficult to detect?
- Is there any change in the amount, distribution, or appearance of the hair?

See Box 11-1 for a list of risk factors for skin, hair, or nail alterations in the elderly.

Nursing Diagnoses

Risk for impaired skin integrity
Impaired skin integrity
Impaired tissue integrity

Nursing Goals/Outcomes

The nursing goals for elderly individuals with or at risk for impaired skin or tissue integrety are (1) to remain free from excessive skin dryness or skin breakdown; (2) to display timely healing of wounds, lesions, and ulcerations; and (3) to maintain optimal nutritional status to promote tissue integrity and healing.

Nursing Interventions

The following nursing interventions should take place in hospitals or extended-care facilities:

1. **Assess the level of impairment and the contributing factors.** Perform a daily skin inspection; measure the location, size, and depth of the affected area or areas; and identify any conditions or changes that may have caused the problem. Changes in skin condition can occur rapidly in the elderly. All problem areas must be measured and documented so that improvement or further breakdown can be evaluated. Nurses should explore any possible causes for the problem and institute nursing measures to prevent or reduce further tissue damage.

2. **Institute measures to reduce the risk of skin and tissue breakdown.**
   Reduce the frequency of complete bathing. The type and frequency of baths or showers will depend greatly on the individual. The condition of the skin and the presence of perspiration or other body wastes must be considered. Some individuals require a complete bath or shower daily; others will benefit more from a complete bath on a biweekly

A   **B**   **C**

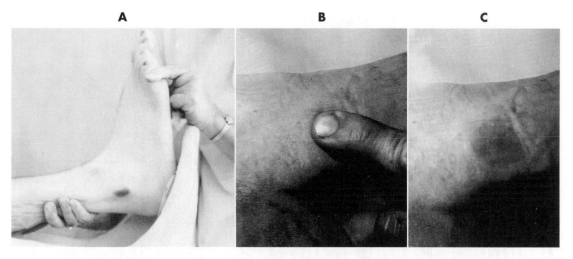

FIG. 11-8 **A,** Abnormal reactive hyperemia. **B** and **C,** In abnormal reactive hyperemia, the affected area is much darker than the surrounding skin and does not blanch with fingertip pressure. (From Pires M, Muller A: *Progressions* 3:3, 1991.)

or weekly basis. On days when total baths are not taken, partial or sponge baths of the face, axilla, and perineum will provide adequate cleanliness and prevent body odors.

Keep skin free from wastes and exudates by using mild nondetergent soaps. Reducing the frequency of bathing is suggested if dryness is a problem. Use of mild, nondetergent, nonperfumed, superfatted soaps (e.g., Basis, Caress, Dove, Neutrogena) for cleansing will decrease excessive skin dryness.

Use emollients, lotions, and oils to maintain skin moisture. Emollients help keep moisture in the skin and reduce dryness. A variety of preparations are available at a wide range of costs. Studies have shown that a light application of mineral oil is effective and inexpensive. Caution should be used, however, because mineral oil may stain clothing. Lotions containing alcohol should be avoided because these can contribute to drying. It may be necessary to try various emollients and lotions to find the one (or the combination) that provides the most relief to the elderly individual (Box 11-2).

Rinse skin carefully. Soaps tend to dry the skin and should be completely rinsed off before drying. If using a basin, complete rinsing may require frequent water changes.

Dry skin tissue gently and thoroughly. Dry the skin by patting rather than rubbing to decrease skin irritation. If the skin is severely irritated, soft towels that have been rinsed carefully to remove all detergents may be necessary.

Turn and position the person frequently, and reduce sources of pressure by keeping bed linen tight and clear of foreign objects. Pressure over bony prominences restricts blood flow to the tissues that are being compressed (Fig. 11-8). These areas are most likely to become ischemic or necrotic. Frequent position changes allow blood flow to become reestablished and reduce the risk of skin breakdown. The maximum amount of time a person is in one position should not exceed 2 hours. More frequent turning is necessary for individuals at high risk for skin problems. The frequency of position changes should be based on assessment of pressure points after the person is turned. A 30° lateral position (Fig. 11-9) is preferred to a full lateral position.

Pressure points over bony prominences are most susceptible to breakdown, but anything that exerts resistance against the skin can become a pressure point. Foreign objects such as large wrinkles, personal belongings (rosary or prayer beads), or needle caps trapped under the body can also contribute to skin breakdown.

Each time the person is repositioned, the skin should be inspected for signs of circulatory reduction such as blanching or hyperemia. If these signs are present, a more frequent turning schedule should be established. Reddened areas should be treated with caution and should *not* be massaged because massage is likely to increase the risk of ulcer formation.

Wash the skin and supply clean, dry linens after episodes of incontinence. Urine and stool contain waste products that are highly irritating to the skin and must be removed promptly. Elderly persons who are known to be incontinent of stool or urine must be checked frequently to reduce the chance of prolonged exposure to moisture and body wastes. Special absorbent pads or garments that wick moisture away from the skin are appropriate in some situations. Problems of incontinence are addressed in greater depth in Chapter 12.

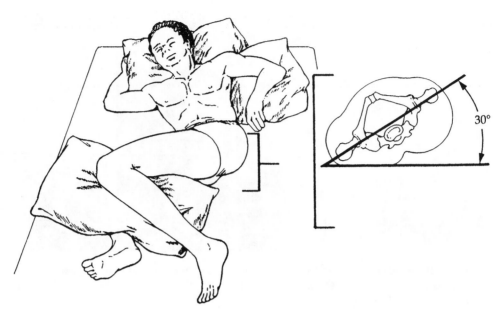

FIG. 11-9 A 30° lateral position is best to avoid pressure points. (From Bryant RA: *Acute and chronic wounds: nursing management,* St Louis, 1991, Mosby.)

Once the skin is thoroughly washed and dried, moisture barriers (e.g., A & D ointment) can be applied to protect the skin. These types of preparations must be removed from the skin at regular intervals to prevent bacterial overgrowth.

Keep the skin dry after episodes of diaphoresis; check skin surfaces where moisture due to normal perspiration can become trapped. Moisture on the skin surface can cause maceration and tissue breakdown. Moisture caused by perspiration usually evaporates and causes few problems unless perspiration is excessive or is trapped between skin surfaces (e.g., under pendulous breasts). Frequent sponging with clear water and thorough drying, exposure to air, or use of a drying substance such as cornstarch will help reduce the amount of moisture and reduce friction between skin surfaces.

Move and transfer the person carefully. The skin of elderly individuals is thinner, less elastic, and has less subcutaneous padding than in younger people. This makes it particularly vulnerable to shearing forces during movement. When the head of the bed is elevated, it is recommended that the elevation should be kept at or below 30° to reduce the shearing force that may occur when a person slides down in bed. To reduce the friction that occurs when tissue is dragged over bed linens, transfer sheets or other assistive devices should be used when turning, repositioning, or transferring a frail elderly person.

Provide appropriate pads, cushions, mattresses or beds designed to reduce pressure. Many types of beds and mattresses designed to distribute weight over a larger area and reduce pressure on body tissues are available. The advantages and disadvantages of some of these are presented in Table 11-5. Wheelchair pads made of gel or inflated with air help reduce pressure on the ischial tuberosities. Only full chair cushions should be used. Inflatable donuts are not recommended because while they reduce pressure on one area they increase pressure on surrounding tissues. This can lead to more ischemia and result in extending the area of tissue damage.

3. **Institute measures to promote tissue healing.**

Promote adequate nutritional intake. Tissue regeneration occurs more slowly in the elderly. Increased intake of calories with emphasis on protein and vitamin C is particularly important because these nutrients are necessary for tissue repair.

Encourage adequate rest. Tissue healing uses energy and places additional physiologic stress on the aging body. For this reason the elderly may require additional rest periods during the day.

Check wounds daily for signs of inflammation or infection, and obtain cultures of wound drainage if appropriate. The typical signs of inflammation or infection may be absent or diminished in the elderly; therefore, special attention should be paid to any open areas. Wound cultures are indicated if any purulent or foul-smelling drainage is observed. Infection will delay healing and place additional stress on the elderly.

Follow aseptic technique when cleansing wounds, changing dressings, or applying medications. When treatments are ordered for skin breakdown such as pressure ulcers, it is essential that good aseptic technique be used to prevent the introduction of pathogenic microorganisms into the area. Good handwashing between patient contacts and strict adherence to body substance precautions are essen-

TABLE 11-5

Surface Types by Purpose and Advantages

Type	Examples	Purpose	Advantages	Disadvantages	Notes
Foam overlay	Geomatt, Biogard	Pressure reduction, comfort	Low cost; ease of use; many sizes	Hot; traps moisture; life is limited; loses pressure reduction with use	Usually one-client use; washing removes flame-retardant chemicals; ease of use at home
Foam replacement	MaxiFloat, DeCube, Comfortex	Pressure reduction, comfort	Reduced bed height; reduces nursing time; multiple client use	High initial cost; difficult to evaluate when effectiveness is lost	Some have removable sections (cubes); may be rented or purchased
Fluid overlay	Lotus	Pressure reduction, comfort	Easily cleaned; multiple client use; readily available	Heavy; leaks with puncture; cannot raise head of bed	May be rented or purchased; baffled systems control motion
Air overlay	Sofcare, Roho, KoalaKare	Pressure relief	Ease of setup; single- or multiple-use products available	Lack of comfort; damaged by sharp objects; requires monitoring for inflation	May be rented or purchased; adapts to multiple settings
Low air loss	KinAir, Flexicair, Mediscus	Pressure relief	Ease of use; seat deflates for transfer; company offers support staff	Portable blowers are noisy; surface may be slippery; noisy	Generally rented; home unit is available
Air fluidized	Clinitron, Fluidair, Skytron	Pressure relief	Reduced friction and shear; facilitates control of high drainage; company offers support staff	Coughing may be less effective; heavy, circulating air may dehydrate; transfers are difficult	Available for home, but may be too heavy
Kinetic	Rotokinetic treatment table	Movement, skeletal stability	Mobilizes secretions; skeletal stability; supports traction; company offers support staff	Must be kept in rotation or no pressure reduction; shearing if client position is not correct	Must be in rotation 21 hours/day, now available as low air loss version
Bariatric	Burke	Management of the morbidly obese, staff safety	Facilitates client independence; converts to a chair	Width is standard so surface may not accommodate turning	Requires addition of special mattress and overlay for pressure relief

From Potter PA, Perry AG: *Basic nursing: theory and practice,* ed 3, St Louis, 1995, Mosby.

tial. All personnel should have their own supply of dressing materials, which are kept apart from other people's supplies. Multipatient treatment carts should not be taken to the bedside. All supplies used for wound care should be protected from environmental contamination by dust, water, or other such substances.

Dead tissue is typically cleansed from a wound by rinsing or irrigating with normal saline. Harsh cleansers, povidone-iodine, and hydrogen peroxide should be avoided because they can damage under-

lying healthy tissues. Excessive force during irrigation can also cause tissue damage.

Clean rather than sterile dressings are used in most situations as long as they comply with the institutional infection-control guidelines. A wide variety of preparations is available for wound care; the particular type selected by the physician or wound care specialist will depend on the location and stage of the lesion (Table 11-6). Individuals with severely compromised immune systems may require use of sterile technique and supplies.

TABLE 11-6

Treatment Options by Ulcer Stage

Ulcer stage	Ulcer status	Dressing*	Comments	Expected change	Adjuvant
1	Intact	None	Allows visual assessment	Resolves slowly without epidermal loss over 7 to 14 days	Turning schedule
		Film, adherent Hydrocolloid	Protects from shear May not allow visual assessment		Support hydration Nutritional support
					Silicone-based lotion to decrease shear Pressure relief mattress or chair cushion
2	Clean	Composite	Viasorb, film plus telfa; exudry; limits shear	Heals through reepithelialization and epithelial budding Manage incontinence	See previous stage
		Hydrocolloid Hydrogel sheet	Change every 7 days if occlusive seal Absorbent, requires secondary dressing of gauze or adherent film		
3	Clean	Hydrocolloid	See Stage 2	Heals through granulation and reepithelialization (NOTE: does not become a stage 2 ulcer as it heals)	See previous stages Electric stimulation Evaluate pressure relief needs
		Hydrogel	Apply 1/4-inch thick, cover with gauze or hydrocolloid		
		Exudate absorbers calcium alginate wound pastes	Change when strike through is noted on secondary dressing; cover with gauze or hydrocolloid		
		Gauze, fluffy Growth factors Adherent film	Use with normal saline Use with gauze Will facilitate softening of eschar	Eschar will lift at the edges as healing progresses; crosshatching central area of eschar with a small blade will facilitate release from center	See previous stages Surgical consult for debridement Surgical consult for closure
	Eschar	Hydrocolloid	Will facilitate softening of eschar	Gauze plus ordered solution	Absorb drainage
		None	Rarely, if eschar is dry and intact, no dressing is used, allowing eschar to act as physiologic cover		

TABLE 11-6

Treatment Options by Ulcer Stage—cont'd

Ulcer stage	Ulcer status	Dressing*	Comments	Expected change	Adjuvant
4	Clean	Hydrogel	See Stage 3 Clean	Heals through granulation and reepithelialization	See Stages 1, 2, and 3 Clean
		Hydrocolloid plus hydrocolloid paste/beads	See Stage 3 Clean; critical to treat areas of undermining	Because of contraction, surface may close more rapidly than base, leaving wound cavity	
		Calcium alginate Gauze Growth factors			
	Eschar	See Stage 3 Eschar	See Stage 3 Clean; pack deeply undermined ulcers; use with gauze	See Stage 3 Eschar	See Stage 3 Eschar

From Potter PA, Perry AG: *Basic nursing: theory and practice,* ed 3, St Louis, 1995, Mosby.
*As with *all* occlusive dressings, wound should *not* be clinically infected.

If a patient has more than one lesion, the most contaminated wound (e.g., one near the perineum) should be cleaned last. Dressings should be kept clean in order to prevent cross-contamination between lesions.

4. **Provide good foot care.** The feet of the elderly are particularly susceptible to problems. Poor circulation, increased incidence of problems such as bunions, excessively thick toenails, and the results of years of wearing poorly fitted shoes all contribute to foot problems in the elderly. The feet should be soaked on a regular basis to remove old, dry skin. After a good soaking, the feet should be dried by patting rather than rough rubbing. Be sure to dry the feet thoroughly, paying careful attention to the areas between the toes. If permitted, the toenails should be cut straight across and the sharp edges filed off. The toenails of diabetics and other elderly persons with circulatory problems should be cared for by a foot specialist. Emollients should be used if the skin on the feet is very dry. When emollients are used on the feet, the elderly need to be aware of the importance of wearing socks to prevent slipping. A daily change into clean socks or stockings is preferable and should be encouraged because clean footwear reduces the risk of infection. Elderly persons with diabetes or circulatory impairment of the lower extremities should be encouraged to wear white, cotton socks to promote cleanliness and provide early recognition of any injury or drainage. Caution should be used that the socks fit properly and do not cause excessive constriction around the ankles or calves.

Any signs of foot irritation, color change, or skin breakdown should be documented and reported promptly.

The following interventions should take place in the home:

1. **Encourage adequate fluid intake and good nutrition.** Good nutrition and adequate fluid intake are needed to maintain healthy tissue. Inadequate intake of nutrients such as protein, vitamin A, and vitamin C can result in fragile tissue that is more susceptible to bruising, shearing force injuries, and breakdown. When inadequate intake is suspected, a more complete assessment (including a food and fluid diary) is appropriate. This will help nurses to determine the cause or causes (e.g., depression, illness) and plan suitable interventions.

2. **Maintain adequate humidity in the environment.** Exposure to hot, dry air, whether in the desert or in overly warm living quarters, will result in excessively dry skin. An excessively dry environment will intensify the tendency toward dryness that is already a problem in the elderly. The result is skin that is rough, dry, cracked, irritated, and more susceptible to breakdown and infection. Dry mucous membranes usually accompany dry skin, increasing the risk of epistaxis (nosebleeds). Living spaces should be maintained at a temperature of approximately 70° F to 72° F. Relative humidity between 40% and 60% is most comfortable and beneficial for the skin and mucous membranes. Commercial humidifiers or even open pans of water set around the house will help increase the amount of moisture in the room.

3. **Avoid excessive exposure to the sun.** Older adults have fewer melanocytes, which are unevenly distributed over exposed body areas. Excessive exposure to sunlight can cause irregular, blotchy, and cosmetically unacceptable tanning. Sunblocks are recommended when significant sun exposure is expected. The elderly are encouraged to wear loose, lightweight, light-colored clothing to prevent exposure to the ultraviolet rays in sunlight that increase the risk of skin cancer.

4. **Obtain regular professional foot care.** Elderly persons, particularly those living alone, often find that foot care is difficult due to the loss of flexibility. Regular appointments with a foot care specialist will reduce the risk of trauma or infection. Professional foot care is essential for diabetics and those with impaired peripheral circulation.

5. **Use any appropriate interventions that are used in the institutional setting.**

NURSING PROCESS

ALTERATION IN ORAL MUCOUS MEMBRANES

Problems in the oral cavity may render an elderly individual unable to chew certain foods. Inspection of the oral cavity is needed to determine the status of the individual's teeth, tongue, and oral mucous membranes. Changes in the condition of the gums and oral mucous membranes may be related to several factors.

Dental care was not readily available to many of today's elderly during their youth because of the cost and the associated discomfort. As a result, many elderly individuals who neglected their teeth now suffer tooth loss. Even those who maintained good dental practices were likely to experience tooth decay and loss due to the fact that preventive dental techniques were not as advanced as they are today (Fig. 11-10).

Tooth decay, loose teeth, and lost teeth are ongoing problems in the elderly population. Poor nutrition and decreased appetite in the elderly can often be attributed to dental problems. Decay, or **caries,** is caused by the action of bacteria that penetrate through the enamel shield of the tooth and cause destruction. If caries is not recognized early, a significant amount of the tooth structure may be destroyed. If the caries extends deep into the tooth, a nerve may be exposed and painful neuritis (toothache) may result. Replacement of the lost tooth material with amalgam restorations (fillings) can help rebuild the tooth, but this leaves a weakened structure that remains susceptible to problems. Lost restorations leave rough edges that cause irritation of the oral mucous membranes, particularly the cheek and tongue.

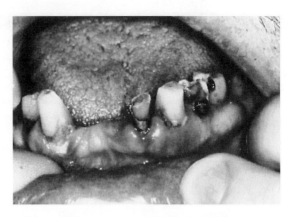

FIG. 11-10 Extensive dental caries in an older adult. (From Papas AS, et al: *Geriatric dentistry: aging and oral health,* St Louis, 1991, Mosby.)

Food debris and plaque build up in the mouth and on the teeth when oral hygiene is inadequate. Activity of bacteria on this debris causes **halitosis,** or bad breath, which is often disturbing to the elderly person and to anyone who has close contact. Periodontal disease is a less obvious but potentially more serious complication of poor oral care. One form of periodontal disease is **gingivitis,** or inflammation of the gums. Gingivitis causes gum swelling, tenderness, and bleeding and eventually leads to recession of the gum tissue away from the tooth. As the gums recede the teeth lose support, become loose in the sockets, and eventually fall out. When a tooth is lost, a gap is created. Healthy teeth shift position or move into the space, resulting in an uneven bite. Chewing becomes increasingly difficult when significant numbers of teeth, particularly the molars needed for chewing and grinding food, become loose or lost.

If only a few teeth are missing, the dentist may attempt to bridge the gaps by attaching artificial teeth to the good teeth. If too many teeth are missing, a partial plate may be required. When all of the upper or lower teeth are removed, a complete set of dentures is required. Both partial plates and dentures can cause problems for the wearer. Partial plates tend to catch particles of food and may weaken the healthy teeth to which they are attached. Complete dentures are expensive and difficult to fit.

Dentures that fit properly at one time may not fit properly if the elderly person loses or gains a significant amount of weight. Fit is also a problem when dentures are left out of the mouth for prolonged periods of time. Many older adults refuse to wear their dentures because of the discomfort caused by an improper fit. This is because the arch of the jaw changes to compensate for the edentulous state. Professional dental attention is needed to repair or rebuild the dentures in these cases.

Dentures can cause irritation, inflammation, and ulceration of the gums and oral mucous membranes. The elderly should inspect their mouths regularly and promptly report any problems to the dentist. Sometimes a minor adjustment of the denture or use of a fixative agent or cushion is all that is required to prevent painful problems.

Xerostomia, or dry mouth, is commonly observed with aging. Dryness may be due to the normal age-related reduction in saliva secretion, inadequate hydration, or disease conditions such as diabetes. Medications such as diuretics, antidepressants, sedatives, hypnotics, antihistamines, and anticholinergics also contribute to problems with xerostomia. In turn, xerostomia makes chewing and swallowing more difficult, promotes tooth decay, and alters the sense of taste.

Inspection of the mouth can reveal a number of abnormalities. White patches in the mouth, called **leukoplakia,** are often precancerous and require prompt medical attention (Fig. 11-11). Lesions on the posterior third or the sides of the tongue are frequently abnormal and should also be brought to the attention of the physician.

Vitamin deficiencies, particularly deficiencies of riboflavin, niacin, and vitamin C, can affect the oral mucous membranes. A smooth, purplish, sore tongue may be related to riboflavin deficiency. Complaint of a burning sensation or soreness of the mouth may be related to niacin deficiency. Multiple painful ulcers of the oral mucous membranes with enlargement of the cervical lymph glands, difficulty swallowing, and foul odor may indicate Vincent's angina. Vincent's angina is a condition caused by opportunistic microorganisms that normally live in the mouth but only cause infection when the individual becomes malnourished.

Superinfections of the mouth are relatively common in elderly individuals who receive broad-spectrum antibiotic therapy for some other infection. Antibiotics destroy the normal mouth flora and allow opportunists or yeast colonies to become established and grow. Candidiasis, a yeast infection (also known as thrush), appears as white patches that adhere to the tongue, lips, and gums. Attempts to remove these patches may result in sore, bleeding tissue. A hairy tongue is the result of enlargement of the papillae on the tongue; this often follows antibiotic therapy. Black or brown discoloration on the tongue may be due to tobacco use or to a chromogenic (color-producing) bacteria. These conditions are more commonly observed in malnourished elderly and those with poor oral hygiene practices. Yeast infections are usually treated by direct oral application or swishes of prescription medication. Hairy tongue usually resolves without medical treatment.

Alcohol and tobacco, even in small amounts, can harm the mucous membranes. Alcohol is chemically

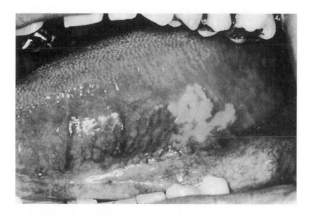

FIG. 11-11   Leukoplakia. Note the formation of white spots. These lesions may become malignant. (From Wood NK: *Review of diagnosis, oral medicine, radiology, and treatment planning,* ed 3, St Louis, Mosby.)

irritating and drying to the mucous membranes. Tobacco, whether smoked, chewed, or taken as snuff, increases the risk of oral cancer.

Good oral hygiene practices are part of routine health maintenance, but meeting oral hygiene needs may be difficult for elderly individuals who have lost strength, coordination, or cognitive processes. Neurologic conditions such as stroke, multiple sclerosis, or Parkinson's disease decrease coordination and strength, making it difficult for the person to manipulate the equipment needed for oral hygiene. Severe arthritics may not only find the equipment difficult to manipulate, but they may also find it difficult to open the mouth adequately for good, thorough cleaning. Elderly persons who take medication for epilepsy or other seizure disorders need to use special precautions because these medications frequently cause hyperplasia of the gingiva. Oral hygiene with soft toothbrushes or swabs is recommended to prevent excessive trauma and bleeding from the tender, swollen tissues. Providing oral hygiene to person's with Alzheimer's disease can be a challenge because affected people do not understand the need for oral hygiene and are likely to resist care.

Assessment of the Oral Cavity

- Does the person have his or her own teeth?
- If so, how many? What is the condition of the teeth?
- Are any teeth loose or decayed?
- Does the person have halitosis?
- Does the person wear dentures? Upper dentures, lower dentures, or both? Partial plates or bridges?
- Are dentures worn during meals or removed? Why?
- How do the dentures fit?
- Are there any signs of irritation in the mouth?

BOX 11-3

Risk Factors for Problems with Oral Mucous Membranes in the Elderly

- Impaired cognitive, neurologic, or musculoskeletal function
- Inadequate fluid intake
- Medication that affects the oral mucous membranes
- Complete or partial artificial teeth
- Tobacco use (smoking or chewing)
- Poor health maintenance practices

- Are food particles trapped under the dentures at meals?
- How good is the person's appetite?
- What is the condition of the oral mucous membranes?
- Are the mucous membranes moist or dry?
- Is any residual food or debris evident in the mouth?
- What is the condition of the tongue?
- Is the tongue clean, coated, pale, red, or irritated?
- Does the person use tobacco or have a history of tobacco use?
- What medications is the person receiving?
- Does the person have any physical conditions that interfere with performing his or her own oral hygiene?

See Box 11-3 for a list of risks for problems with oral mucous membranes in the elderly.

Nursing Diagnosis

Alteration in oral mucous membranes

Nursing Goals/Outcomes

The nursing goals for elderly individuals diagnosed with alterations in the oral mucous membranes are (1) to obtain regular professional dental care; (2) to demonstrate techniques for maintaining or restoring the integrity of the mucous membranes; (3) to inspect the oral cavity on a regular basis and seek care promptly if any symptoms occur; (4) to experience no complaints such as irritation, inflammation, or ulceration; (5) to ingest foods and fluids without discomfort; and (6) to verbalize specific actions that will promote healthy oral mucous membranes.

Nursing Interventions

The following nursing interventions should take place in hospitals or extended-care facilities. In a hospital or extended-care setting, individuals who are able to provide their own oral hygiene should be encouraged to do so. When individuals are not capable of meeting their own oral hygiene needs, nurses or nursing assistants must provide the care. When performing oral hygiene, gloves and other appropriate protective devices should be worn to maintain universal precautions.

1. **Complete a thorough assessment of the oral mucous membranes.** Individuals who require intermediate or skilled nursing care are likely to have more oral hygiene problems and greater oral hygiene needs. If one wishes to judge the quality of nursing care provided in an extended-care facility, the first place to look is in the mouths of the patients or residents. For whatever reason, oral hygiene seems to be the area of hygiene that is most often neglected. This is troubling because oral care is a very important component of nursing care. Good oral hygiene promotes comfort, enhances appetite, and fosters a sense of well-being.

2. **Initiate referral to a dentist or dental hygienist.** If any problems with the teeth or oral mucous membranes are observed, the individual should be seen by a dentist. Hospitals may have outpatient dental clinics that will see in-house patients if necessary. If the problem is not urgent, the individual should be encouraged to make an appointment with his or her own dentist after discharge. Extended-care facilities should have a clinic or dentist on staff who will see residents on a scheduled or referral basis. If there is no dentist on the premises, transportation will need to be arranged with the family or a transport service. It is important that nurses refer individuals as soon as a problem is detected to prevent the development of more serious conditions. Problems related to ill-fitting dentures should be referred to the dentist for prompt follow-up. Be sure to send the improperly fitting dentures along on the visit.

3. **Provide oral hygiene.** Thorough oral hygiene should be provided a minimum of once a day. Brushing after each meal and at bedtime is more desirable and is probably necessary for individuals suffering from halitosis, xerostomia, or gingivitis. Individuals who have poor nutritional intake due to "funny tastes" in the mouth should have additional oral hygiene prior to meals. Frequent oral hygiene is also necessary for individuals with upper respiratory infections. Excessive respiratory secretions coat the mouth and tongue, leaving a bad taste. The frequency of oral hygiene should be determined by the nurse and stated specifically in the care plan (e.g., "oral hygiene q2h and prn").

   Dentures should be cleansed using warm water and a nonabrasive cleanser. The dentures should be brushed over a basin of water or a towel to prevent the possibility of breakage. Ultrasonic cleaning devices are available in some facilities and are very effective at removing particles of debris, particularly from the wire clasps on partial plates. The oral cavity should be thoroughly cleaned and inspected before dentures are reinserted.

Elderly denture wearers should be discouraged from removing and wrapping their dentures in paper napkins or tissue. Many dentures have been thrown away in this manner. It is also wise for anyone who wears dentures to have his or her name (or social security number) etched into each plate. This can prevent permanent loss of these costly items if for some reason the client is separated from them.

Dentures should be removed from the mouth before sleep to prevent slippage, which could result in trauma to the mouth or problems with breathing.

When performing oral hygiene on an unconscious patient, nurses must take special care to prevent aspiration. Unconscious individuals should be placed in a side-lying position, and adequate towels should be used to protect the bedding and clothes. The mouth is propped open with gauze or padded tongue blades. All surfaces of the teeth, tongue, and oral mucous membranes should be cleansed with a soft brush; damp gauze; sponge-tip swab; or clean, moistened washcloth. Special toothbrushes that attach to suction machines are available in some facilities. Lemon-and-glycerin swabs should be used with caution because they may be irritating to open areas on the mucous membranes and because they may ultimately cause drying (glycerin tends to draw moisture away from tissues).

Dry lips may require application of Vaseline, mineral oil, or Carmex. These petroleum-based products should be used with extreme caution because of the potential for aspiration and resulting pneumonia.

4. **Promote adequate intake of nutrients and fluids.** If the individual is avoiding certain foods or fluids because of dental problems, it may be necessary to contact the physician or dietary department to obtain a change in food consistency. Soft, chopped, or pureed foods may be necessary for persons who are unable to chew because of loose teeth or improperly fitting dentures. If food tends to become trapped under the dentures, dentures should be removed promptly after each meal and cleansed. Excessively hot or cold foods may irritate the mucous membranes or teeth and should be avoided if they cause problems. Any temperature modification should be documented in the care plan so that consistent approaches can be used. For example, if the individual tolerates beverages at room temperature, all fluids—including the water at the bed-

side—should be provided this way. Fluids should be kept at the bedside and offered to the individual at planned intervals throughout the day.

5. **Provide lozenges or topical analgesics as prescribed.** If severe or painful lesions are present in the mouth, the physician may order the use of topical analgesics in lozenge or viscous form (viscous lidocaine). Drinking and eating should be avoided for 1 hour after administration of these preparations.

6. **Communicate suspected oral side effects of medication therapy to the physician and dentist.** If the nurse suspects that a drug may be causing untoward side effects on the oral mucous membranes, this information should be communicated promptly to the physician so that any necessary adjustments in dosage or drugs can be made.

The following interventions should take place in the home:

1. **Complete a thorough assessment of the oral mucous membranes.** A thorough assessment is necessary to detect the presence and severity of any problems. Specific interventions will be based on the information gathered.

2. **Stress the importance of regular dental visits.** Dental hygiene is essential for aging individuals. Periodic dental visits should be part of ongoing health maintenance practice, even for edentulous individuals. Those living at home should be encouraged and reminded to make regular dental appointments. If cost is prohibitive, dental clinics as well as schools of dentistry and dental hygiene may offer care at reduced rates. Some dentists will also give price reductions to elderly people if requested.

3. **Review the person's oral hygiene practices.** Elderly persons who have their own teeth should be taught to brush, floss, and irrigate the mouth at least once daily. If problems of halitosis, plaque formation, "bad taste," or gingivitis are present, more frequent brushing may be required.

Brushing is best done with a soft- to moderate-bristle brush. Too firm a bristle may scratch or irritate the oral cavity. Commercial fluoridated toothpastes are available at a reasonable cost. Special toothpastes such as Sensodyne are available for individuals with sensitive teeth and gums. Elderly individuals who have been in the habit of using salt or baking soda as a dentifrice should be counseled to avoid ingesting these products because they are high in sodium.

Flossing between the teeth helps remove trapped food and maintain healthy gums. If the elderly person has difficulty holding the floss, a loop tied at each end of the string will help provide a better grip.

Irrigation of the mouth is best accomplished

with a commercial irrigator. If a commercial irrigator is too costly, a bulb syringe can be used. Even the swish-and-swallow technique of rinsing the mouth with water is better than doing nothing. The person should also be instructed to gently brush the tongue and to inspect the entire oral cavity for signs of irritation.

Individuals who wear dentures should also be instructed in proper oral hygiene. Dentures should be cleaned thoroughly every day. In some people, food debris tends to become trapped under the dentures. If this is a problem, the person should be instructed to remove the denture and rinse it after each meal to prevent irritation. Thorough cleansing can be done by brushing with a commercial dentifrice or by using a soaking cleanser. Some people choose to use both. Many individuals use a powder or pad to help the dentures adhere to the gums. It is important that all of the fixative be removed at each cleansing. If it is not removed, an uneven surface may result and irritate the gums. Dentures should be cleaned and stored in tepid water because hot water may cause them to warp. When the dentures are out of the mouth, the entire oral cavity should be cleansed with a soft- to moderate-bristle brush and the entire oral cavity inspected for signs of irritation. If there are signs of irritation from the dentures, the individual should see the dentist. Dentures can be reworked until they fit comfortably.

4. **Provide assistive devices as needed.** If the individual has difficulty holding the toothbrush because of arthritis or a weakened grip, modifications may be needed. Wrapping tape, aluminum foil, a small sponge, a polystyrene ball, or other padding around the handle of the brush may make it easier to grasp. Handle extenders made of a ruler or dowel rod may help those who are unable to reach the mouth easily (Fig. 11-12).

5. **Obtain the assistance of family members, friends, or community agencies.** Some elderly may require transportation or other help in getting to dental appointments. The assistance of family members, friends, or transportation services may be needed to keep dental appointments. Family and friends can also help by purchasing and setting up oral hygiene equipment. A family member or friend can be shown how to modify a toothbrush or prepare floss for use by the elderly person.

6. **Explain the need to avoid alcohol and tobacco.** Because alcohol and tobacco are likely to irritate the mucous membranes and cause significant health problems, it is important that nurses stress the importance of eliminating, or at least restricting, their use.

7. **Promote adequate intake of nutrients and fluids.** Nurses should explain how nutrients, particularly vitamins, can contribute to healthy mucous membranes. Instruction about diet may be necessary if inadequacies are detected. The importance of fluid intake for saliva formation and its use as a rinse for the mucous membranes should be stressed. The elderly should be encouraged to keep a glass of water available by the chair or bedside as a reminder to drink adequate fluids. Highly sugared beverages should be avoided because they encourage tooth decay. Many elderly with altered mucous membranes prefer to avoid ice in beverages, which can stimulate toothache. If

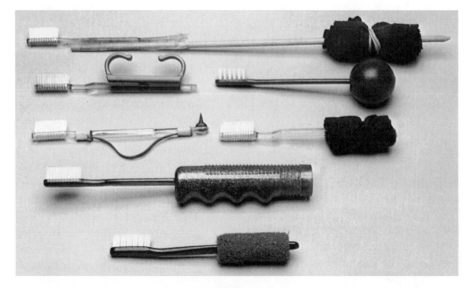

FIG. 11-12   Adaptive aids for brushing. (From Papas AS, et al: *Geriatric dentistry: aging and oral health*, St Louis, 1991, Mosby.)

the individual has difficulty chewing food because of loose or missing teeth, a food processor, grinder, or blender can be used to change the food's consistency.

8. **Discuss the benefits of adequate moisture in the environment.** If the environment is dry or if the individual is a mouth-breather, an additional source of moisture may be needed. A freestanding humidifier or one attached to the furnace will increase the moisture present in the air so that less will be drawn away from the mucous membranes.

9. **Suggest use of hard candy, chewing gum, or artificial saliva to increase moisture in the mouth.** Sucking on hard candy or chewing gum will stimulate the production of saliva. If a sugar-based candy or gum is used, the teeth must be brushed more frequently to avoid tooth decay. Those on sugar-restricted diets should use only sugar-free candy or gum. Artificial saliva preparations may be used according to package directions if there is no medical contraindication.

10. **Discuss the relationship between medications and oral hygiene.** If the individual is receiving any medications that could affect the mucous membranes, he or she should be taught any necessary observations or precautions. For example, people who are taking phenytoin (Dilantin) for epilepsy or people who are on antibiotic therapy should know the possible side effects that indicate the necessity to contact the physician.

11. **Use any appropriate interventions that are used in the institutional setting.**

SUMMARY

Under normal conditions the aging skin and mucous membranes are more susceptible to damage than are the comparable tissues of younger individuals. When disease factors are present the risk for damage is even greater. Careful assessment allows nurses to recognize normal changes and identify any abnormalities that may indicate more serious problems. Nursing interventions are designed to reduce the risk of damage or trauma to fragile tissues.

READINGS AND REFERENCES

Allman, et al: Pressure ulcer risk formation among hospitalized patients with activity limitation, *JAMA* 273:865, 1995.

Bergstrom N, et al: Assessing risk and preventing pressure ulcers, *Patient Care* 27:36, 1993.

Bergstrom N, et al: The Braden scale for predicting pressure sore risk, *Nurs Res* 36:205, 1987.

Berkey DB, et al: The old-old dental patient: the challenge of clinical decision making, *J Am Dent Assoc,* 127:321, 1996.

Berlowitz DR, et al: Rating long-term care facilities on pressure ulcer development: importance of case mix adjustment, *Ann Intern Med* 124:557, 1996.

Brandeis GH, Powell JW: Preventing and treating pressure ulcers, *Brown University Long-Term Care Quality Letter* 6:1, 1994.

Carroll P: Bed selection (beds for pressure sores), *RN* 58:44, 1995.

Chernoff R: Policy: Nutrition standards for treatment of pressure ulcers, *Nutr Rev* 54:S43, 1996.

Daouiche RO, et al: Osteomyelitis associated with pressure ulcers, *Arch Intern Med* 154:753, 1994.

Hermosillo D: Bare facts on skin care, *Independent Living* 8:28, 1993.

Hofman A, et al: Pressure sore and pressure-decreasing mattresses: controlled clinical trials, *Lancet* 43:568, 1994.

Huber J: Latest development and practices in the treatment of pressure ulcers, *Palaestra* 9:64, 1993.

Jeter KF, Lutz JB: Skin care in the frail, elderly, dependent, incontinent patient, *Adv Wound Care* 9:29, 1996.

Kayser-Jones J, et al: An instrument to assess the oral health status of nursing home residents, *Gerontologist* 35:814, 1995.

Ketch LL: Pressure sores, *West J Med* 158:403, 1993.

Krasner D: Managing pain from pressure ulcers, *Am J Nurs* 95:22, 1995.

Maklebust J: Pressure ulcers: what works, *RN* 58:46, 1995.

Marsh R: Care of decubitus ulcers, *Independent Living* 9:21, 1994.

Mor V: Documenting pressure ulcer care using the MDS, *Brown University Long-Term Care Quality Letter* 7:3, 1995.

National Pressure Ulcer Advisory Panel: Pressure ulcer research: etiology, assessment and early intervention, *Dermatol Nurs,* 8:41, 1996.

Nursing home-based skin care: where we are and where we're headed: an overview, *Nursing Homes* 42:25, 1993.

Patterson D: Advances in pressure relief and reduction, *Nursing Homes* 43:44, 1994.

Paules SJ, Levisohn D, Heffron W: Persistent scabies in nursing home patients, *J Fam Pract* 37:82, 1993.

Perez D: Pressure ulcers: updated guidelines for treatment and prevention, *Geriatrics* 48:39, 1993.

Pressure sores, *Ostomy Quarterly* 32:68, 1995.

Pressure ulcer treatment, *Am Fam Physician* 51:1207, 1995.

Schubert V, Heraud J: The effects of pressure and shear on skin microcirculation in elderly stroke patients lying in supine or semi-recumbant positions, *Age Aging* 23:405, 1994.

Spoelhof GD, Ide K: Pressure ulcers in nursing home patients, *Am Fam Physician* 47:1207, 1993.

Van Rijswijk L: Moist wound healing with occlusive dressings, *Nursing Homes* 43:27, 1994.

Whittington K: Debunking wound care myths, *RN* 58:32, 1995.

ELIMINATION

LEARNING OBJECTIVES

1. Describe the normal elimination processes.
2. Describe age-related changes in bladder and bowel elimination.
3. Discuss methods for assessing elimination practices.
4. Identify the older adults who are most at risk for problems with elimination.
5. Identify selected nursing diagnoses related to elimination problems.
6. Describe interventions used to prevent or reduce problems related to elimination.

In order to function properly, the body must be able to rid itself of waste products effectively. The two major systems involved in waste elimination are the urinary system and the gastrointestinal (GI) system. Small amounts of urea (a by-product of protein metabolism) and sodium chloride can be eliminated through the skin, but the skin is not considered a major site of elimination.

NORMAL ELIMINATION PATTERNS

Adults develop patterns for bowel and bladder elimination that are somewhat unique to themselves. As long as the pattern is within normal limits and is effective for the individual, no special intervention is required. Diet, fluid intake, activity, and lifestyle influence these patterns. Even in young adults, elimination patterns can be disrupted by illness, medications, or changes in daily routine.

The typical adult bowel movement consists of a moderate amount of formed, brown stool that is passed without difficulty. The normal frequency of bowel elimination varies from several stools per day to only two or three per week. Most adults experience bowel elimination every 1 to 2 days. The urge to defecate most commonly occurs 30 to 45 minutes after a meal, when the gastrocolic and defecation reflexes stimulate peristalsis. Another common time for defecation is first thing in the morning after consumption of a warm beverage. Many people develop a daily routine or establish rituals over their lifetimes that are designed to promote normal elimination. Attempts to change these habits late in life can create problems.

Urine elimination in adults also follows patterns. The typical adult experiences the urge to urinate when the bladder contains about 300 ml of urine. Voluntary control of the external sphincter muscles enables healthy adults to hold larger amounts within the bladder until urination is convenient. Most adults void between 6 and 10 times a day, but this may vary greatly depending on fluid consumption, personal habits, and emotional state.

ELIMINATION AND AGING

A large percentage of the elderly population suffers from problems with elimination. The most common elimination problems experienced by the elderly are constipation, diarrhea, and incontinence of bladder and/or bowel. These problems may result from changes in the function of the GI system or the urinary system, or they may be related to changes in other body systems such as the musculoskeletal and nervous systems.

Incontinence of bladder and/or bowel is one of the most common reasons that older adults are institutionalized. Many families who can cope with other problems are unable to deal with incontinence.

Constipation

Constipation means different things to different people. It is not a disease but a symptom of some other problem. Constipation is defined as hard, dry stools that are difficult to pass. Because bowel elimination patterns can differ widely from person to person, the frequency of elimination is not a good measure. For some people, regularity means more than one bowel movement a day; for others it means three bowel movements a week. Elderly people who were raised with the idea that a daily bowel movement is essential to health tend to spend undue amounts of time worrying about their bowels.

Constipation, both real and perceived, is a common complaint of the elderly. Changes related to aging or chronic illness increase the risk for constipation. Factors that increase the risk of constipation include decreased abdominal muscle tone, inactivity, immobility, inadequate fluid intake, inadequate dietary bulk, disease conditions, medications, dependence on laxatives or enemas, and various environmental conditions.

Peristalsis normally slows somewhat with aging. Loss of abdominal muscle tone and inadequate physical activity contribute to even slower peristalsis. Elderly individuals with weak abdominal muscles and those who are inactive or immobile are highly likely to become constipated.

Water is absorbed as waste products pass through the large intestine. Inadequate fluid intake or excessive fluid loss through perspiration, emesis, or wounds increases the body's need to recover as much fluid as possible. Because many of the elderly suffer from some degree of fluid volume deficit, the body attempts to reabsorb as much fluid from the stool as possible. The physiologic need to absorb water combined with a slower rate of peristalsis results in stools that are drier, harder, and more difficult to pass. Fluid volume deficit also leads to a decrease in urine production.

Dietary fiber plays an important role in promoting normal bowel elimination because this indigestible substance is very effective at trapping moisture and providing bulk to the wastes. Foods such as whole grains, fruits, vegetables, and lean meats are high in fiber. Fiber-rich foods are often lacking in the elderly person's diet because these foods are more difficult to chew, particularly when teeth are loose or missing. Foods such as dairy products, eggs, refined breads, desserts, and many convenience foods consumed by the elderly contain very little fiber. When the diet lacks adequate fiber, less stool is produced. This small amount moves more slowly through the intestine, further contributing to excessive dryness. The small mass of stool produced without fiber is inadequate to stimulate the normal defecation reflex, resulting in infrequent elimination with as many as 4 or more days between bowel movements.

The risk for constipation is increased with a number of disease processes, including stroke, diabetes, metabolic imbalances, dementia, and depression. Cancerous tumors located in the GI tract can result in a partial or total obstruction that can be mistaken for constipation or impaction.

Medications often contribute to constipation in the elderly. The more medications an elderly person takes, the greater his or her risk is of medication-induced constipation. Medications identified as increasing the risk of constipation include narcotic analgesics, particularly those containing codeine; anticholinergics, including many tricyclic antidepressants and antipsychotics; diuretics; iron supplements; calcium-channel blockers; antacids containing aluminum carbonate or aluminum hydroxide; some anticonvulsants; some nonsteroidal antiinflammatory agents; and possibly some antihypertensive agents, such as the angiotensin-converting enzyme (ACE) inhibitors.

Many elderly individuals who have had problems with constipation over the years may have dealt with them by taking laxatives or enemas. It is estimated that about 30% of healthy elderly persons take laxatives regularly. Some started taking laxatives when they were quite young because "regularity" (having a daily bowel movement) was at one time considered important for good health. Some elderly people have been taking laxatives or enemas daily for 50 or 60 years. We now recognize that this is dangerous because the body can become dependent and require this assistance to stimulate elimination. Reestablishing normal bowel elimination in a laxative-dependent elderly person is almost impossible because the body has "forgotten" how to work on its own.

Repeatedly ignoring the urge to defecate can lead to suppression or even extinction of the defecation reflex. Changes in neurologic sensitivity or fear of pain may cause the elderly to ignore or delay defecation. Those with neurologic disorders may not be aware of the need to defecate because the strength of nerve impulses transmitted to and from the sphincter muscles is decreased. With no urge to defecate, individuals may go for many days unaware of the fact that their bowels have not emptied. Elderly individuals who encounter pain with defecation are more likely to avoid or deliberately delay what they know will be a painful experience. Pain can originate from the decreased production of mucus in the intestine that is typical with aging. Without the lubrication provided by mucous, the stool becomes excessively dry and irritating to the rectal tissues. The presence of hemorrhoids or anal fissures further contributes to the likelihood of pain. Delaying defecation creates a vicious circle. When defecation is delayed the stool becomes harder, dryer, and more difficult to pass. This in turn leads to more painful defecation, which results in further avoidance of defecation. Active interventions are needed to break this cycle.

Delays in defecation are not always chosen by the elderly person. An aging person who requires assistance may need to suppress the defecation reflex while waiting for help getting to the bathroom. If this occurs repeatedly, the individual may lose sensitivity to the urge to defecate and become constipated. If unable to suppress the urge, he or she runs the risk of being considered incontinent.

Environmental factors can play a role in constipation, particularly with the institutionalized elderly. The aging person may be embarrassed by the sounds or odors involved with bowel elimination. Lack of privacy may cause anxiety or may result in the person's ignoring or suppressing the urge to defecate.

Difficulty assuming an anatomically suitable or comfortable position can also interfere with effective bowel elimination. Sitting upright or squatting are the preferred positions for defecation because it is easier to bear down in these positions, and gravity assists elimination when the body is upright. People confined to bed find that bedpans are particularly uncomfortable and difficult to use. Although they may be necessary, bedpans should be avoided whenever the use of a toilet or commode chair is possible.

Fecal Impaction

Fecal impaction, the presence of a mass of hardened feces that is trapped in the rectum and cannot be expelled, is a result of unrelieved constipation. In severe cases, the fecal mass may extend up into the sigmoid colon. Individuals who have a history of chronic constipation are most at risk for impaction.

Symptoms of impaction include a longer than usual delay in defecation. More than 3 days without a bowel movement warrants close attention. Passage of small amounts of liquid stool without any formed fecal material can also indicate impaction. This liquid stool is fecal material from higher in the colon that is able to pass around the hardened mass. It typically oozes from the rectum and differs from a diarrheal stool, which passes with normal force.

Aging persons suffering from fecal impaction are likely to complain of cramping or rectal pain. Abdominal distention and loss of appetite are common. Digital examination of the rectum typically reveals the presence of a hardened mass of feces. This procedure should be done with extreme caution because it is uncomfortable and traumatic to the rectal tissues. Particular caution must be used when examining elderly persons with a history of cardiac problems because rectal examination can stimulate the vagus nerve and result in a sudden decrease in heart rate, syncope, or even loss of consciousness. Some facilities require physician's orders before a digital examination of the rectum is performed.

Before deciding that an elderly person has a problem with bowel elimination, nurses should thoroughly assesses the total situation, including the frequency, amount, and consistency of stools. Assessment should also include identification of factors that contribute to the development of bowel elimination problems. This will enable development of a plan that promotes sound elimination patterns.

Constipation is the most common problem in the elderly, but diarrhea and fecal incontinence are fairly common occurrences. Information regarding these conditions is presented later in this chapter.

NURSING PROCESS

ALTERATIONS IN BOWEL ELIMINATION

Assessment of Bowel Elimination

- How often does the person have a bowel movement?
- Is there any pattern to when bowel elimination occurs?
- Is the person continent or incontinent of stool?
- What is the consistency of the stool?
- What is the amount of stool?
- What is the color of the stool?
- Are blood, mucus, undigested food, or other unusual substances evident in the stool?
- Has the stool been checked for occult blood?
- Does the person have to strain to have a bowel movement?
- Is the stool expelled with excessive force or does it ooze from the body?
- Do you observe or does the person report any particular foods that affect bowel movements?

BOX 12-1
Risk Factors Related to Bowel Elimination in the Elderly

- Neurologic problems that decrease the ability to sense the need for elimination or to control the sphincter muscles
- Reduced mobility
- Inadequate intake of dietary bulk
- Tube feedings
- Gastrointestinal obstructions or disease (Crohn's disease, diverticulosis)
- Inadequate fluid intake
- Cognitive impairment (Alzheimer's disease, dementia)

- Do these foods cause diarrhea or constipation?
- Does the elderly person rely on any aids for bowel elimination (suppositories, laxatives, or enemas)?
- How long has the person been using this aid?
- Is the abdomen distended?
- If the person cannot speak, does he or she rub the abdomen?
- Has the person's appetite decreased?
- If the person cannot sense rectal fullness, what does digital examination of the rectum reveal?
- Does the person's diet have adequate bulk?
- Does the person take any bulk enhancers?
- What does the person say about his or her bowel habits?
- Has the person's bowel pattern changed recently?
- Does the person report any concerns related to bowel elimination?

See Box 12-1 for a list of risk factors for problems with bowel elimination in the elderly.

Nursing Diagnosis

Constipation

Nursing Goals/Outcomes

The nursing goals for elderly individuals diagnosed with constipation are (1) to exhibit regular patterns of bowel elimination, (2) to identify behaviors that promote normal bowel functioning, and (3) to modify behaviors to enhance regular bowel elimination.

Nursing Interventions

The following nursing interventions should take place in hospitals or extended-care facilities:

1. **Assess bowel elimination patterns and contribut-**

ing factors. It is important to determine whether the aging person actually has a problem with constipation or only perceives a problem. Because many elderly people cling to the idea that daily bowel elimination is necessary, they may consider themselves constipated when no real problem exists. If this is the case, nurses should explain the normal range of variation. If the person is experiencing constipation, the causes should be determined and the plan of care directed toward eliminating or reducing the causative factors. Aging persons with a history of constipation or risk factors for constipation must be assessed regularly to avoid fecal impaction.

2. **Increase physical activity.** Physical mobility—even as little as twisting the body, turning from side to side, flexing the trunk, or lifting the legs to the abdomen—can help stimulate peristalsis. If possible, the elderly should be encouraged to participate in more vigorous activity such as walking, bending, and stretching.

3. **Increase intake of dietary fiber and fluids.** Increased fluids and dietary bulk will enhance the normal process of defecation. Cereal fiber is more effective at preventing constipation, and most older adults find it palatable. Some foods such as bran or prunes have bulk *and* a natural laxative effect. Many elderly will accept these foods if they are offered as part of the breakfast meal.

   An increase in fluid intake will reduce the risk of constipation from excessive absorption in the large intestine. Fluid intake of 2000 ml/day is recommended. More fluid is necessary during hot summer months or when illness results in excessive fluid loss. Elderly people who take diuretics should be encouraged to consume adequate fluids as long as their cardiovascular status is stable.

4. **Schedule or encourage toileting at times when the person's defecation urge is strongest.** If the individual suppresses the urge to defecate, he or she is at greater risk for constipation. Encouraging the elderly to use the toilet (or taking them there) at a time when defecation is likely will enable a healthy pattern to develop. The most likely times are early in the morning, after drinking the first warm beverage of the day, and shortly after meals. Some elderly persons go through established rituals that support normal elimination. The existence and nature of these rituals should be determined by talking with the person, and this information should be used in care planning.

5. **Position the person to facilitate ease of elimination.** Use of a toilet is most conducive to normal elimination. If this is not possible, a bedside commode where the person can be seated is the next best option. Positioning a small footstool under the feet of the elderly person who has weak abdominal muscles increases intraabdominal pressure and may make defecation easier. A bedpan is the least desirable option. Bedpans are uncomfortable, and their use makes it difficult for the person to achieve the normal "bearing down" force that is necessary for defecation.

6. **Provide privacy for elimination.** Privacy will reduce the risk of constipation that results from suppressing elimination to prevent embarrassment. To prevent unpleasant odors, soiled bedpans should be removed promptly and an air freshener supplied.

7. **Administer stool softeners or bulk-forming laxatives as prescribed by the physician.** Stool softeners keep fecal material moist and reduce the chance of irritation to the anus when stool is passed. Bulk-forming substances such as psyllium (Metamucil) expand and trap moisture in the feces. Care must be used to administer these bulk-forming laxatives with adequate amounts of fluid. If adequate fluid is not ingested, these substances can cause constipation or bowel obstructions (Table 12-1).

8. **Administer prescribed suppositories or enemas if other methods have not been effective.** If other methods of stimulating defecation have not been effective, it may be necessary to administer suppositories or enemas. Glycerine suppositories are usually well tolerated by the elderly. They enhance elimination by drawing fluid into the bowel through osmosis. Biscodyl suppositories are fairly well tolerated but are more likely to cause cramping. The elderly are more likely to accept suppositories because they are generally less traumatic and less invasive than are enemas. Enemas should be used with caution because they can lead to damage of the rectal mucosa and contribute to electrolyte imbalance. If performed incorrectly, enemas increase the risk of rectal perforation.

The following interventions should take place in the home:

1. **Provide information regarding high-fiber foods, and encourage increased consumption of these.** Many elderly individuals prefer processed foods that are easy to prepare and chew. Providing information about the value of foods that are easily obtained such as cereals, whole wheat breads, bran muffins, and prunes can help the elderly select foods that will reduce the incidence of constipation. If family members prepare the meals, the importance of fiber in preventing constipation should be discussed.

2. **Encourage adequate fluid intake.** Approximately 2000 ml of fluid should be taken each day. This should include approximately six glasses of water, juice, and other beverages such as tea or coffee.

TABLE 12-1

Considerations Related to Certain Laxatives

Type	Considerations
Stimulant laxatives Phenolphthalein Castor oil Bisacody Senna	Use with caution in the elderly; can cause cramping or vomiting; may lead to electrolyte imbalance, altered fat absorption, fat-soluble vitamin deficiency, and dependency; less expensive than some other forms
Bulk laxatives Psyllium Calcium polycarbophil Methyl cellulose	Work effectively; safe for long-term use in the elderly; can cause flatulence; resistance or noncompliance is common due to taste; risk of worsened constipation or impaction if fluid intake is inadequate
Hyperosomolar laxatives Lactulose Sorbitol	Safe and effective even in frail elderly
Fecal softeners Docusate sodium	Do not have a laxative action so are not effective for chronic constipation; result in softer stool allowing easier passage when straining is dangerous

Some individuals drink senna tea, which has laxative properties.

3. **Encourage adequate activity and exercise.** Activity enhances peristalsis and, along with good dietary practices, is most important in preventing constipation. Walking after meals may very effectively stimulate the urge to defecate. Aging persons should stay near toilet facilities so that they can act immediately when the urge arises. Suppressing the urge to defecate can increase the risk of constipation.

4. **Discuss the risks involved with the use of laxatives without medical supervision.** Many older adults are unaware of the side effects and problems related to laxative use. These concerns should be discussed, and the elderly should be encouraged to discuss any bowel elimination problems with the physician before using laxatives.

5. **Use any appropriate interventions that are used in the institutional setting.**

A nursing care plan for constipation is presented on p. 198.

Diarrhea

Diarrhea is defined as the frequent passage of liquid, unformed stools. The stools are liquid because they pass through the large intestine too rapidly and are expelled before sufficient water can be absorbed in the large intestine. Diarrhea is a symptom and can have many causes in the elderly, such as malabsorption syndromes, tumors of the GI tract, lactose intolerance, diverticulosis, and pathogenic organisms. Aging persons who receive large amounts of concentrated tube feedings often experience diarrhea.

Many elderly persons with diarrhea complain of nausea, vomiting, and abdominal cramps in addition to frequent stools. Rectal pain and skin irritation of the anus and buttocks are common because fecal material is very irritating.

Diarrhea can easily result in excessive fluid loss. This is a major concern in the elderly, who are already at risk for fluid volume deficit. Because diarrhea can quickly result in dehydration, the physician should be notified promptly so that the cause can be isolated and treatment begun.

Nursing Diagnosis

Diarrhea

Nursing Goals/Outcomes

The nursing goals for elderly individuals diagnosed with diarrhea are (1) to exhibit regular patterns of bowel elimination, (2) to identify behaviors that promote normal bowel functioning, and (3) to modify behaviors to enhance regular bowel elimination.

Nursing Interventions

The following nursing interventions should take place in hospitals or extended-care facilities:

1. **Assess the elimination pattern and suspected causative factors.** Diarrhea in the elderly can result from many factors. It is important that nurses pay close attention to the frequency and nature of stools. Time of day of the onset as well as any factors that appear related to the onset of loose stools

---

NURSING CARE PLAN

ELIMINATION

Mrs. Port is an 85-year-old woman who resides at Shady Grove Nursing Home. She has mild osteoarthritis, and she prefers to sit and visit or do crafts. She can move about using a walker. When her osteoarthritis pain is severe, she takes acetaminophen with codeine #3.

She eats with friends in the dining room and prefers to eat meat, white bread, and desserts. She eats very little of the fruits or vegetables served, and she consumes about 1200 ml of fluid per day.

Mrs. Port reports that she has bowel movements about every 2 or 3 days. "I used to have a bowel movement every other day. Now I really have to push and it hurts to have a BM." The nursing assistant reports that the stool is hard and dry.

NURSING DIAGNOSIS

Constipation

DEFINING CHARACTERISTICS

- 2 to 3 days between bowel movements
- Complaints of straining at stool
- Hard, dry stools
- Less than normal frequency of bowel movements

GOALS/OUTCOMES

Mrs. Port will have regular bowel movements at 1- to 2-day intervals; experience no difficulty passing stool; and describe diet changes that promote regular elimination.

NURSING INTERVENTIONS

1. Assess bowel elimination pattern for the frequency, amount, consistency, and effort required.
2. Explain the importance and effect of adequate fluid intake on bowel elimination.
3. Design a plan for increasing fluid intake to 2000 ml per day, including beverages favored by Mrs. Port.
4. Encourage consumption of fruits, vegetables, and whole grain breads or cereals.
5. Discuss alternative measures for pain control to decrease reliance on codeine-based medication.
6. Encourage increased physical activity.

EVALUATION

Mrs. Port has increased her fluid intake to 1800 ml/day. She reports eating bran cereal, whole wheat toast, and prune juice for breakfast and a fruit or vegetable with lunch and dinner. Formed, soft bowel movements have been reported every other day and documented in Mrs. Port's chart. She states, "It feels so much better when I don't have to strain." Continue the plan of care.

---

should be assessed. For example, a loose stool that follows a meal, a tube feeding, or administration of a medication is significant and should be reported. Additional complaints such as pain, cramping, fever, and force of expulsion should be assessed. If the liquid stool seeps from the rectum, fecal impaction must be suspected. Removal of the impaction will correct this problem.

2. **Maintain adequate fluid intake.** Diarrheal stools lead to an excessive loss of body fluid. Fluid re- placement to prevent dehydration is essential. In addition to simple fluid balance, electrolyte levels may be disturbed if the episodes of diarrhea are severe or prolonged. Oral fluids should be provided within dietary restrictions. Fluids that are rich in electrolytes (e.g., juices, Gatorade, or broth) are better than plain water. Fluids that are high in fiber, caffeine, and milk should be avoided because they tend to induce diarrhea. If the individual is unable to take fluids orally, intravenous infusions

may be necessary. The elderly should be watched carefully for signs of dehydration, such as decreased skin turgor, postural hypotension, tachycardia, and altered laboratory values.

3. **Institute measures to maintain skin integrity.** Clean the skin immediately after each episode of diarrhea. Diarrheal stool is very irritating to the skin and can rapidly lead to skin breakdown. The anal area should be washed after each stool, and a protective ointment or lotion should be applied to provide a barrier against the caustic body wastes. If the skin becomes excessively irritated and tender to touch, sitz baths followed by air drying or heat lamp treatments may help promote healing. Care must be taken to prevent further trauma to the tissue. Bed linens must be kept clean and dry at all times.

4. **Promptly report observations to the physician, and follow-up on physician's orders regarding medications that decrease intestinal motility.** Diarrhea in the elderly is a serious concern. Because it can have many causes, diarrhea should be reported to the physician promptly so that its origin can be determined. The physician will probably prescribe not only fluid maintenance but also medications to decrease the rate of intestinal motility and increase water absorption. The timing for administering these medications is usually related to the frequency of diarrheal stools. It is important that nurses administer the medications as prescribed.

   If diarrhea persists, diagnostic tests on stool specimens may be ordered to determine whether the diarrhea is parasitic or bacterial in origin. Precautions, including gloves and proper hand washing, must be followed when obtaining or handling stool specimens.

The following interventions should take place in the home:

1. **Explain the importance of seeking medical attention if the person is experiencing diarrhea.** Many elderly persons become severely dehydrated from diarrhea before they seek medical attention. Nurses should stress the importance of calling a physician if diarrhea is severe or lasts more than 1 day. Any additional complaints such as abdominal pain, cramping, or fever also indicate the need to call a physician immediately. Many prescription and nonprescription medications can cause diarrhea. Because many elderly persons have prescriptions from more than one physician, it is important that they tell each physician all of the medications they are taking, including over-the-counter preparations.

2. **Explain the importance of proper food preparation and storage in preventing bacterial diarrhea.** Many cases of diarrhea are related to improper food preparation or storage. Many elderly people do not pay close attention to the length of time food sits on the table or stove. If not refrigerated, food becomes a good medium for the growth of bacteria, many of which can cause diarrhea. Nurses should stress the importance of refrigerating all dairy products, meats, and other prepared foods immediately after purchase or after the meal. Food should not be allowed to "warm up" on the counter for hours before preparation.

3. **Use any appropriate interventions that are used in the institutional setting.**

Bowel Incontinence

Bowel incontinence is the inability to control the passage of fecal material from the anus. Aging persons who suffer from neurologic or cognitive problems are likely to experience bowel incontinence. Because they are unable to perceive the need to defecate or control the sphincter muscles, they are unable to prevent the defecation process. Some persons are cognitively aware of the need to defecate but are physiologically unable to control the process. Incontinence is highly embarrassing to these individuals and may result in their withdrawal from social activities. Bowel incontinence can lead to tissue damage if wastes are not promptly removed from the skin.

Nursing Diagnosis

Bowel incontinence

Nursing Goals/Outcomes

The nursing goals for elderly individuals diagnosed with bowel incontinence are (1) to exhibit regular patterns of bowel elimination, (2) to identify behaviors that promote normal bowel functioning, and (3) to modify behaviors to enhance regular bowel elimination.

Nursing Interventions

The following nursing interventions should take place in hospitals or extended-care facilities:

1. **Assess patterns of elimination and causative factors.** It is important to know how often and when the individual is incontinent. If these episodes have a regular pattern, nurses can use this information to plan nursing care. For example, many individuals have a pattern of defecating 30 to 45 minutes after a meal. If the person is taken to the bathroom at that time, an episode of incontinence will be prevented. Unfortunately, not all individuals have such a regular pattern of defecation.

2. **Establish a toileting schedule.** If a defecation pattern is detected, the person should be taken to the bathroom at the time they are most likely to defe-

cate. If there is no detectable pattern, the physician may order the use of digital stimulation or glycerin suppositories. When repeated on a daily or every-other-day basis, these measures may establish a regular pattern of defecation. When planning a toileting schedule, nurses should consider the elderly person's daily routines and scheduled appointments (e.g., physical therapy). To be effective, all individuals and departments that have contact with the individual should be aware of the plan and follow through with it.

3. **Take measures to prevent or reduce episodes of constipation.** It is difficult to prevent incontinence when an individual is constipated. Measures used to prevent constipation will increase the likelihood of regular elimination.

4. **Use appropriate aids or garments.** It is best if episodes of incontinence can be prevented by regular toileting or other methods discussed previously. If these measures are not completely successful, use of special pads or garments can reduce the embarrassment of soiling the bed or clothing. These aids should not be used in place of other nursing measures that promote bowel control.

5. **Clean the person promptly after each episode of incontinence.** Incontinence can easily lead to skin breakdown. It is essential that any soiled linens or garments be removed as soon as possible to reduce skin irritation. This care should be provided tactfully to reduce damage to the self-esteem of the elderly, most of whom are acutely embarrassed by their incontinence and will be sensitive to any negative verbal or nonverbal communication from the nursing staff. All soiled materials should be removed from the room and put into appropriate containers to reduce environmental odors.

The following intervention should take place in the home:

1. **Use any appropriate interventions that are used in the institutional setting.**

NURSING PROCESS

ALTERATIONS IN URINARY ELIMINATION

Urinary Retention

Urinary retention is an abnormal accumulation of urine in the bladder because the bladder is unable to empty completely. Normally, no more than 50 ml of urine remains in the bladder after voiding. The person experiencing urinary retention often has several hundred milliliters remaining after voiding. Urinary retention in the elderly can result from decreased muscle tone in the bladder wall, decreased fluid intake, prostate gland enlargement, trauma to the muscles of the perineum, neurologic damage, medications, or anxiety.

Symptoms of retention include a feeling of fullness, discomfort or tenderness in the bladder, restlessness, and diaphoresis. Persons experiencing urinary retention may complain of a total inability to void or of passing small amounts (between 25 and 50 ml) of urine at frequent intervals. This pattern is called **retention with overflow.** Severe retention results in bladder distention that can be detected by inspecting or palpating the area over the symphysis pubis. Treatment of urinary retention depends on the cause. If retention is due to perineal trauma or anxiety, noninvasive measures such as medications or a sitz bath may be enough to stimulate effective voiding. If severe retention is due to an obstruction such as an enlarged prostate, catheterization or surgery may be necessary to prevent serious bladder damage that may result from persistent or excessive bladder distention.

Urinary Incontinence

Urinary incontinence is the involuntary loss of urine in sufficient amount or frequency to be a social or hygiene problem. Urinary incontinence is a major problem in the aging population. It is estimated that nearly 30% of independent-living and 50 % of institutionalized elderly have problems with incontinence (Box 12-2).

Incontinence has medical, emotional, social, and economic consequences for the elderly. Incontinence can result in skin irritation or breakdown and can contribute to pressure ulcers; it can lead to guilt and frustration; it can lead to social isolation; and it can be costly because of the need for expensive undergarments, extra laundry expenses, or even the cost of institutional care.

BOX 12-2

Reversible Causes of Incontinence

D—Delirium
I—Infections
A—Atrophic vaginitis
P—Psychologic causes (depression, psychosomatic)
P—Pharmaceutical agents
E—Endocrine conditions (particularly diabetes mellitus)
R—Restricted mobility (including environmental barriers)
S—Stool impaction

The elderly may hesitate to discuss incontinence problems with the physician or nurse because they are embarrassed or because they think that incontinence is simply a problem of aging that they must endure. The topic must therefore be introduced in a sensitive manner by caregivers. In some cases incontinence is curable using surgery, medications, or other treatments. In other cases it can be managed to allow the elderly person a more normal lifestyle.

A number of normal physiologic changes that occur with aging and common diseases seen with aging can cause or contribute to incontinence. Different forms of incontinence (i.e., stress, urge, overflow, functional, and total incontinence) are recognized as problems in the elderly.

Stress incontinence

Stress incontinence is leakage of urine during conditions that increase intraabdominal pressure such as exercise, lifting heavy objects, laughing, coughing, or sneezing. When a full bladder is compressed against weakened urinary sphincters, incontinence occurs. This problem is most commonly observed in women, particularly those who have weakened perineal muscles due to aging and childbearing.

Urge incontinence

Urge incontinence is characterized by a sudden, strong urge to void. Individuals suffering from urge incontinence are often unable to hold back the urine long enough to reach a commode or toilet. Urge incontinence is often seen in older individuals who suffer from diseases that affect nerve transmission to the bladder (e.g., Parkinson's disease, multiple sclerosis, stroke, and dementia). Urge incontinence is also observed when there is increased bladder stimulation due to lower urinary tract infections, concentrated urine, and irritating chemicals such as caffeine or alcohol. Atrophic urethritis, uterine prolapse, fecal impaction, or prostate enlargement also increases the likelihood of urge incontinence. Even healthy elderly individuals with no known medical problems may experience occasional episodes of urge incontinence.

Urge incontinence has its basis in the physiologic changes seen with aging. With aging, the bladder decreases in size; it can hold less volume (often 200 ml or less) and needs to be emptied more often. This results in the increased urinary frequency seen with aging. When larger volumes of urine are produced in response to excessive fluid intake or increased use of diuretics, the problem of urinary frequency is magnified. In addition, many elderly experience involuntary spasms of the muscles of the bladder wall called **detrusor spasms.** These spasms can occur even when the

bladder contains small volumes, resulting in a sense of urgency to empty the bladder. When the need to void is frequent and urgent, the result is urge incontinence.

Urge incontinence is likely to occur after removal of an indwelling catheter. Use of an indwelling catheter results in diminished bladder capacity. Frequency, urgency, and incontinence are likely to occur when a catheter is removed suddenly without incremental clamping, which allows the bladder muscles to stretch gradually to accommodate larger volumes.

Overflow incontinence

Overflow incontinence is defined as leakage of small amounts of urine from an overly full bladder. The bladder cannot hold the amount of urine being produced so it overflows. Overflow incontinence is a common problem for diabetics suffering from loss of bladder muscle tone due to neuropathy or experiencing polyuria related to hyperglycemia. Overflow incontinence is also common in elderly men with benign prostate hyperplasia. Enlargement of the prostate restricts the flow of urine so that the bladder never empties completely. This contributes to overflow problems (see the section on urinary retention). Women who have an obstruction at the outlet of the bladder due to a prolapsed uterus, cystocele, or rectocele may experience similar problems. Those with neurologic disorders such as multiple sclerosis or spinal cord injuries above the sacral area are also prone to overflow incontinence.

Functional incontinence

Functional incontinence is seen in older adults who have normal urethral and bladder function. It is caused by a poor relationship between the aging person's abilities and his or her environment. Changes in functional ability may be cognitive or physical in nature. The inability to recognize a toilet, perform simple tasks such as using a zipper or pulling down underwear, walk to the bathroom, transfer to the toilet, or ask for assistance can result in functional incontinence. Environmental factors contribute to the problem of functional incontinence and increase its likelihood. Functional incontinence is likely to occur when there is an insufficient number of toilets, when toilets are difficult to access because of their location or height, when there is an insufficient number of caregivers to provide needed assistance, and when physical restraints prevent free movement. Medications that interfere with cognition or mobility, alter bladder tone, and increase urine production often contribute to functional incontinence (Box 12-3).

BOX 12-3

Medications that Affect Continence

- Diuretics—Cause rapid filling of the bladder due to the rapid increase in urine production
- Anticholinergics—Interfere with normal contraction of the muscles of the bladder wall
- Sedatives and hypnotics—Interfere with alertness and recognition of the need to urinate
- Narcotics—Interfere with normal contraction of the muscles of the bladder wall; decrease awareness of sensations from the bladder
- α-adrenergic agonists—Increase tone of the internal sphincter muscle
- α-adrenergic antagonists—Decrease tone of the internal sphincter muscle
- Calcium-channel blockers—Decrease tone of the muscles of the bladder wall

---

Total incontinence

Total incontinence is a condition in which the elderly experience continuous and unpredictable loss of urine. Total incontinence can be caused by neurologic changes, bladder muscle spasms, trauma, or diseases affecting the bladder or sphincter muscles.

Some incontinent elderly appear to have more than one form of incontinence. This problem is sometimes called **mixed incontinence.** For example, many older adults report that when they have the urgent need to urinate, they cannot respond quickly enough because of decreased functional ability and environmental limitations. Incontinence can be a continuous and ongoing problem or may only occur occasionally. Careful history taking and medical examination are needed to determine the specific type of incontinence and the underlying causes so appropriate medical treatment and nursing interventions can be initiated.

Assessment of Urine Elimination

- Is the person continent or incontinent?
- Is the person incontinent at any specific time of day or under any special conditions?
- Does the person have a history of any medical conditions that would interfere with urine elimination (neurogenic bladder)?
- Does the person have a history of any medical condition that would decrease awareness of the need to void?
- What is the volume of a typical voiding?
- How much urine is produced each day?
- What is the odor, color, and consistency of urine?
- Are there any signs of a urinary tract infection (burning, pain with urination, frequency)?

BOX 12-4

Risk Factors Related to Bladder Elimination in the Elderly

- Neurologic problems that decrease the ability to sense the need for elimination or to control the sphincter muscles
- Endocrine disorders
- Altered structures that interfere with elimination (prostate enlargement or tumors)
- Decreased mobility (especially those on bedrest)
- Inadequate or excessive fluid intake
- Cognitive impairment (Alzheimer's disease, dementia)

- Is there a recent urinalysis? What are the results?
- What is the person's normal pattern of voiding?
- Does the person experience any difficulty starting to urinate?
- Does the person experience any involuntary loss of urine when he or she coughs, laughs, or sneezes?
- Does the person complain of any pain or burning with urination?
- What is the person's pattern of fluid intake?

See Box 12-4 for a list of risk factors for problems with bladder elimination in the elderly.

Nursing Diagnoses

Altered Pattern of urinary elimination
Incontinence: total, stress, urge, functional, reflex
Urinary retention

Nursing Goals/Outcomes

The nursing goals for elderly individuals diagnosed with urinary elimination problems are (1) to exhibit a reduction in episodes of urinary incontinence or retention; (2) to urinate at acceptable times in acceptable places; (3) to identify measures that reduce episodes of urinary incontinence or retention; and (4) to establish a routine to reduce or prevent the occurrence of bladder elimination problems.

Nursing Interventions

The following nursing interventions should take place in hospitals or extended-care facilities:

1. **Assess elimination patterns.** There are a wide variety of urinary problems that the elderly may experience. Careful assessment of elimination patterns and problems will enable nurses to develop a plan that addresses the unique needs of a specific

BOX 12-5

Modified Kegel Exercises

The purpose of the following exercises is to strengthen the pelvic floor muscles, the squeezing action that helps hold back the flow of urine. It is important that these exercises be done faithfully for 3 to 4 months to see improvement. If no improvement is seen in this time, consultation with a urologist is suggested.

A. FOLLOW THESE INSTRUCTIONS TO IDENTIFY THE MUSCLES YOU WILL BE EXERCISING

1. Sit or stand. Without tensing the muscles of your legs, buttocks, or abdomen, imagine that you are trying to hold back a bowel movement by tightening the ring of muscle around the anus. Do this exercise only until you identify the back part of the pelvic floor.
2. When you are passing urine, try to stop the flow, then restart it. This will help you identify the front part of the pelvic floor. Now you are ready to do the complete exercise.

B. DO THIS EXERCISE FOR 2 MINUTES AT LEAST THREE TIMES DAILY (AT LEAST 100 REPETITIONS)

1. Working from back to front, tighten the muscles while counting to four slowly, then release them. You can do this exercise anywhere—sitting or standing, while watching television or waiting for a bus. There is no need to interrupt your normal daily activity. In order to feel only the pelvic muscles, do not tighten the abdominal, thigh, or buttock muscles or cross your legs. Their movement is distinct and separate from that of the other muscles and can be checked by women while they are in the bath or shower by placing one finger inside the vagina and contracting the muscles. Men can only check success through improved urine control.

C. DO THIS EXERCISE EVERY TIME YOU URINATE

1. Start and stop your stream five times each time you urinate. That is, start the flow of urine, squeeze to hold back, then let go to resume the flow. Repeat this sequence several times. Remember, do this every time you urinate. You probably will notice that you have much more control of the flow of urine in the morning than you do in the afternoon. That is because your muscles are not so tired.

With permission: HIP, Help for Incontinent People, Inc., Box 544, Union, SC 29379.

person. Nurses should determine how often the person voids and how much is voided each time. If the elderly person is incontinent, nurses need to know how often and when this occurs. Nurses should also consider whether the person is receiving medications that affect continence. For example, if incontinence only occurs at night when the elderly person is receiving diuretic medications, the time of administration should be considered.

2. **Assess fluid intake patterns.** Fluid intake has a direct effect on urine elimination. Many elderly individuals with urination problems attempt to correct the problem by drinking less. This is likely to increase problems with incontinence because the more concentrated urine that is produced is more likely to irritate the bladder, increasing the risk of an episode of incontinence. Fluid restriction also increases the risk of problems with fluid balance and bowel elimination. The elderly should be encouraged to consume most of the day's fluids early in the day and to reduce fluid intake after 7 PM in order to reduce the incidence of incontinence during sleep. Fluids that irritate the bladder such as alcohol or caffeine should be avoided.

3. **Explain measures that help improve tone of the sphincter muscles.** Kegel exercises are helpful in improving the tone of the sphincter muscles. These exercises include starting and stopping the stream of urine when voiding. Improved muscle tone can help the person hold the urine until he or she can reach a toilet or obtain assistance (Box 12-5). Biofeedback has also shown promise as a method of reducing stress and urge incontinence.

4. **Modify clothing to make toileting easier.** The time that is wasted manipulating buttons or zippers may be long enough to cause incontinence. Use of Velcro closures and elastic waists with loops may speed undressing and reduce functional problems related to toileting.

5. **Reduce environmental barriers by providing grab bars in the bathroom, installing toilet risers, keeping the urinal or bedpan readily available, and providing a call signal for assistance.** Min-

imizing environmental barriers to safe elimination can help the elderly function more effectively and will reduce the incidence of incontinence due to mobility problems.

6. **Answer call signals promptly.** Decreased muscle tone and neurologic changes hinder the ability of many elderly persons to delay urination. An elderly person is less able to wait for assistance to the bathroom than is a younger person. Call signals or other requests for assistance with toileting must be responded to promptly or an episode of incontinence is likely. An occurrence of incontinence caused by lack of staff response is embarrassing for the elderly person and frustrating to all involved because it need not happen. Routine scheduling of trips to the bathroom at regular intervals throughout the day will help reduce the need for the person to call for assistance (Fig. 12-1).

7. **Develop a toileting schedule.** Planning a regular toileting schedule will encourage emptying of the bladder at regular intervals. This reduces the likelihood of urgency and incontinence. The schedule should be based on the individual's urinary elimination patterns; there is no absolute best time schedule. If the person is frequently incontinent, begin by scheduling toileting at 2-hour intervals. Because urine is produced at a rate of approximately 50 to 75 ml/hour and the elderly person's bladder capacity is about 150 to 200 ml, this frequency will reduce episodes of incontinence. Toileting too frequently can actually decrease the ability of the bladder to hold an adequate amount of urine, increasing the risk of incontinence. When a 2-hour schedule is successful, the time should be increased gradually to retrain the bladder to accommodate larger volumes of urine. A regular schedule of every 3 to 4 hours is desirable.

8. **Familiarize the elderly with the locations of bathrooms throughout the facility.** Many elderly persons who experience urgency or incontinence are afraid to leave their rooms because they fear being unable to reach a bathroom when necessary. This may result in isolation and withdrawal from others. Even a short distance may be too far for an elderly person with an urgent need to urinate. Reassurance that toilets are available can reduce these fears.

9. **Provide support and encouragement.** Incontinence is disturbing to alert elderly persons. Episodes of incontinence are embarrassing and can lead to frustration and loss of self-esteem. Even those involved in bladder training programs are likely to have accidents. It is essential to focus on successes and minimize failures.

10. **Initiate actions to maintain skin integrity.** Aging skin is particularly susceptible to damage from moisture and the waste products in urine. Wet clothing and linens must be removed immediately to prevent maceration and irritation. The skin should be thoroughly washed and dried after each episode of incontinence.

11. **Provide incontinence pads or garments when appropriate.** Incontinence pads or garments reduce the need to completely change the bed or clothing after an episode of incontinence (Figs. 12-2 and 12-3). These items tend to trap moisture next to the skin, however, and should be used with caution. Some of the newer incontinence garments are constructed with a barrier that keeps moisture away from the skin. Because newer incontinence garments are also smaller and less conspicuous, they are more acceptable to elderly persons than is the old "diaper." These garments allow the elderly more freedom to move about without fear of embarrassing themselves. Whenever possible, however, these pads and garments should not be used as a replacement for toileting.

The cost of incontinence garments can be significant for persons with limited financial resources. When incontinence pads or garments are soiled, they should be changed promptly and disposed of properly to reduce environmental odors.

12. **Administer medications as prescribed by the physician.** Uroseptic medications such as sulfonamides are often used to treat urinary tract infections. Nurses should be sure to check with the individual for allergies to sulfa before administering these medications. Such medications as ditropan or imipramine may be prescribed to reduce bladder spasms that cause incontinence. Nurses must administer these medications as prescribed and assess the patient for signs of their effectiveness. Many of the medications prescribed to treat incontinence cause side effects such as dry mouth, dry eyes, confusion, constipation, orthostatic hypotension, and tachycardia. Comfort measures and safety precautions are necessary if these side effects occur.

13. **Insert catheter as prescribed by physician.** Catheterization requires a physician's order (Fig. 12-4). Insertion of an indwelling catheter is not a recommended method for treating incontinence. The risk of urinary tract infections increases dramatically with this invasive procedure. Catheters should be used only when the benefits to the patient outweigh the risks involved. It is essential that strict sterile technique be used when inserting an indwelling catheter. When the catheter is in place, good perineal care is essential for reducing the possibility of ascending urinary tract infection. Many elderly persons who have had an indwelling

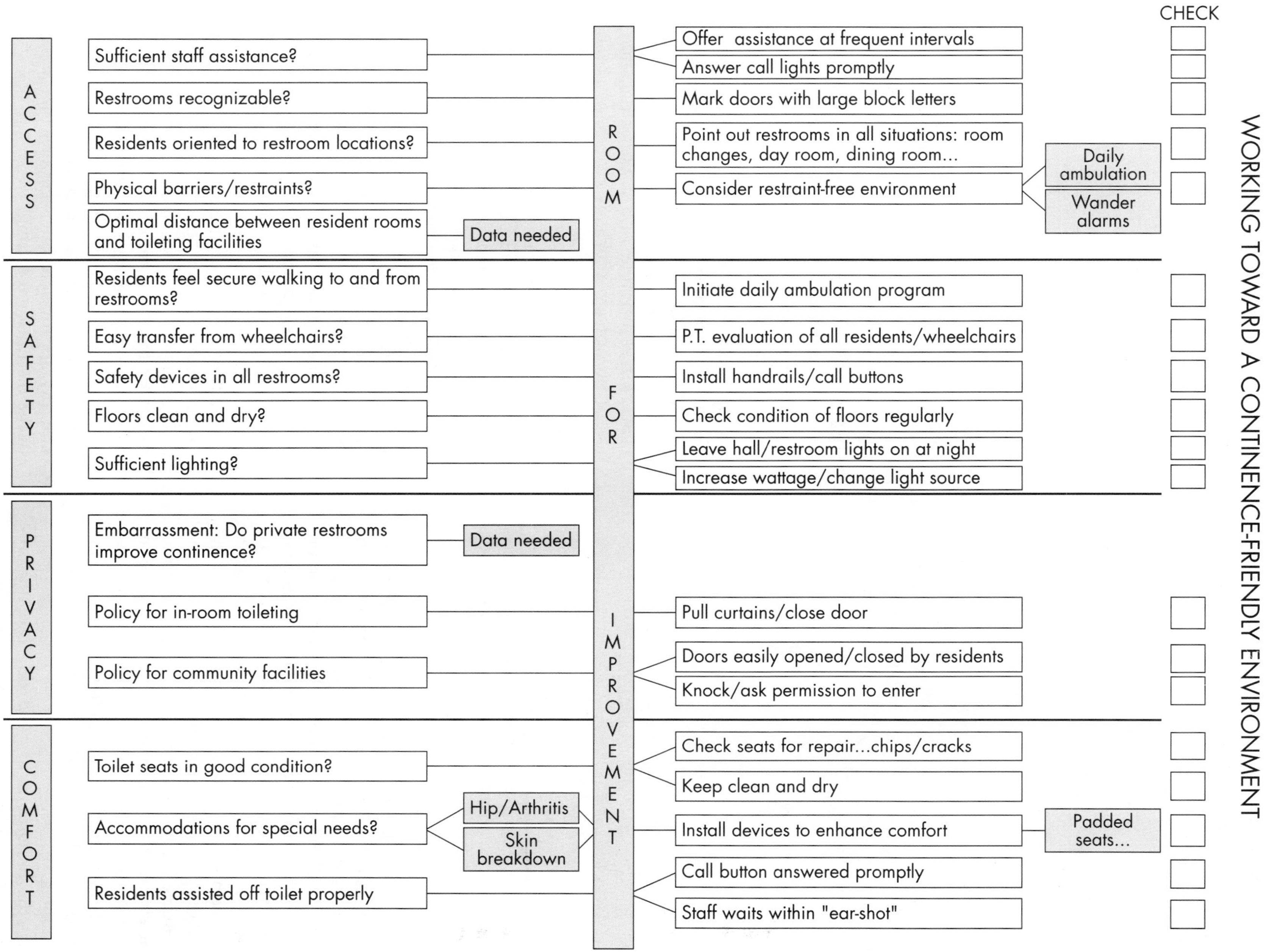

WORKING TOWARD A CONTINENCE-FRIENDLY ENVIRONMENT

FIG. 12-1 Working toward a continence-friendly environment. (Courtesy of Proctor & Gamble, Cincinnati, Ohio.)

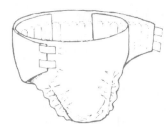

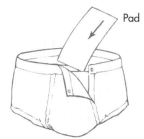

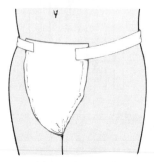

FIG. 12-2 Disposable and reusable incontinence garments for men and women. (From Gray M: *Genitourinary disorders*, St Louis, 1992, Mosby.)

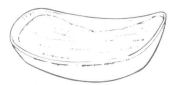

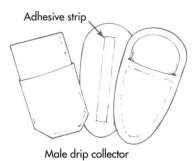

FIG. 12-3 Disposable incontinence pads. (From Gray M: *Genitourinary disorders*, St Louis, 1992, Mosby.)

catheter even for a limited time are at increased risk for incontinence once it is removed. When the catheter is in place, the bladder is decompressed. Once the catheter is removed, the bladder is unable to adapt to holding a significant volume of urine. Before removing the catheter, a procedure in which the catheter is clamped intermittently to increase bladder capacity can reduce this problem.

The following interventions should take place in the home:

1. **Encourage the individual to establish a pattern of urine elimination.** A pattern of voiding on awakening, after meals, before leaving home, before becoming interested in a lengthy activity, before exercise, and before bed can reduce the risk of incontinence.

2. **Stress the importance of good skin care and hygiene after episodes of incontinence.** Poor hygiene increases the risk of skin irritation or breakdown and increases the risk of urinary tract infections. The importance of changing soiled clothing promptly, careful handwashing after toileting, and (for women) proper wiping from front to back should be reinforced.

3. **Encourage discussion of concerns with the physician.** Nurses working in a home setting may be aware of urinary problems that have not been shared with the physician. The elderly should be encouraged to reveal their problems and concerns with a physician so an appropriate diagnosis can be made and treatment initiated. All observations regarding urine elimination should be documented appropriately in the person's record and appropriate notification made to the physician.

4. **Provide encouragement during treatment for urinary problems.** Problems with urinary retention or incontinence do not usually respond quickly to treatment. Weeks or months of treatment may be required before any improvement is noticed. This can easily result in noncompliance with the plan of care. The elderly will need encouragement to take medications, practice exercises, or follow through with other medical recommendations.

5. **Discuss methods for coping with incontinence.** Aging persons are more likely to become socially isolated rather than embarrass themselves in public. Developing strategies for coping (e.g., use of incontinence garments, learning the location of toilets in stores or theaters) can help prevent this.

6. **Use any appropriate interventions that are used in the institutional setting.**

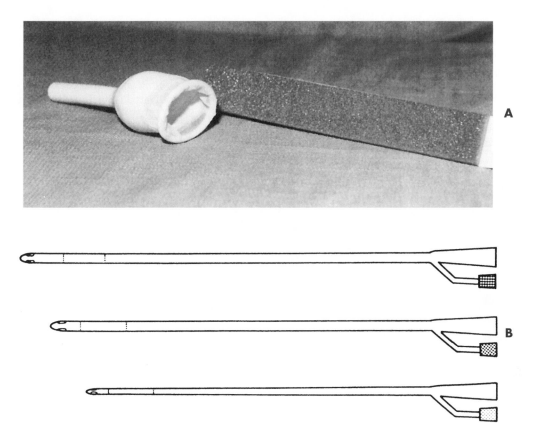

FIG. 12-4   **A,** Condom catheter and adhesive fastener. **B,** Urinary (indwelling Foley) cathe-
ters are available in various sizes and shapes for specific needs of individual patients. (**A** from
Castillo HM: *The nurse assistant in long-term care: a rehabilitative approach*, St Louis, 1992,
Mosby; **B** from Hoeman SP: *Rehabilitation/restorative care in the community*, St Louis, 1990,
Mosby.)

SUMMARY

Both bladder and bowel elimination are essential for
normal body functioning. Unless waste products are
removed effectively from the body, serious consequences will result. Aging results in less effective removal of waste products, but a problem more significant to the elderly is any alteration in the ability to
control the elimination process. Problems related to
elimination are serious concerns for the elderly, and a
great deal of physical and mental energy is devoted
to dealing with changes in elimination function.

READINGS AND REFERENCES

Abyad A, Mourad F: Constipation: common sense care of
the older patient, *Geriatrics* 51:28, 1996.
Agency for Health Care Policy and Research: Urinary incontinence: 80% of cases can be improved AHCPR says, *Geriatrics* 51:18, 1996.
Avorn J, et al: Reduction of bacteriuria and pyuria after ingestion of cranberry juice, *JAMA* 271:751, 1994.
Catanzaro J: Managing incontinence: an update, *RN* 59:38,
1996.

Constipation in the elderly, *Medical Sciences Bulletin* Web site:
http://pharminfo.com/pubs/msb/constip.html, 1994.
Ditsler J: Trends in improved continence management, *Nurs-
ing Homes* 45:28, 1995.
Dodson AL: AHCPR's urinary incontinence caregiver guide,
Nursing Homes 46:28, 1997.
Faller N: Is your facility continence friendly? *Nursing Homes*
43:23, 1994.
Gallo ML, Fallon PJ, Staskin DR: Urinary incontinence: steps
to evaluation, diagnosis and treatment, *Nurse Practitioner*
22:21, 1997.
Greer DS Web site: *Incontinence in the elderly* http://biomed-
cs.biomed.brown.edu/RIMedicine/AugArt.html, 1997.
Hittner P: The fear of incontinence, *Better Homes and Gardens*,
November, 1996.
How one Alzheimer's unit achieved almost complete conti-
nence, *Brown University Long-Term Care Quality Letter* 9:1,
1997.
Jeter KF, Lutz JB: Skin care in the frail, elderly, dependent,
incontinent patient, *Adv in Wound Care* 9:29, 1996.
Managing acute and chronic urinary incontinence, *Am Fam
Physician* 54:1661, 1996.
Mold JW: Pharmacotherapy of urinary incontinence, *Am
Fam Physician* 54:673, 1996.

Mor V: Incontinence severity ratings questioned, *Brown University Long-Term Care Quality Letter* 8:8, 1996.

National institute on Aging Web site: *Age page: constipation,* http://www.agepage.com/constapn.html, 1995.

National institute on Aging Web site: *Age page: incontinence in older adults* http://www.agepage.com/incontin.html, 1997.

O'Keefe EA, et al: Bowel disorders impair functional status and quality of life in the elderly: a population based study, *J Gerontol* 50:M184, 1995.

On cranberry juice and urinary tract infections, *Tufts University Diet & Nutrition Letter* 12:1, 1994.

Ouslander JG: Geriatric urinary incontinence, *Generations* 20:33, 1996.

Resnick NM: An 89-year-old woman with urinary incontinence, *JAMA* 276:1832, 1996.

Resnick NM: Urinary incontinence, *Lancet* 346:94, 1995.

Resnick NM, Gillyatt P: Staying dry, *Harvard Health Letter* 21:3, 1995.

Strange CJ: Incontinence can be controlled, *FDA Consumer* 31:28, 1997.

ACTIVITY AND EXERCISE

LEARNING OBJECTIVES

1. Describe normal activity and exercise patterns.
2. Describe how activity and exercise patterns change with aging.
3. Discuss the effects of disease processes on the ability to participate in exercise and activity.
4. Describe methods of assessing changes in the ability to participate in activity or exercise.
5. Identify the older adults who are most at risk for experiencing problems related to activity and exercise.
6. Identify selected nursing diagnoses related to activity and exercise problems.
7. Describe nursing interventions that are appropriate for elderly individuals experiencing problems related to activity and exercise.
8. Differentiate between a custodial focus and a rehabilitative focus in nursing care.
9. Discuss the impact of nurses' attitudes on care planning.
10. Identify the benefits of a rehabilitative focus on the elderly.
11. Identify the goals of rehabilitation nursing.

NORMAL ACTIVITY PATTERNS

The activity-exercise health pattern deals with behaviors related to exercise, activity, leisure, and recreation. Nurses must consider the wide range of behaviors within this pattern that fall under the general term **activity**. Activity is anything that requires the expenditure of energy. Some activities require only a small expenditure of energy, whereas others require a great deal of energy.

Basic body functions such as breathing, temperature control, and metabolism expend the least amount of energy. Sitting, resting, watching television, reading, and playing cards or bingo are sedentary activities that require little energy. Activities of daily living (ADL) such as dressing, grooming, eating, bathing, and toileting require a greater expenditure of energy. Cooking, cleaning, driving, and shopping require still more effort and expend more energy. Walking can be a mild or vigorous activity, depending on the pace. Running, swimming, dancing, aerobics, and other forms of active exercise require the greatest energy expenditure. Although the amount and type of exercise an individual performs change over the life span, exercise and activity remain an essential part of life. Persons who were not physically active as young adults are not likely to become physically active as they age. A healthy pattern of activity and exercise should be established early in life to ensure that these behaviors become habitual and are carried into old age.

Exercise helps people look and feel better. Physical activity is necessary to maintain normal joint mobility and muscle tone. When people do not participate in regular activity, all body systems suffer. Preventing mobility problems is easier than trying to overcome the problems when they develop. Elderly individuals should be encouraged to be as active and independent as possible. Because existing medical conditions may restrict activity, nurses should be aware of any problems that may affect the individual's ability to participate in activities. The elderly should be assisted to do as much as is permitted.

Many aging individuals remain physically active. Today it is common to see individuals in their sixties, seventies, and eighties leading active, self-sufficient lives. Aging no longer implies that a person must sit forever in a rocking chair or recliner and "vegetate." All one has to do is visit a park or shopping mall early in the morning, where many older adults can be seen walking for their health. Access to golf courses during the season is harder because of the amazing number of senior citizens playing 18 holes. Activity is good for people of all ages. Aging may change the type and amount of participation, but more and more people are realizing that active participation in a wide variety of activities is the best way to maintain high-level function.

Physical activity requires a complex interaction of physiologic processes, primarily those of the neurologic, musculoskeletal, cardiovascular, and respiratory systems. Anything that interferes with the coordination of these systems can alter the ability to participate in physical activity.

Of major importance is the function of the nervous system, which is the primary coordinating system of the body. The brain controls the involuntary activities of the body, including metabolism, respiration, and temperature control. Areas of the brain control the high-level processes of perception and cognition. Before any voluntary activity occurs, individuals must be able to recognize that a need for action exists. Once the need is recognized, the individual must have the desire as well as the ability to perform that action. The brain is also the motor control center of the body, and it communicates with the somatic peripheral nervous system. Any physiologic age- or disease-related change that alters the function of the brain's motor centers or that interferes with the transmission of impulses from the brain to the musculoskeletal system can interfere with activity.

The musculoskeletal system must then be able to respond to these messages from the brain. Normal and pathologic changes in muscles or bones can interfere with normal activity. Even if the nervous and the musculoskeletal systems are intact, problems in the cardiovascular and respiratory systems can lead to alterations in activity. Muscles, including the heart muscle, require an adequate supply of oxygen and nutrients to function properly. Anything that interferes with the oxygen supply to tissues will affect the ability to perform activity.

ACTIVITY AND AGING

With advancing age, most people experience some changes in the ability to perform or tolerate activity, and this ability varies widely among the elderly. In general, the more active a person has been, the more active he or she will remain with aging.

The first change noticed by most aging persons is a decrease in the rate or speed of activity. Things that could be done quickly in the past now take longer. Many elderly individuals complain that it takes them much longer to dress, shop, or do other simple activities than it used to. Normal aging does not interfere with the transmission of nerve impulses, but it does slow the speed of nerve transmission.

A loss of muscle mass can interfere with activities that require muscular strength. Activities such as moving furniture, lifting bags of groceries, shoveling snow, and vacuuming may be increasingly difficult.

Decreased joint flexibility can result in problems with performing ADLs. Reaching for objects on shelves, dressing, bending to put on shoes, and even washing the feet or back may be difficult.

Agility, the ability to move quickly and smoothly, decreases with age. This may cause difficulty when the elderly try to climb ladders or avoid hazards while walking.

Dexterity, the ability to perform fine manipulative skills, is also likely to decrease with age. Gross motor skills remain intact longer than do fine motor skills. However, skills that were perfected when younger, such as playing a musical instrument or sewing, may be maintained at a high level if the skills are used regularly.

Decreased stamina is typically seen with aging. This is most often due to a decrease in oxygen supply to body tissues. Decreased oxygen exchange may be caused by a loss of elasticity in the lungs and a smaller chest cavity. The decreased availability of oxygen may lead to frequent pauses during activity or a slower pace when performing activities.

Coordination of multiple activities is likely to decrease with aging. Activities that require simultaneous perception of many stimuli and quick physical response (such as driving) are often affected. Elderly individuals with impaired vision and hearing, decreased strength, slow reaction time, and decreased coordination may not be able to perform this type of complex activity safely.

Because these changes appear gradually over time, most elderly individuals learn to compensate for or cope with them. Many strategies such as pacing activities, finding alternative methods of performing activities, and simplifying activities demonstrate the capacity of the elderly to adapt and adjust.

EFFECTS OF DISEASE PROCESSES ON ACTIVITY

If, in addition to normal changes, the aging person has health problems that affect the critical body systems, his or her ability to participate in activity is further impaired.

Organic brain syndrome, Alzheimer's disease, and stroke can affect both the high-level thinking functions and the motor functions of the brain. Persons suffering from severe forms of these diseases may not recognize the need for the most basic activities such as moving, eating, dressing, bathing, or toileting. Even if they do recognize these needs, their altered motor function may prevent them from meeting basic needs.

Neurologic damage due to head injury, infection, degenerative disease, Parkinson's disease, or toxic drug reactions can interfere with normal nerve impulse transmission. Elderly persons suffering from these conditions may recognize a need and have the desire to perform an activity yet be unable to carry out the activity. The nervous system does not transmit appropriate messages to the muscles to enable them

to perform the activity. Abnormal nerve transmission can result in difficulty getting started with movement or in uncoordinated muscle activity (e.g., a staggering gait), which further limit the ability to participate in normal activities.

Diseases or injury to the musculoskeletal system can interfere with the ability to perform activity. Fractures can lead to limited or extensive mobility restriction, depending on the part or parts of the body affected. Fracture of a small bone such as a finger results in limited loss of mobility. Fracture of a large bone such as the femur results in severe limitation of mobility. Not only does the fracture itself restrict mobility, but the treatment also further limits mobility. Even after surgical repair, the person with a fractured hip is not permitted to participate in certain activities (e.g., weight bearing on the extremity) until healing has occurred. While waiting for healing to occur, strength and joint mobility can be lost if preventive nursing interventions are not instituted.

Diseases such as gout and arthritis cause joint pain, which leads to restricted activity. A person with severe gout or arthritis is likely to avoid use of the painful joints in order to reduce discomfort. Unfortunately, this inactivity can lead to further loss of joint mobility and muscle strength, which even further reduces the ability to perform activities. Joint degeneration with aging severely restricts mobility, particularly in the weight-bearing joints in the knees and hips. Joint-replacement surgery is an increasingly common option for the elderly. After a period of rehabilitation, most elderly achieve a greatly improved activity level.

Foot conditions commonly seen in the elderly (e.g., bunions, hammertoes, and calluses) may interfere with ambulation, particularly if footwear does not fit properly. Painful feet are a common reason for decreased activity in the elderly.

Any disease condition that interferes with the intake or distribution of oxygen to body tissue will significantly interfere with a person's ability to participate in activity and exercise. These conditions include diseases of the respiratory system that prevent adequate gas exchange in the lungs (e.g., asthma, emphysema, bronchitis, and pneumonia) and diseases of the cardiovascular system that prevent adequate distribution of oxygen to body tissues and heart muscle (e.g., myocardial infarction, congestive heart failure, heart block, arteriosclerosis, and hypertension).

Inadequate oxygenation places additional stress on the cardiovascular and respiratory systems. Pulse and respiratory rates increase in an attempt to compensate for the decreased amount of oxygen. If additional demands for oxygen occur, as they do with even moderate activity, the elderly may experience additional symptoms. Fatigue with minimal activity is common with oxygen deprivation. Pain may be reported with activity. Most common are angina (when the heart muscle does not receive adequate amounts of oxygen) and intermittent claudication (when the tissues of the lower extremities are deprived of oxygen). Initially this pain only occurs with activity; in severe cases of deprivation, it will also occur at rest. Severe oxygen deprivation can result in cardiac or respiratory distress.

To compensate for these symptoms, elderly persons spontaneously restrict their activities. Individuals may become housebound because the effort of dressing is too much for them. Some are unable to eat or perform basic hygiene because it is too exhausting. Sometimes the activity limitation is so severe that individuals are able to maneuver around the house only by placing chairs at 10-foot intervals. They move that short distance, then sit and rest until they are able to move to the next chair.

Malnourishment can also contribute to the reduced ability to perform activity. Inadequate intake of nutrients can result in muscle atrophy. Malnourished individuals lack adequate protein to build muscle tissue, an adequate supply of glucose to fuel the muscles, and adequate iron to form hemoglobin. Inadequate iron intake can result in anemia, which leads to a decrease in the oxygen available to tissues and further reduces the ability to perform activity.

Although not physiologic in origin, emotional disorders such as severe grief, anxiety, or depression can lead to decreased participation in normal activity. Individuals who are emotionally disturbed may be directing all of their energy inward and may not be willing or able to summon the energy required for physical activity. It is important to remember that these people need to continue to use their bodies to prevent loss of physical function.

NURSING PROCESS

ALTERATIONS IN PHYSICAL MOBILITY

Most older adults experience some changes in their ability to perform physical activities. These changes may result from the normal changes of aging or from some pathologic changes.

Assessment of Physical Mobility

- Does the individual have full range of motion in the joints?
- Are there any contractures or deformities?
- Does the person experience any pain or tenderness in the joints?
- Is there any particular motion that aggravates joint pain?
- What relieves discomfort?

- How is the muscle tone of the arms and legs?
- Is muscle strength equal on both sides of the body?
- Is there any muscle tenderness?
- Is the person bedridden, wheelchair-bound, or ambulatory?
- If ambulatory, what is the pattern of the gait? (Steady? Shuffling? Ataxic? Slow? Rapid?)
- Is the person able to lift his or her feet when walking, or does he or she shuffle?
- Does the person maintain an upright posture when walking?
- Do both sides of the body move evenly?
- How well can the person maintain balance?
- What kind of footwear does the person wear for walking?
- Does the person have any foot problems (e.g., bunions or calluses) that interfere with walking?
- How far can the person ambulate without discomfort?
- Does the person require any assistive devices (walkers or canes) for ambulation?
- Does the person know how to use these assistive devices properly?
- Does the person feel comfortable and confident using these aids?
- Does the person require the assistance of another person to ambulate?
- If not ambulatory, what is the person's activity level?
- Does the person use a wheelchair?
- Can the person operate the wheelchair himself or herself?
- Does the person receive passive range-of-motion exercises?
- Is the environment safe for the individual?

See Box 13-1 for a list of risk factors for impaired physical mobility in the elderly.

BOX 13-1

Risk Factors Related to Impaired Physical Mobility in the Elderly

- Intolerance of physical activity because of medical conditions that decrease endurance or strength
- Pain
- Neuromuscular or musculoskeletal conditions
- Cognitive impairment (Alzheimer's disease or dementia)
- Severe anxiety or depression
- Prescribed bed rest
- Restrictive devices (restraints, casts, splints, immobilizers)

Nursing Diagnosis

Impaired physical mobility

Nursing Goals/Outcomes

The nursing goals for individuals with impaired physical mobility are (1) to increase participation in physical activities that maintain strength and mobility, (2) to maintain normal anatomic position and function in all joints, (3) to remain free from joint contractures and foot drop, and (4) to maintain or increase strength and mobility using assistive devices.

Nursing Interventions

The following nursing interventions should take place in hospitals or extended-care facilities:

1. **Identify the prescribed activity level.** The activity level is established by the physician based on the elderly person's overall health status. It is important that the patient be as active as possible yet not exceed the prescribed activity level. It is particularly important that the nurse be aware of any weight-bearing restrictions related to fractures or joint replacements. Failure to take proper precautions can lead to serious and permanent harm.

2. **Continue to assess strength and joint mobility.** Strength and joint mobility are not always consistent in the elderly. Changes may be caused by something as simple as a change in the weather, or they may be an early indication of a change in the elderly person's health status. Nurses should pay special attention to mobility if the elderly person has experienced weakness or falls. Significant changes such as one-sided weakness or severe pain should be reported promptly to the physician.

3. **Perform physical mobility activities in conjunction with daily care.** Passive range-of-motion exercise can be provided in conjunction with the bath. Active exercise can become part of dressing, meals, grooming, toileting, and other ADL. Even minimal participation in ADL can increase physical mobility. Any exercise performed by the elderly individual during bathing, hair combing, and oral hygiene that uses the joints and muscles can be beneficial.

4. **Provide good body alignment and frequent position changes.** The bedridden elderly are at high risk for loss of joint mobility. Poor alignment can result in muscle fatigue, which enhances the likelihood of contractures. Flexion contractures of the hip, knee, and foot occur when the stronger flexor muscles dominate. These contractures can result in permanent loss of the ability to stand or ambulate. To prevent this, good alignment and position-

ing are important. Positioning devices (pillows, trochanter rolls, foot supports) should be used when needed to maintain proper alignment.

5. **Avoid unnecessary restraint that limits physical mobility.** By definition, restraints limit mobility. Any device that restricts mobility is a restraint, including vests, wheelchair tables, foot pedals, and safety bars. Many of these devices that historically have been used to "protect" the elderly from falls have actually increased the likelihood of injury. An elderly person who is prevented by these devices from using joints and muscles loses strength and function and becomes increasingly susceptible to injury. Ensure that splints or other devices do not unnecessarily restrict joint movement.

6. **Consult with the physical therapist to determine a suitable activity/exercise plan that maintains muscle strength and joint mobility.** The physical therapist may be able to suggest exercises that will benefit a specific individual. These exercises should become part of the nursing care plan and be included in the day's activities (Fig. 13-1). Passive range-of-motion exercises will help keep the joints flexible, but they do little to maintain muscle strength. Passive range of motion should be provided a minimum of twice a day for immobile elderly individuals. Active range of motion will help with both joint flexibility and muscle toning. Elderly persons with hemiplegia or hemiparesis can be taught to use the stronger side of the body to exercise the weaker extremities. Many facilities provide exercise programs that are adapted to meet the ability levels of the residents. Exercise is often done to music because the rhythm encourages motion. Isometric exercises, such as alternately tightening and relaxing the muscles of the arms, abdomen, or buttocks, may benefit some older adults by helping to maintain the strength of the abdominal and gluteal muscles and quadriceps. Isometric exercise does not affect the joints. Isotonic exercise, which helps improve muscle strength, muscle tone, and joint mobility, includes such movements as lifting the body off of the bed with a trapeze (Fig. 13-2), pressing against a footboard, or pushing against the bed to lift the buttocks off of the mattress. Isometric and isotonic exercises should be used with caution by persons with cardiac problems because they increase stress on the cardiovascular system. They may result in elevation of the blood pressure and use of the Valsalva maneuver, which can lead to cardiac overload or cardiac arrest. To prevent this problem, the elderly should be instructed to breathe through the mouth while exercising.

7. **Verify that the individual is suitably dressed for activity and that he or she has the proper foot-**

LYING DOWN

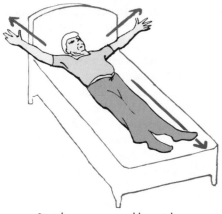

Stretch your arms and legs; take a deep breath.

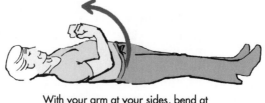

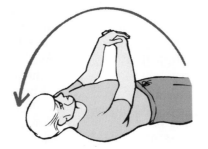

With your arm at your sides, bend at the elbow and curl your arms as if "making a muscle."

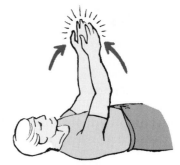

Clap your hands directly above your head.

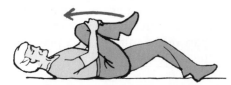

Grab each leg with both hands below the knee and pull toward your chest slowly.

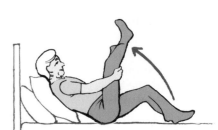

Fold your hands on your stomach; raise your arms over your head toward the headboard.

Lift each leg off the bed, but try not to bend your knee. Use an arm to help.

SITTING

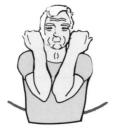

Touch your elbows together in front of you.

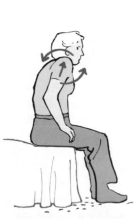

Shrug your shoulders forward, then move them in a circle, raising them high enough to reach your ears.

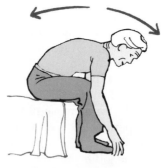

Twist your whole upper body from side to side with your hands on your hips.

Bend forward and let your arms dangle; try to touch the floor with your hands.

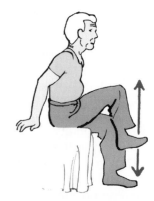

While still sitting, move each of your knees up and down as if you are walking; each time your right foot hits the ground, count it as one. Lift your knee high.

FIG. 13-1   Various exercises that can done while lying down, sitting, standing up, and walking. (From Johnson-Paulson JE, Kosher R: *Geriatr Nurs* 322, 1985.)

STANDING UP

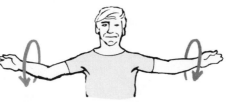

Hold your arms out and turn them in big circles.

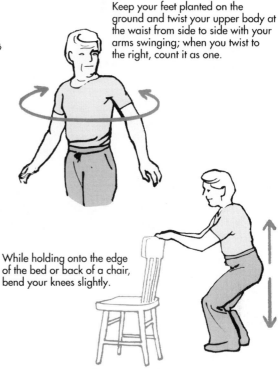

Keep your feet planted on the ground and twist your upper body at the waist from side to side with your arms swinging; when you twist to the right, count it as one.

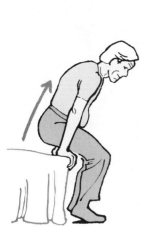

Using your arms, push off from the bed and stand up; if you get dizzy, sit down and try again.

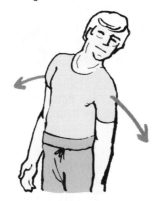

With hands at your side bend at the waist as far as you can to the right side, then to the left.

While holding onto the edge of the bed or back of a chair, bend your knees slightly.

WALKING PLACES

Walking is good exercise. It helps in toning muscles, maintaining flexibility of joints, and also is good exercise for the heart and circulatory system. Walking briskly for 20 minutes a day, 3 times a week can be as effective a heart conditioner as jogging, but it does take a longer time to achieve the same effect as jogging. For those who cannot walk rapidly for long periods, walking to the point of muscular fatigue also helps maintain good muscle tone.

There are signs your body may give you to indicate you are overdoing exercise. Stop, rest, and if necessary call your physician if you experience any of these symptoms:

- SEVERE SHORTNESS OF BREATH
- CHEST PAIN
- SEVERE JOINT PAIN
- DIZZINESS OR FAINT FEELING
- HEART FLUTTERS

In all walking exercises, go only as fast as you are able to walk and still carry on a conversation. If you cannot, slow down.

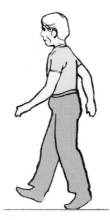

INSIDE

It is important to maintain walking ability. Determine how far you can walk and each day walk to ¾ of that distance, building endurance. Wear supportive shoes and use whatever aids are necessary.

OUTSIDE

Wear soft-soled shoes with good support, i.e., jogging shoes. When walking, push off *from* your toes and land on your heels. Swing arms loosely at your sides. Begin with 10-minute walks and build to 20 to 30 minutes.

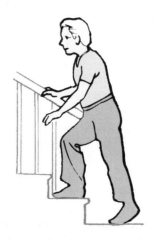

Walking upstairs requires effort. Place one foot flat on a step, push off with the other and shift your weight. Use a railing for balance if necessary.

FIG. 13-1, cont'd   For legend see opposite page.

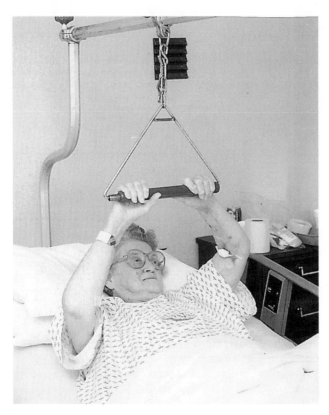

FIG. 13-2 Patient using a trapeze bar. (From Potter PA, Perry AG: *Basic nursing: theory and practice,* ed 3, St Louis, 1995, Mosby.)

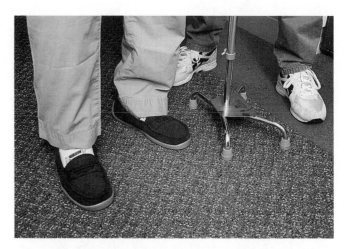

FIG. 13-3 Quad cane. Note that proper footwear is being worn. (From Potter PA, Perry AG: *Basic nursing: theory and practice,* ed 3, St Louis, 1995, Mosby.)

wear. Proper clothing and footwear should be selected for exercise. Clothing should be nonconstricting (to allow freedom of movement) and suitable to the environment. Many elderly choose comfortable footwear over footwear that provides proper support. Most slippers do not provide adequate support and are intended for rest periods, not ambulation. Shoes should be worn whenever possible. Shoes should fit well and support the foot to decrease the likelihood of falls. If the individual has foot problems, special footwear may be necessary. Gait changes, particularly the inability to lift the feet freely, increase the risk of falls. If footwear is too loose or is not supportive, the risk of falls increases. Shoes should fit snugly enough that they do not slip off the heel when walking. Elderly women, particularly those with kyphosis, should be encouraged to wear low heels when walking to provide for balance.

8. **Provide pain medication in a timely manner so that maximum benefits from the medication occur when greatest physical effort is expected.** Pain is a common reason for decreased physical mobility. Nurses should be aware of particular activities that intensify or relieve an individual's pain. Pain increases with fatigue; therefore, activi-

ties should be paced so that they do not overly fatigue the individual. Antiinflammatory medications or analgesics should be administered so that the elderly person is as comfortable as possible when physical activity is scheduled.

9. **Verify that the individual knows the correct method for using assistive devices and that he or she does in fact use them for activity. Explain proper use if needed.** If assistive devices such as wheelchairs, walkers, or canes are needed, nurses should verify that the elderly know how to use them properly (Figs. 13-3 and 13-4). Verify that the elderly person knows how to use the walker, particularly when climbing stairs. Verify that the person holds the cane in the correct hand when walking. Remind the person to lock the wheelchair wheels before sitting down to prevent falls. Ensure that the assistive devices are kept nearby so that they are easily available to the elderly person. If the individual suffers from one-sided weakness, ensure the device is placed on the stronger side. Remember that many elderly do not like to use these devices because they are cumbersome and because they are a constant reminder of failing health. Nurses must continue to stress the importance of using the devices if they are needed for safety.

10. **Encourage wheelchair-bound clients to move using their arms or feet whenever possible.** If unable to walk, the elderly may still be able to move about in a wheelchair, which involves using either the arms to turn the wheels or the legs and feet to propel the chair.

11. **Provide adequate assistance during ambulation.** Gait belts and the assistance of one or two helpers may be needed to provide safety and a sense of security. The loss of balance seen in some elderly

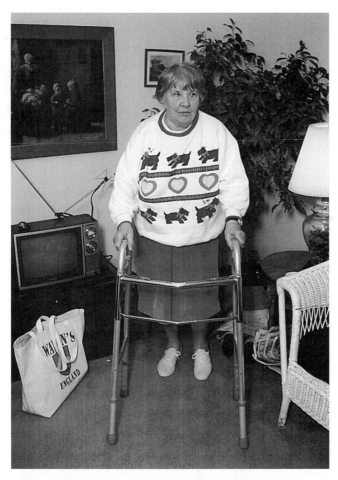

FIG. **13-4** Patient using a walker. (From Potter PA, Perry AG: *Basic nursing: theory and practice,* ed 3, St Louis, 1995, Mosby.)

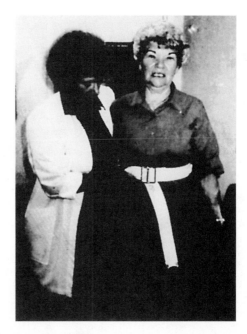

FIG. **13-5** When helping an elderly patient to ambulate, grasp the gait belt in back and use the other hand to steady the patient. (From Castillo HM: *The nurse assistant in long-term care: a rehabilitative approach,* St Louis, 1992, Mosby.)

BOX 13-2

Benefits of Exercise for Senior Citizens

- Maintain independence
- Retain mobility
- Prevent or reduce depression
- Encourage sleep
- Improve self-esteem
- Improve appetite
- Improve cardiovascular status
- Maintain or improve musculoskeletal function
- Prevent obesity
- Decrease stress level
- Expand social network
- Enhance appreciation for life

---

persons increases the risk of falls. A gait belt should be used when assisting an unsteady person. Gait belts that are properly secured around the person's waist allow the caregiver to prevent injury to the individual. The belt is near the person's center of gravity; thus the caregiver can sense subtle balance changes and anticipate problems (Fig. 13-5). If the belt is too loose, it may slide up under the rib cage and cause injury. Regular belts on trousers or dresses may be used, but only with caution because they are usually narrower and may not fasten as securely as a proper gait belt. Holding the arm of the elderly person to provide support is inadequate in most cases and should be avoided. If the elderly person starts to fall, the caregiver could dislocate the shoulder or cause other severe trauma to the elderly person.

The following interventions should take place in the home:

1. **Teach or reinforce the benefits of regular activity and exercise.** Many articles in senior citizen magazines and the popular press address the benefits of exercise (Box 13-2). Sedentary senior citizens may need to be reminded or encouraged to take this information to heart. Important information to communicate to the elderly includes the fact that moderate or higher levels of physical activity are associated with lower mortality rates. Physical activity has been associated with many beneficial physiologic effects, including improved cardiovascular status, decreased risk of colon cancer, beneficial effects on non-insulin-dependent diabetes mellitus, maintenance of normal muscle strength and joint function, reduced risk of falling, and decreased incidence of obesity. Activity also has psy-

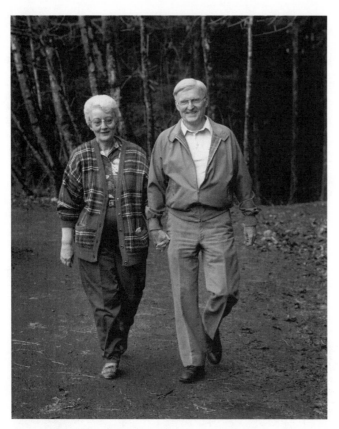

FIG. 13-6 Healthy aging. (Courtesy of Rod Schmall, West Linn, Ore.)

chologic benefits, including a decreased incidence of depression, improved mood, and an enhanced sense of well-being.

2. **Assess the home for safety hazards or conditions that may interfere with mobility.** The home may present conditions that interfere with mobility or increase the risk of falls. Modifications of the environment may be required to prevent accidents or injury. Chapter 9 addresses assessment of home safety in greater detail.

3. **Help the elderly develop a schedule for regular physical activity that is appropriate for their prescribed activity level.** The physician should be consulted before an elderly person who has chronic disease or has lived a sedentary lifestyle starts an exercise program. Once an appropriate target level is established, the individual should be taught to start slowly and build up to the optimal level over time.

   Active elderly persons should be encouraged to participate in regular physical activity. Exercise should be planned into the day's activities. If exercise is not viewed as important enough to plan for, it will not get done. Three 20- to 30-minute sessions a week on nonconsecutive days are good; daily exercise is even better. Midmorning is a good

time for exercise, but afternoon and early evening are also good times. Much will depend on the individual's peak energy time. Blood supply may be diverted to digestion for up to 2 hours after large meals; therefore, intense physical activity should not be scheduled immediately after meals. Walking is one of the best exercises for the elderly (Fig. 13-6). Swimming and cycling are also recommended. Exercise programs, including aerobics classes, are sponsored by many senior citizen centers. Before joining this type of exercise program, the elderly should see their physicians to ensure that the program is appropriate and safe. In addition to providing exercise, these programs provide an opportunity for social interaction. Exercising with others provides motivation and makes the effort more worthwhile and pleasant.

4. **Explain the importance of warm-up and cool-down exercise.** Before starting an exercise session, the individual should warm up for about 5 minutes. Simple exercises that make the joints limber and slowly stretch the muscles are recommended. Exercises that do not put undue stress on bones and joints are tolerated better by the elderly. The elderly must also be aware of the importance of a cool-down period after exercise. Five minutes of slower activities (similar to the warm-up activities) will help blood return from the muscles to the central circulation. If an elderly person stops exercise too suddenly, he or she may experience fainting (syncope) because of inadequate blood flow to brain tissue.

5. **Explain the importance of proper dress for environmental conditions and proper footwear for safety.** Environmental conditions, including heat, cold, high humidity, and air pollution, must be considered when planning activity. Elderly persons should try to minimize exercise on excessively hot or cold days. On very hot days, activity is best planned for early in the day or later in the evening when the temperature is cooler. Some large cities experience ozone alerts due to excessive air pollution. On ozone alert days, it is wise for all individuals, particularly the elderly, to minimize their activity. On warm days, lightweight, loose clothing should be worn to allow the body to cool through evaporation. On extremely cold days, it is wise for the elderly to exercise indoors. Cold weather can be extremely stressful for individuals with cardiac or respiratory conditions. If the elderly must go outside in cold weather, clothing should be layered to trap heat. A mask or scarf worn over the face and mouth will help warm the air before it enters the respiratory tract.

6. **Review signs and symptoms that necessitate**

contacting the physician. The elderly should be aware that any new or unusual pain, weakness, or other untoward symptoms that are experienced during activity should be reported promptly to the physician.

7. **Use any appropriate interventions that are used in the institutional setting.**

A nursing care plan on impaired physical mobility is presented on p. 220.

A nursing care plan on impaired physical mobility is presented on p. 220.

NURSING PROCESS
ACTIVITY INTOLERANCE

Activity intolerance is a state in which the aging individual has insufficient physiologic or psychologic energy to accomplish necessary or desired daily activities. Activity intolerance is a common problem for elderly who live a sedentary lifestyle.

Assessment of Ability to Tolerate Activity

- Does the person complain of shortness of breath, fatigue, or weakness?
- How much exertion can the person tolerate before shortness of breath or fatigue is noticed?
- Has the person's participation in normal or routine activities decreased?
- Does the person complain of decreased interest in activities?
- What are the person's pulse and blood pressure?
- Do the vital signs remain within normal limits with activity?
- Does the person experience orthostatic hypotension?
- Is the person's nutritional intake adequate?

See Box 13-3 for a list of risk factors for activity intolerance in the elderly.

Nursing Diagnosis

Activity intolerance

Nursing Goals/Outcomes

The nursing goals for elderly individuals with activity intolerance are (1) to demonstrate an increased ability to tolerate activity and (2) to identify factors that contribute to activity intolerance.

Nursing Interventions

The following nursing interventions should take place in hospitals or extended-care facilities:

1. **Identify factors that contribute to activity intolerance.** People can stop participating in physical activity for a variety of reasons. The approaches that nurses should use depend on the nature of the problem. For example, an elderly person who stops participating in activities because of depression after the death of a spouse has a very different problem from that of the person who is physically unable to tolerate activity because of cardiac problems. Some aging persons have no real reason for declining activity level other than a belief that it is expected and accepted with old age. As they age, the elderly become increasingly sedentary and consequently lose functional abilities. Nurses should be aware of the specific concerns and problems experienced by the individual in order to develop an effective plan of care.

2. **Identify the activities that the elderly view as essential or desirable.** The activities nurses feel are important are often different from those the elderly value. The elderly should be consulted and included in the planning and structuring of activities. It is easier to motivate a person to work toward goals or activities that they consider important.

3. **Plan activities so that the elderly progress from easier activities to those that are more demanding.** Activities should build from the least strenuous toward those requiring more physical exertion. Those who are unable to tolerate low levels of activity will need to progress slowly because progression that is too rapid will lead to exhaustion, a feeling of failure, and loss of motivation. Once mild activities are tolerated, then activities that are more physically demanding can be attempted. The pace at which activities are introduced will depend on the specific needs and abilities of the individual. Some elderly will be able to resume near-normal levels of activity; others will always experience some amount of activity intolerance.

4. **Encourage the elderly to pace activities throughout the day, alternating periods of activity with periods of rest.** Attempting to do too much in too short a period of time is a common cause of activity intolerance in the elderly. Most elderly will benefit from a planned approach to activity that includes periods of activity and periods of rest. By pacing activities, the individual will usually find that he or she can accomplish more and feel better.

5. **Monitor vital signs to assess the physiologic response to activity.** Vital signs are good indicators of the elderly person's ability to tolerate activity. Individuals who have been immobile or sedentary may experience significant changes in vital signs as they increase their activity. Tachycardia is a common occurrence when beginning an activity program. Once it is elevated, it takes longer for the

NURSING CARE PLAN

ACTIVITY-EXERCISE

Mrs. King is a 73-year-old woman who lives at Poplar Bluff Nursing Home. She was diagnosed 3 years ago with Parkinson's disease. She has bilateral tremors in both arms. She is able to walk but does so very slowly with a rigid, flexed posture. Her coordination and balance are poor. She has experienced occasional falls when ambulating in the hall. She states, "I get tired so easily. My bones and muscles ache all of the time, and recently I've noticed that my fingers and toes tingle." The physician has ordered physical therapy three times a week to maintain her strength and flexibility. Mrs. King participated in pottery activities until recently. She states that "they're just too hard for me now."

NURSING DIAGNOSIS

Impaired physical mobility

DEFINING CHARACTERISTICS

- Impaired coordination and balance
- Muscle rigidity
- Altered posture
- Slowed movements
- Tremors

GOALS/OUTCOMES

Mrs. King will participate in mobility activities and exercises, and maintain mobility at the highest level possible.

NURSING INTERVENTIONS

1. Provide passive range-of-motion exercises twice daily.
2. Encourage Mrs. King to perform active range-of-motion exercises whenever possible.
3. Encourage participation in activities of daily living.
4. Consult with occupational therapy regarding assistive devices for feeding and dressing.
5. Discuss the exercise program with physical therapist so that exercises can be incorporated into the daily routine on nursing unit.
6. Have Mrs. King ambulate with the help of an assistant using a gait belt.
7. Provide massage for tight muscles.
8. Schedule daily or every-other-day tub baths for muscle relaxation.
9. Provide adequate periods of rest on a scheduled basis.
10. Encourage continued participation in activities such as music therapy or other relaxing pastimes.
11. Provide positive encouragement for successes.

EVALUATION

Slight tremors are still noted in both arms, and Mrs. King moves slowly but with slightly less rigidity than noted previously. No falls have been reported in the past 2 weeks. She states, "I feel stronger since I've been getting the therapy and doing exercises. I even helped get myself dressed today." Continue the current plan of care.

pulse of an aging individual to resume its normal rate than it does in a younger person. Changes in blood pressure, particularly orthostatic hypotension, may pose safety risks to the elderly. Those who are sedentary and those who have been on bed rest often experience dizziness or lightheadedness when changing position. This may result in falls if the person is not careful. Changing position more slowly and waiting after each position change will help prevent injuries or falls.

6. **Teach methods of conserving energy.** Simple modifications in activity can help the aging person con-

BOX 13-3

Risk Factors Related to Activity
Intolerance in the Elderly

- Sedentary lifestyle
- Decreased sense of self-worth, self-esteem, or independence
- Generalized weakness, immobility, restriction to bed rest
- Problems related to oxygenation
- Cognitive impairment (Alzheimer's disease or dementia)
- Malnourishment

serve energy. Sitting while dressing requires less energy than does standing. Dressing in clothing with Velcro grips and zippers is less exhausting than dressing in clothing with small buttons or other difficult fasteners. Slip-on shoes require less energy than do laced shoes. Occupational therapists can provide assistance in modifying the environment so that a maximum amount of activity can be performed with a minimum amount of exertion.

7. **Teach older adults and their families methods of reducing stress.** Both psychologic and physiologic stress place extra demands on the body and decrease the elderly person's ability to tolerate activity. Methods for reducing stress are discussed in Chapter 18.

The following interventions should take place in the home:

1. **Modify the environment to reduce energy expenditure and promote safety.** All frequently used objects should be kept close at hand. Remote controls for the television, stereo, or lights are desirable. Furniture should be arranged to provide easy access to resting places. Care should be taken to ensure that the environment is safe. Hazards such as scatter rugs and other clutter on the floor should be removed.

2. **Identify family or community resources to assist with energy-intensive activities.** The family should be encouraged to assist the aging person in energy-intensive activities such as cleaning, cooking, and laundry. If this is not possible, service agencies such as Meals on Wheels may be available.

3. **Use any appropriate interventions that are used in the institutional setting.**

A nursing care plan on impaired physical mobility is presented on p. 220.

A nursing care plan on impaired physical mobility is presented on p. 220.

NURSING PROCESS

PROBLEMS RELATED TO OXYGENATION

In order to survive, body tissues and organs must have an adequate supply of oxygen. The respiratory and cardiovascular systems work together to meet the oxygen needs of the body. If either system functions inadequately, a variety of physiologic changes will be observed.

The aging heart and lungs are generally able to meet the demands of a normal activity level. Under conditions of emotional or physical stress, however, they may not be able to supply the physiologic needs of the body.

Assessment of Oxygenation of Tissues

- Does the person experience excessive fatigue?
- What level of activity causes this fatigue?
- Does the person have any complaints of nausea, vomiting, or anorexia?
- Does the person complain of dyspnea? Is this worse at any specific time of day, such as during the night?
- Does the person complain of chest pain?
- Is the person experiencing tachycardia?
- What is the respiratory rate?
- Is breathing silent and effortless? If not, describe.
- Does the chest expand evenly with respiration? Is breathing deep or shallow?
- Does the person adopt a posture that is more comfortable for breathing?
- Is there a cough?
- Is the cough productive?
- What is the appearance of the sputum?
- Does the person have an order for supplemental oxygen?
- Does the person have a history of exposure to air pollution?
- Does (or did) the person smoke?
- Are there any signs of cyanosis? Cold, clammy skin? Diaphoresis?
- Is the skin cool to the touch?
- Are the jugular veins distended? At what angle: 30°, 45°?
- Are the peripheral pulses palpable? Are pulses equal on both sides of the body?
- What color are the nail beds and fingers?
- What is the capillary refill time?
- Is there a normal amount of body hair over the feet and lower legs?

- Does the person experience any leg pain with ambulation?
- How severe is the pain? Is it relieved by rest?
- Does the person complain of cold hands and feet?
- Are there signs of peripheral edema?
- Is the person's urinary output low despite normal fluid intake?
- Has the person had a rapid weight gain of more than 10 lbs?
- Has the person shown signs of confusion?
- Does the person complain of anxiety, loss of ability to concentrate, or insomnia?
- Are there any changes in relevant laboratory values (e.g., hemoglobin, hematocrit, cardiac enzymes, electrolytes)?
- If an electrocardiogram was done, are there any changes?
- If chest radiography was done, are there any signs of heart enlargement or congestion?

See Box 13-4 for a list of risk factors for problems related to decreased cardiac output in the elderly.

Nursing Diagnoses

Decreased cardiac output
Impaired gas exchange
Ineffective airway clearance
Ineffective breathing pattern

Nursing Goals/Outcomes

The nursing goals for elderly individuals with gas exchange problems are (1) to maintain an open, patent airway; (2) to exhibit an effective respiratory pattern; (3) to experience fewer episodes of dyspnea, angina, and cyanosis; (4) to demonstrate an increased ability to tolerate activity; (5) to identify methods to reduce physical and psychologic stress; and (6) to manifest signs of improved cardiac function (stable vital signs, adequate urinary output, adequate tissue perfusion).

Nursing Interventions

The following nursing interventions should take place in hospitals or extended-care facilities:

1. **Assess pulse and respiration before, during, and after activity.** Vital signs are good indicators of the ability to tolerate activity. These should be assessed while the individual participates in various levels of activity to determine which specific activities cause the greatest problems. Tachycardia is a common sign of decreased cardiac output. In order to compensate for the decreased volume, the heart beats more rapidly. This increased rate places increased stress on the heart muscle and can make the problem worse. Once elevated, it takes longer for the heartbeat of older adults to return to a normal resting rate. Consistent tachycardia or an excessive delay in return to a normal rate indicates serious cardiac problems. The respiratory rate is likely to increase with the heart rate because the body is attempting to meet oxygen needs. With severe cardiac problems, fluid may build up in the lungs, interfere with oxygenation, and further stress the heart.
2. **Monitor laboratory values, radiograph reports, and other diagnostic studies.** Laboratory tests, including hematocrit and arterial blood gases, will provide information regarding the oxygen-carrying capability of the blood. Results of cardiac enzyme studies (e.g., elevated levels of creatinine phosphokinase and lactate dehydrogenase) can indicate cardiac damage from a myocardial infarction. Electrolyte levels should be evaluated, particularly if the person is receiving diuretics. Chest radiographs can reveal the presence of pulmonary congestion, which could indicate respiratory tract infection or pulmonary edema.

   Other diagnostic tests (e.g., electrocardiography) may reveal cardiac pathology before other symptoms are obvious. Any abnormal test results should be reported to the physician immediately.
3. **Observe respiratory effort, including the use of accessory muscles.** An individual who has difficulty breathing will appear to labor when breathing. Use of the accessory muscles of the abdomen and shoulders is an indication that the individual is working harder than normal to breathe.
4. **Evaluate oxygenation by observing for signs of cyanosis and by checking capillary refill time.** In order to meet the life-sustaining needs of the body, blood flow to the extremities may be reduced. This results in cold, clammy skin; slow capillary refill time; pallor; and cyanosis. These changes are most often observed in the lips and fingertips. Delayed capillary refill time indicates that blood supply to the extremities is restricted.
5. **Assess the peripheral pulses, particularly in the**

lower extremities. Assessment of peripheral pulses will reveal any areas of the body that are not receiving adequate oxygen. The lower extremities are most at risk because of the arteriosclerotic changes of aging.

Inadequate oxygen can result in ischemia and necrosis. Mild ischemia can result in hair loss from the lower extremities. Severe ischemia may result in stasis ulcers and in necrosis of the toes, which often necessitates amputation.

6. **Position the person to maximize chest expansion, and encourage frequent changes of position.** Age-related changes tend to reduce the size of the chest cavity. To maximize oxygen exchange, the person should be encouraged to stand or sit in a position that is as upright as possible. Bedridden individuals should change position frequently to prevent stasis and pooling of respiratory secretions within the lungs.

7. **Clear secretions and teach effective coughing.** The elderly may find it difficult to cough effectively due to loss of muscle strength and tone. The inability to remove secretions from the respiratory tract can increase the risk of respiratory tract infections. If the elderly person is very weak and unable to remove secretions, suction may be necessary. When suctioning, care should be used to avoid excessive stimulation of the respiratory tract, which increases production of secretions.

8. **Administer medication as ordered to promote cardiovascular and respiratory function.** Medications such as cardiotonics may be ordered to strengthen the pumping ability of the heart. Mucolytics, bronchodilators, and expectorants may be ordered to enhance the person's ability to remove respiratory secretions. All precautions regarding these medications must be observed, particularly careful monitoring of vital signs.

9. **Administer supplemental oxygen as ordered.** Increasing the amount of available oxygen by using supplemental oxygen may make breathing easier. Oxygen should be prescribed by the physician and administered at the prescribed rate. Low doses are normally used because high oxygen concentrations will decrease respiratory effort. Supplemental oxygen is most commonly administered through a nasal cannula (Fig. 13-7). When oxygen is being administered, good care of the nasal passages is essential. The nares should be kept free of secretions, and the skin should be inspected regularly for breakdown where the plastic tubing presses at the nares and over the ears. Safety precautions such as posting of no smoking signs are important when oxygen is in use.

10. **Use spirometers to improve ventilation.** Spirometers are often ordered by the physician to im-

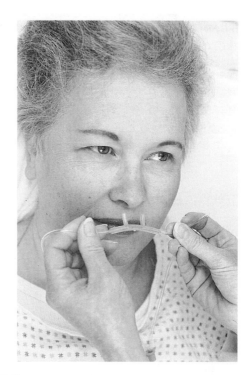

FIG. **13-7**   Nasal cannula.   (From Potter PA, Perry AG: *Basic nursing: theory and practice,* ed 3, St Louis, 1995, Mosby.)

prove respiratory effort. Many elderly persons are unfamiliar with these devices and need clear explanations regarding their use. Many elderly find these devices unpleasant and therefore avoid using them. Nurses should continue to reinforce the importance of these devices and encourage the patient to use them at regular intervals.

11. **Assess for the presence, location, and duration of pain.** Pain that occurs during activity should be assessed and reported. Its location, severity, and whether it radiates or stays in one area should be determined. It is important to know whether the pain occurs during an activity or afterward. Anginal pain originates in the heart and occurs when the heart muscle is deprived of oxygen because of coronary artery narrowing or increased oxygen demand. This pain classically starts in the upper left chest and radiates down the left arm. In some individuals, the pain is referred to the jaw. Coronary vasodilators such as nitroglycerin are used to improve blood flow and decrease the pain.

Intermittent claudication is a specific type of pain that is described by some as cramping, tightness, or aching. This pain is most commonly in the foot or calf, but it may extend to the thigh or buttock. It typically occurs during activity and disappears with rest. Intermittent claudication is an indication of inadequate oxygen supply to the tissues of the leg, and the pain is a result of ischemia. Most physicians recommend daily walking

TABLE 13-1

Home Oxygen Systems

Primary use	Advantages	Disadvantages
COMPRESSED GAS CYLINDERS		
Intermittent therapy, such as for exercise or sleep only	100% oxygen, relatively inexpensive, no loss of gas during storage, relatively portable, delivery of up to 15 L/min	Bulky, possibly unsightly, frequent refilling necessary with continuous use
LIQUID OXYGEN SYSTEMS		
High liter flows for active patients	100% oxygen, conveniently portable, portable units refilled at home, delivery of up to 6 L/min	Usually weekly delivery necessary for refill, evaporates if not used, potential for frostbite at connections and if spilled
CONCENTRATORS		
Moderate liter flows for patients with limited mobility inside or outside home	Fixed monthly cost, minimal interruption of household by supplier, no refills of "main tank," most units with delivery of up to 4 or 5 L/min	Oxygen concentration decreases as liter flow increases (usually 85% to 90%), power supply necessary, electric bill increase of $15 to $20 a month, second system for portability necessary (usually gas cylinders)

From Dettenmeier PA: *Pulmonary nursing care,* St Louis, 1992, Mosby.

for 60 minutes, pausing when pain occurs. Any activity that causes vasoconstriction (e.g., smoking) must be stopped. Cold environments should also be avoided because cold will further aggravate the condition.

12. **Administer sedatives and painkillers with caution.** Many sedatives and analgesics affect the rate or depth of respiration. Respiratory rate and depth should be assessed before these medications are administered to verify that the initial rate is adequate for safety. Respirations should be assessed again after administration.

13. **Maintain a calm, restful environment, and provide emotional support.** Stress places additional oxygen demands on the body. A calm, restful environment will decrease the effects of stress. Decreasing the number of interruptions, closing doors, playing soft music, or making other environmental changes may benefit an individual who is experiencing stress. If the stress is severe or if it is made worse by interaction with unpleasant roommates, a private room may be medically indicated. Time spent listening to the concerns of the elderly is very beneficial in reducing their stress.

14. **Explain stress reduction techniques.** Stress can be controlled by means of nonmedical interventions, including meditation, guided imagery, biofeedback, and relaxation techniques. These techniques are particularly helpful to older adults because they enable the individuals to control their own behavior and lack the side effects of antianxiety medications.

15. **Promote good fluid and nutritional intake within medical restrictions.** Adequate fluid intake will keep respiratory secretions liquefied, making them easier to expectorate. If the elderly person has congestive heart failure or other disease processes that lead to fluid retention, it is important to give fluids with caution and assess for signs of fluid overload. Adequate nutrition, particularly adequate iron intake, is essential for production of adequate hemoglobin, which is necessary for oxygen transport.

The following interventions should take place in the home:

1. **Explain how to use oxygen equipment safely.** Ensure that the elderly person and his or her family know how to operate the equipment. If oxygen is required, the family should be taught safety precautions related to its use. Teaching should include the reasons that smoking and open flames are dangerous. All persons having contact with the oxygen should know the proper precautions to use when handling oxygen tanks and equipment (Fig. 13-8). They should know how to verify that adequate oxygen is available and whom to call if any equipment problems arise. (Table 13-1)

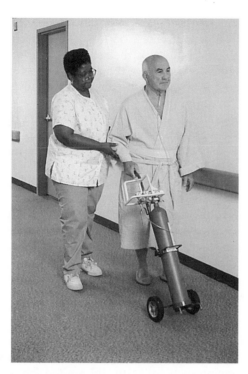

FIG. 13-8   Portable oxygen cylinder used during ambulation. (From Sorrentino SA: *Mosby's textbook for nursing assistants,* ed 4, St Louis, 1994, Mosby.)

Power outage may present a problem to individuals who use an oxygen concentrator. It is wise to keep a backup tank of oxygen for use in such an emergency. It is also wise to notify the power company in advance that the resident needs power returned quickly. Persons needing oxygen or other medical equipment are usually a priority for power companies.

2. **Explain the signs and symptoms of possible complications and the measures to take if these occur.** The elderly and their families should be aware of the signs and symptoms of a change in condition that may indicate complications. The telephone number of the physician and emergency services should be prominently displayed next to the phone so that help can be summoned rapidly if needed.

3. **Use any appropriate interventions that are used in the institutional setting.**

NURSING PROCESS

SELF-CARE DEFICITS

When a person is partially or totally restricted in his or her ability to perform the most basic ADL (i.e., bathing, dressing, grooming, eating, and toileting), a self-care deficit is present. With advanced age or the onset of disease, many individuals experience some degree of problem with self-care. Problems related to self-care can be devastating to the elderly, because of their effect on self-esteem. People who cannot meet these needs become dependent on others and lose much control over the most basic elements of their lives. Older adults who cannot feed themselves must eat what they are fed. Those who cannot dress themselves must wear what another person chooses. Those who cannot bathe or groom themselves will only be as clean and well-groomed as another person allows. Those who cannot go to the bathroom alone are likely to become incontinent. Nurses must be able to recognize the individual's specific difficulties and degree of limitation with self-care so that appropriate nursing interventions can be planned. These interventions should be directed toward maintaining the individual's functioning at the highest possible level. The previously discussed concepts of rehabilitation form the basis for working with older individuals with self-care deficits.

Assessment of Self-Care Deficits

- Can the person feed himself or herself? If not, what level of assistance is required? (0-4)
  0 = completely independent
  1 = requires devices or equipment
  2 = requires help, supervision, or teaching from another person
  3 = requires devices and help from another person
  4 = totally dependent
- Can the person toilet himself or herself? If not, what level of assistance is required? (0-4)
- Can the person bathe himself or herself? If not, what level of assistance is required? (0-4)
- Can the person dress himself or herself? If not, what level of assistance is required? (0-4)

See Box 13-5 for a list of risk factors for self-care deficits in the elderly.

Nursing Diagnoses

Feeding self-care deficit
Bathing/hygiene self-care deficit
Dressing/grooming self-care deficit
Toileting self-care deficit

Nursing Goals/Outcomes

The nursing goals for elderly individuals with self-care deficits are (1) to perform self-care at the highest possible level within limitations; (2) to demonstrate the use of modified techniques and assistive devices to accomplish self-care; (3) to verbalize improved self-esteem related to self-care abilities; and (4) to identify resources that are available to provide assistance.

Nursing Interventions

The following nursing interventions should take place in hospitals or extended-care facilities:

1. **Assess the individual to determine the factors that cause or contribute to the deficit such as age-related changes, disease processes, medications, and cognitive or perceptual changes.** Each aging individual will present a unique set of problems to which nurses must respond when planning care. Unless the specific needs of each person are identified, the plan of care is meaningless. Some individuals will be able to regain many skills and become less dependent; others will remain at lower levels of function. A good assessment covers the person's strengths and limitations so that the most appropriate care plan can be developed.

2. **Include the elderly in problem identification and care planning.** A plan that does not include the individual is likely to fail. Overcoming a self-care deficit requires the person's total commitment and cooperation. The only way nurses can hope to get this level of commitment is by including the elderly person in the entire process. If he or she is unable to communicate verbally, nurses should observe nonverbal communication. Many individuals who cannot express their needs verbally will respond to simple directions and positive encouragement.

3. **Allow adequate time for completion of activities.** With aging, even healthy, active persons require more time than younger individuals to accomplish a task. Those experiencing self-care deficits will require even more time than the well elderly. Most facilities and nurses are geared toward getting things done as quickly as possible. In many facilities, elderly individuals who are perfectly capable

of completing self-care activities are not allowed to do so because it takes too long. This practice is in opposition to those of the rehabilitative focus. Encouraging and allowing the elderly to perform self-care does take more time than having the care provided by the nursing staff. This fact must be taken into consideration when assignments are made so that adequate time is available. If these adjustments are not made, the staff can actively undermine any chance of success.

4. **Develop a plan that moves in stages toward the highest possible level of function, and give positive feedback to reinforce positive changes.** The plan to increase self-care ability should be structured in stages so that the individual achieves some successes. If too much is expected, the individual may become frustrated and give up. It is better to work toward and build on small successes. For example, if the person has not been doing any personal hygiene, successfully washing the face is a major accomplishment. Success of this nature should not be ignored but should be reinforced by a comment such as, "You did a good job washing your face." A simple checklist that enables the person to see that he or she is making progress may be helpful. Reinforcing the positives and minimizing the negatives is the best way to achieve the desired goals and increase motivation.

5. **Consult with occupational and physical therapists to identify alternative methods and equipment that would most benefit the individual.** Occupational and physical therapists are specialists in rehabilitation. They have extensive knowledge of the techniques and equipment available to improve self-care ability. Modification of an activity (such as sitting instead of standing) may enable an individual to perform self-care activities (Fig. 13-9). Modified clothing or eating utensils may mean the difference between complete dependence and independence.

6. **Modify the environment with assistive devices designed to meet the specific needs of the individual.** Once the need for special assistive devices is identified, nurses should ensure the availability of these devices (Figs. 13-10 to 13-12). Identifying that a toilet riser, grip rail, or special spoon is needed does no good if the item is not available. The staff may have to wash special eating utensils so that they are not lost. Residents sharing a bathroom may have to adjust to the presence of a toilet riser. They must either use the riser or be willing and able to remove and replace it when they use the toilet. In some situations, modification of the environment with assistive devices may necessitate room changes so that individuals with common needs are grouped together.

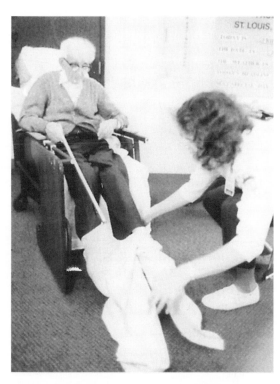

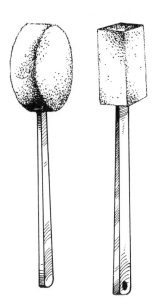

FIG. 13-10   Long-handled bath sponges. (From Dittmar S: *Rehabilitative nursing: process and application*, St Louis, 1989, Mosby.)

FIG. 13-9   An occupational therapist watches an elderly man put on pajama bottoms with the help of an assistive device as part of a daily exercise or skill regimen. (Courtesy of Barnes Extended Care, St Louis.)

The following interventions should take place in the home:

1. **Assess the ability of the family or significant others to provide safe care.** Many totally dependent elderly are being cared for today in the home setting. Nurses may make regular visits, but much of the responsibility for care falls on spouses or other family members. These caregivers may have little or no training for the tasks involved. Often the caregiver is elderly or infirm. Nurses are responsible for seeing that no harm comes from the home care situation. If the care needs exceed the ability of the caregivers, nurses may have to contact other family members or social services to ensure the elderly individual's safety. If the caregiver is capable of providing care, he or she will probably need additional teaching related to providing care.

2. **Assess the home environment to determine safety and the need for modifications such as grip rails, bath chairs, or toilet risers.** Depending on the level of self-care deficit, the home may require major modification. Individuals with minimal self-care deficits may only require a few assistive devices to function adequately (Fig. 13-13). Those with serious self-care deficits will require more modifications.

3. **Identify community resources available to help obtain the necessary equipment.** Special assistive devices can be costly and may require special skill for installation. Many communities have agencies or volunteer groups that help provide the necessary assistance.

4. **Inform the families or significant others of the necessity to allow the elderly to do as much as possible for themselves.** Family members are often too helpful and do not expect the elderly individual to do anything for him- or herself, which can lead to a loss of functional ability. Nurses should explain the importance of allowing and encouraging the aging individual to do as much as possible. Nurses should stress that this is the best thing caregivers can do for their loved ones, and that they are not being thoughtless or neglectful.

5. **Discuss respite care and other options with caregivers.** Anyone who provides long-term care in the home places him- or herself at risk. Home care is often exhausting for the caregivers. It is advisable for nurses to discuss the possibility of some form of respite care so caregivers are able to maintain their own health and mental well-being.

6. **Assist the family with arrangements for hospitalization or extended-care placement.** When the aging individual becomes completely dependent, the spouse or family may have to consider alternative methods of providing care. This is a very difficult area financially and emotionally. Nurses may be able to provide some guidance or may be able to contact other social service agencies that can help the family through this difficult process.

7. **Use any appropriate interventions that are used in the institutional setting.** A nursing care plan

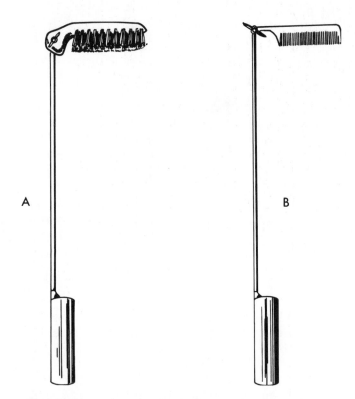

FIG. 13-11 **A,** Adapted hairbrush. **B,** Adapted comb. (From Dittmar S: *Rehabilitative nursing: process and application,* St Louis, 1989, Mosby.)

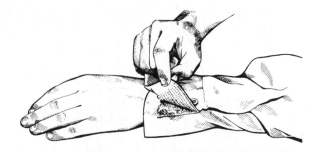

FIG. 13-12 Velcro shirt sleeve to facilitate closures. (From Dittmar S: *Rehabilitative nursing: process and application,* St Louis, 1989, Mosby.)

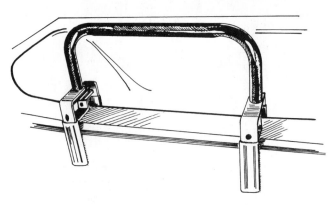

FIG. 13-13 Bathtub with grab bars. (From Dittmar S: *Rehabilitative nursing: process and application,* St Louis, 1989, Mosby.)

for impaired physical mobility is presented on p. 220.

NURSING PROCESS

DIVERSIONAL ACTIVITY DEFICIT

Diversional activities play an important role in the lives of older adults. Diversional activities can help fill time and provide creative outlets, particularly when they are meaningful to the elderly person.

Assessment of Participation in Diversional Activities

- What activities does the person enjoy?
- How often does the person participate in these activities?
- Does the person prefer solitary or social activities?
- How much time does the person spend alone?
- Does the person interact with other individuals? Who? How often?
- What is the nature of these interactions?
- Can the person financially afford to participate in the activities he or she enjoys?
- Is the person able to get to the desired activities, particularly if they require transportation?

- Do the person's sensory or cognitive changes interfere with interests?
- Do the person's physical changes interfere with interests?
- Is the person napping because of boredom? How often?
- What is the person's psychologic state of mind (e.g., depressed)?

See Box 13-6 for a list of risk factors for diversional activity deficit in the elderly.

Nursing Diagnosis

Diversional activity deficit

Nursing Goals/Outcomes

The nursing goals for elderly individuals with diversional activity deficit are (1) to identify activities that might be of interest; (2) to express interest in participating in diversional activities; (3) to participate in selected diversional activities; and (4) to demonstrate socially acceptable behaviors while participating in activities.

Risk Factors Related to Diversional Activities in the Elderly

- Restricted in mobility
- An environment with limited activities
- Anxiety, depression, or grief
- Limited financial or transportation resources
- Cognitive or perceptual problems

Nursing Interventions

The following nursing interventions should take place in hospitals and extended-care facilities:

1. **Assess current and past hobbies, activities, and interests.** The best way to prepare for a good old age is to have as many interests as possible when you are young. Young people are so busy raising families and working that they often neglect to develop hobbies or interests outside of family and work. Those individuals who have developed a wide range of interests seem to adjust to aging better than those with few interests. After their families have grown and they have retired from work, many men and women finally get the opportunity to participate in hobbies and other activities that they desire. Some elderly persons have a steady stream of activities that keep their days full. Others complain that there is nothing to do and that they are bored. Lack of interests and diversions makes time seem to pass slowly and may lead to depression and social isolation.

2. **Include the individual in selecting and planning diversional activities.** The elderly should have the right to choose the activities they find most meaningful. Purposeful activity is good for maintaining self-esteem; busywork is not. Older adults who reside in extended-care facilities because of illness or infirmity may have fewer opportunities and diversions available. Nurses can help these individuals maintain active interests by exploring those activities that were enjoyed at an earlier age. The nurse's interest and a little creativity can go a long way toward meeting the social and diversional needs of the elderly.

3. **Provide suitable reading materials such as large-print books or books on tape.** Many elderly persons enjoy books but are not able to read because of visual changes. Books with large print may be usable and are available through most libraries. If visual impairments are severe, audiotapes of favorite books are also available.

4. **Focus on what the individual can do, not on what he or she cannot do.** Positive successes are likely to lead to more successes. It is often depressing to the elderly to focus on activities that they can no longer do. Directing attention to positive accomplishments will help the person maintain a more positive attitude.

5. **Suggest activities that are occurring in the facility, such as music or discussion groups, occupational therapy, activity therapy, or religious activities.** Many elderly persons will not be able to leave the care setting to participate in certain activities. Physical or economic changes may interfere with normal diversional activities. Hospitalization or change of living accommodations can lead to a variety of restrictions and inconveniences. Nurses can help individuals maintain social contacts and interests by exploring other activities. Occupational and activity therapists may suggest activities and provide assistance in learning new skills. Activity and occupational therapy are provided in most residential care settings. Therapists can help individuals learn new activities or ways to modify existing interests. For example, if physical changes make knitting too difficult, lap weaving may be possible. Music therapy provides another form of diversion and allows individuals to express their feelings nonverbally. Music is often combined with exercise because rhythm seems to enhance activity.

6. **Work with the activities department to plan new or different activities based on client input.** Many facilities tend to fall into habits or patterns of repeating the same activities. Many elderly are very creative and should have input into decision making. Some facilities are very progressive and offer a wide variety of activities; others do not. Nurses play a more important role in extended-care facilities.

7. **Encourage social interaction among residents with similar interests.** People of all ages find shared activities enjoyable. Those who share common interests are more likely to want to spend time together (Fig. 13-14).

8. **Spend time with individuals to demonstrate interest in their personal interests.** Each of us needs to know that we are special. Even a few minutes spent with an elderly person will help nurses know that person better and will enable more personal responses. Commenting on their latest craft projects or asking how they are enjoying a television show demonstrates interest and caring.

9. **Change the physical environment to increase stimulation and interest (bulletin boards of currently scheduled activities, seasonal themes, flyers about topics of interest).** Lack of stimulation can lead to loss of interest and disengagement from others. Any device that helps maintain inter-

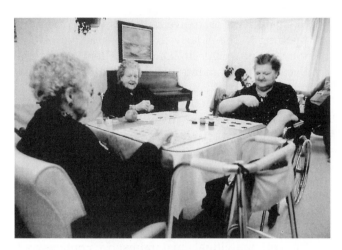

FIG. 13-14   Recreational activities are important for the elderly. (From Sorrentino SA: *Mosby's textbook for nursing assistants,* ed 4, St Louis, 1996, Mosby.)

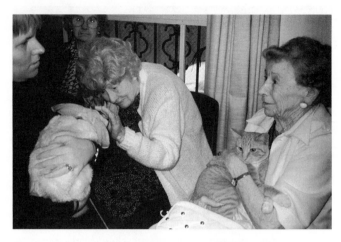

FIG. 13-15   Pets can be great comfort to the elderly. (Courtesy of Priscilla Ebersole.)

est and contact with the rest of society will help the aging person remain alert and interested.

10. **Enlist the help of volunteers to read, play games, or just talk with residents.** There is not enough time for nursing staff to meet the needs of all of the patients in an institution. Many groups such as Scouts, social clubs, and school groups are interested in providing community service. Volunteering to work with the elderly is a very rewarding activity. The intergenerational mix is often a learning experience for both old and young.

11. **Display the results of residents' activities in a prominent place and give recognition to all participants.** Displaying what residents have created (e.g., craft work, creative writing, or other achievements) recognizes their positive accomplishments and enables the staff and visitors to realize that creativity and productivity do not end with old age.

12. **Explore the possibility of new activities such as pet therapy to stimulate interest of withdrawn individuals.** Pet therapy is becoming increasingly common. The benefits of association with animals have been documented in many studies. Elderly individuals who have pets are healthier and live longer than those without pets. Institutionalized individuals—even those who have isolated themselves from most human contact—seem to respond to the unquestioning affection given by animals. Some residential care centers have pets that live in the home (Fig. 13-15).

13. **Ensure that physical needs are met before and during diversional activities. Make sure assistance is available for toileting, snacks, and transfers.** Many elderly with physical deficits are reluctant to leave their rooms or care units because of fear. Many are afraid that they will not get to a bathroom in time and will embarrass themselves. Others are afraid that no one will be available to help them move from place to place or meet other physical challenges. Nurses should ensure that there is adequate help to meet physical care needs before and during activities. Aging persons should be given the opportunity to use the toilet before leaving the care unit and at regular intervals during the activities. Even diversional activities require increased energy expenditure, so snacks that are in keeping with the prescribed diets should be made available.

The following interventions should take place in the home:

1. **Provide information regarding community resources for the elderly, including senior citizen centers, libraries, museums, and volunteer activities.** Many senior citizen centers offer a variety of craft programs, including painting, weaving, woodworking, and pottery. Participation in these activities may provide exposure to crafts that the individual never had the opportunity to try before. Some individuals find real talents that they never suspected they had. Travelogs, movies, or speakers on topics of current interest help the elderly maintain interest in world events. Activity centers can provide an opportunity for social interaction that reduces the sense of isolation. Aging individuals whose friends have died or moved often find new friends at these centers.

   Some senior citizen centers also offer classes in such subjects as foreign languages, history, and even computers. Some colleges allow senior citizens to audit classes on a space-available basis. The senior citizen benefits from the stimulation of the course, and the younger students benefit from the different perspective of the elderly individual. Elder Hostel is a program through which older adults can travel around the world by staying in hostels and expanding their knowledge. Some older adults are interested in volunteer activities such as foster grandparenting or literacy programs.

2. **Identify community resources that provide transportation to desired activities.** Lack of transportation is a common cause for social isolation and failure to participate in activities. Many communities have special programs that provide buses or vans to transport the elderly to shopping centers or activities for a nominal fee. The elderly should be made aware of these services and be assisted with making contact if they are hesitant to call for help.

3. **Explore and identify options for meaningful use of time.** Many elderly persons look only at the things that they are unable to do and do not consider all of the options available. Spending time exploring interests and possible activities can help expand their outlook.

4. **Encourage participation in new and meaningful activities.** Many elderly persons need encouragement to seek diversional activities. Many are interested in participating in new activities but are afraid to try because of their age. They often fear that others will not accept them or will laugh at their inexperience. Information that familiarizes the person with the activity can be provided beforehand. Knowledge about the activity can reduce fear of the unknown. Exploration of past successes in facing new or different challenges may provide the necessary encouragement to try something new.

5. **Use any appropriate interventions that are used in the institutional setting.**

REHABILITATION

Our attitudes affect our expectations, and our expectations affect our plans. If caregivers do not expect much from the elderly, we will not get much; if we keep our expectations high, much is possible.

The attitudes held by nurses regarding aging and the elderly will have a significant impact on their planning of nursing care. Attitudes about the value of elderly persons and about their potential for leading active, meaningful lives will influence the priorities, the goals, and the interventions selected during the planning process. Attitudes will also influence how much

nurses include and involve the elderly in the planning process.

Low expectations for older adults lead to a low-level, or custodial, focus in care planning. High expectations of the elderly lead to a high-level, or rehabilitative, focus.

NEGATIVE ATTITUDES— THE CONTROLLING OR CUSTODIAL FOCUS

Nurses who take a negative view of aging sees it as a process of deterioration and loss. With this negative perspective, older adults are viewed as helpless, passive, dependent, and incapable of making decisions regarding their care. Nurses who have these negative attitudes generally see little potential for improvement in the elderly. While this may be true for a small percentage of the elderly, it is not the norm.

If nurses have predetermined that older adults are incapable of making their wishes known or that they are not interested in what happens, then the nurses will not consider their input important or necessary for care planning. Preferences or desires often go unnoticed, merely because the nurse chose not to listen to verbal or nonverbal communication.

Once nurses predict or anticipate little potential for improvement, their expectations are kept low. With a negative attitude toward aging and the elderly, priority is given to slowing the process of physical deterioration. Maintenance of function is supported, but no improvement or higher level of functioning is expected or encouraged. Little if any attempt is made to reverse or undo any functional losses. Goals are limited to maintaining the existing level of function or the status quo.

With maintenance as the goal, the care plan is often limited to physiologic and safety concerns. Interventions generally address the lowest level of needs according to Maslow. The elderly are kept clean, groomed, clothed, and fed. Basic elimination needs are met. Accommodations are clean and reasonably comfortable. Medications are administered, and treatments are performed. Higher-level needs such as security, love, and a sense of belonging, however, are minimized or ignored.

Nurses then control all aspects of the planning process and take total responsibility for determining what is best for the elderly person. The care plan requires the nurse to be active and the older adult to be passive. By its very nature, this type of care plan promotes helplessness, loss of function, and dependence on nurses and other caregivers. Little is expected; even less is achieved. A few elderly persons are severely impaired and have experienced a profound loss of mental and physical capabilities because of aging and disease. Some are so severely affected that they are truly unable to communicate their wishes or do anything for themselves. However, it is amazing how much even severely impaired persons can and will communicate about their care, often nonverbally, if nurses pay attention.

If functional losses are so severe that the person is unaware of reality or absolutely unable to function, then and only then should all needs be anticipated and provided by nurses or other caregivers. However, this determination should not be made quickly. Many seemingly hopeless and helpless elderly have more ability and potential than we give them credit for. Often the potential remains hidden because we do not expect to find it.

Negative attitudes that older adults themselves have may lead to declining function. They may feel helpless, hopeless, or afraid to try. If nurses reinforce these negative feelings, nothing positive will occur. Elderly persons who have potential for improvement but are given only custodial care are likely to lose hope. Loss of the will to fight and of the ability to strive for something better is the most destructive attitude.

POSITIVE ATTITUDES—THE REHABILITATIVE FOCUS

When nurses have a positive attitude toward aging and feel that the elderly are able and willing to participate in their care, the outcome is very different. These nurses recognize that as the elderly experience the normal physiologic changes of aging or the impact of disease, they are more likely to require nursing care. This care may be given in the home, in the hospital, or in an extended-care facility. Nurses who have a positive attitude toward aging recognize that most elderly people have a great deal of unused and often unrecognized potential. Nurses with a positive attitude toward aging recognize that most aging persons want to retain control of their lives. A rehabilitative care focus addresses both the actual and potential problems the elderly are likely to experience. A rehabilitative focus does not wait until problems occur. It is a proactive approach to nursing care planning that deals with *prevention* of problems—not just reactions to them.

Most aging persons will benefit from a rehabilitative focus in care planning. In order to plan care with a rehabilitative focus, nurses must (1) acknowledge that older adults have intrinsic worth that exceeds their limitations; (2) accept that older adults have the right to make informed decisions regarding their care; (3) recognize that loss of function or disability has a serious impact on older adults, as well as on their fam-

ilies and significant others; and (4) recognize that older adults and their families and significant others are important members of the health team and that all should play a role in decision making whenever possible.

The long-term goal of rehabilitative nursing care is to help older adults achieve and maintain maximum physical, psychosocial, and spiritual health. When planning care with a focus on rehabilitation, nurses must (1) attempt to prevent complications of physical disability, restore optimal functioning, and help the individual adjust to alterations in lifestyle; (2) attempt to minimize the impact of physical changes or disease processes that interrupt or alter functioning and life satisfaction; (3) focus on maintaining the highest achievable level of independent function; (4) provide for comfort needs and adjustments in lifestyle that are conducive to health; (5) support the ability of older adults to adapt to change; (6) help aging persons reestablish and maintain control over their lives; and (7) work to reduce the impact of societal factors that restrict the elderly person's ability to maintain independence.

Under these guiding principles, nurses work with older adults and establish priorities based not on the nurse's values, but on the older adult's values. Goals that are challenging yet realistic are established *with* the aging patient. The nursing interventions most likely to help these persons achieve their goals are then selected and communicated as the plan of care.

When planning care with a rehabilitative focus, nurses look beyond the nursing interventions and act as coordinators for all of the various disciplines that enable the aging person to achieve the highest level of physical, mental, psychosocial, and spiritual functioning. Nurses seek input from a wide range of specialists, including (but not limited to) physicians, pharmacists, dietitians, physical therapists, occupational therapists, speech therapists, activity therapists, dentists, podiatrists, chaplains, and social workers. For elderly individuals residing in their own homes, nurses consider the environmental impact of the surroundings and the community services available.

All of these specialists, along with the older adult and his or her family, should have input into the development of the care plan. When a formal meeting is held in a hospital or extended-care facility, it is frequently referred to as a "staffing." Regular reviews of the plan of care should be scheduled to determine whether any modifications are necessary. Information should be shared by all concerned parties and communicated clearly. Interventions should be spelled out in enough detail that all parties are aware of their roles. The elderly should be reminded of their rights to change or modify the plan of care.

A rehabilitation focus is not limited to the care provided in institutional settings. Rehabilitation is also directed toward improving or maintaining the capability of the disabled elderly to function in society. Like other healthy, capable adults, nurses are often unaware of environmental barriers that prevent the disabled from accessing goods and services. Box 13-7 provides a good way of assessing the world through the eyes of a disabled person. Nurses who believe that older adults have the desire and ability to maintain high-level function at home and in the community must become social activists and work to make others aware of the needs of the disabled. Much work is needed to make the everyday world accessible to them.

BOX 13-7

Access Checklist for the Physically Disabled

Accessible means "the condition of being approachable." For the physically disabled, this term means not only approachable, but usable. The questions here will help you determine beforehand whether your destination is likely to be accessible. Call ahead and ask these questions plus any of your own.

RESTAURANTS

- Are there designated parking spaces for the disabled?
- Are there any steps or curbs between the parking area and the front door? If yes, how many?
- Are there steps to get in the front door? If yes, how many?
- If the front door is not at ground level, are there any alternative entrances (e.g., ramp, side door at ground level) or alternative methods of entry (e.g., restaurant personnel willing and able to assist)?
- Are doorways to public areas at least 28 inches wide (32 inches for an electric wheelchair)?
- Are public rest rooms accessible? This means there are no steps leading from the dining area to the rest room, doors at least 28 (32) inches wide, wider stall (3' × 5'), and grab bars.
- How many doors are there at the restaurant entrance? The restroom entrance? If there are consecutive sets of doors, how much space is there between them?
- Are there Braille menus?
  If you are attending a meeting or social event in the restaurant's banquet hall, inquire about the accessibility of that facility as well.

HOTELS/MOTELS

Ask all of the "restaurant" questions plus the following:
- Are there steps leading to the hotel/motel restaurant, lounge, bar, gift shop, meeting rooms, etc?

- Do elevator doors open at least 28 (32) inches?
- What are the internal dimensions of the elevator?
- Are elevator buttons set lower?
- Are there Braille elevator buttons?
- Are public telephones set lower?
- Are specially adapted rooms available for the disabled? If yes, how many? Can the rooms be reserved?

If no specially adapted rooms are available, ask the following:
- Are the doorways to hotel rooms at least 28 (32) inches wide?
- Is there a sill or step at the door entering the room? At the door entering the bathroom?
- Are bathroom doors at least 28 (32) inches wide?
- Does the bathroom door swing in or out? If the door swings in, does it block any of the plumbing?
- Does the room have a bathtub or shower stall? If there is a shower stall, what is its width and depth?
- Are there grab bars by the toilet, tub, shower?
- Are there handheld showers?
- Can a wheelchair fit under the bathroom sink? (This requires at least 29 inches of clear space under the sink.)
- Are there amplified telephones?
- Is there a teletypewriter or teletypedisplay reservations system?
- Are guide dogs allowed?

Because of the number of questions involved in checking a hotel/motel's accessibility, you may want to write ahead if time permits.

Share this checklist with travel agents and others you meet. It will help spread awareness of accessibility as well as let others know what features are needed to meet your needs.

From Sacred Heart Rehabilitation Hospital, Milwaukee, Wis.

SUMMARY

The ability to perform activity and exercise requires that the musculoskeletal, respiratory, cardiovascular, and nervous systems work together effectively. Age- and disease-related changes in these systems contribute to the decreased level of activity that is common with aging. Any problems with activity and exercise can result in lifestyle changes for the elderly. Careful assessment and prompt initiation of appropriate nursing interventions will help the elderly achieve and maintain the highest level of function possible.

READINGS AND REFERENCES

Administration on Aging Web site: *Don't take it easy—exercise: National Institute on Aging AgePage,* www.aoa.dhhs.gov/agepages/exercise.html, 1995.

Allison M, Keller C: Physical activity in the elderly: benefits and intervention strategies, *Nurse Pract* 22:53, 1997.

Brechtelsbauer DA: Managing rheumatologic disease in nursing home patients, *Postgrad Med* 96:91, 1994.

Brown EW: New hope for old exercisers, *Medical Update* 19:2, 1996.

Buckwalter JA: Decreased mobility in the elderly: the exercise antidote, *Physician Sports Med* 25:126, 1997.

Campbell AJ, Buchner DM: Unstable disability and fluctuations of frailty, *Age Aging* 26:315, 1997.

CIGNA HealthCare of Colorado Web site: *Aging, exercise and depression: separating myths from realities,* http://www.coolware.com/health/joel/exercise.html, 1997.

Exercise can benefit physically restrained, *Brown University Long-Term Care Quality Letter* 8:6, 1996.

Exercise promotes health—and slows aging—in the elderly, *Brown University Long-Term Care Quality Letter* 9:1, 1997.

Fiatarone MA, O'Brien K, Rich B: Exercise: Rx for a healthier old age, *Patient Care* 30:145,1996.

Fiatarone MA, Garnett LR: Keep on keeping on, *Harvard Health Letter* 22:4, 1996.

Fontane PE: Exercise, fitness and feeling well *American Behavioral Scientist* 39:288,1996.

For the young at heart: exercise tips for seniors, http://geriatricspt.org/consumer/Young.html, 1997.

Henry L: Feel young and look young again, *Muscle Fitness* 58:182, 1997.

Murgueytio AM, Barney KF: Bathroom independence, *Independent Living Provider* 11:24, 1996.

Physical activity and health: a report of the Surgeon General, http://www.cdc.gov/nccdphp/sgr/chapcon.html, 1997.

Potera C: Choosing the best exercise for seniors, *Physician Sports Med* 25:21, 1997.

Potera C: Helping frail, older adults build strength, *Physician Sports Med* 22:36, 1994.

Roberts BL, Palmer R: Cardiac response of elderly adults to normal activities and aerobic walking, *Clin Nurs Res* 5:105, 1996.

Sowden A, et al: Preventing falls and subsequent injury in older people, *Effective Health Care* 2:4, 1996.

Tempkin T, Tempkin A, Goodman H: Geriatric rehabilitation, *Nurse Pract Forum* 6:173,1995.

Weight training restores mobility in frail elderly, *Executive Health's Good Health Report* 30:6, 1994.

Williams BD, et al: Activities of daily living and costs in nursing homes, *Health Care Financing Rev* 14:117, 1994.

Yusef HR, et al: Leisure-time physical activity among older adults: United States, 1990, *Arch Intern Med* 156: 1321, 1996.

SLEEP AND REST

1. Describe normal sleep and rest patterns.
2. Describe how sleep and rest patterns change with aging.
3. Discuss the effects of disease processes on sleep.
4. Describe methods of assessing changes in sleep and rest patterns.
5. Identify the elderly who are most at risk for experiencing sleep pattern disturbances.
6. Identify selected nursing diagnoses related to sleep or rest problems.
7. Describe nursing interventions that are appropriate for elderly individuals experiencing problems related to sleep pattern disturbance.

SLEEP-REST HEALTH PATTERN

The sleep-rest health pattern describes the patterns of sleep, rest, and relaxation that are exhibited throughout the 24-hour day. Individual perceptions, rituals, and aids used to promote sleep and rest are included.

No one knows exactly why we sleep, but it is a fact that we all require sleep to function normally. Sleep apparently allows the body time to rejuvenate and to respond to the stresses of daily living. Lack of adequate sleep can affect health and behavior. Studies have connected sleep deprivation and insomnia to altered appetite; fatigue; decreased ability to perform tasks that require high-level coordination; increased traffic accidents, home accidents, falls, and irritability; emotional instability; difficulty with concentration; and impaired judgment.

Many elderly people experience problems related to sleep. It is estimated that as many as half of all independent-living elderly and two thirds of institutionalized elderly have sleep disturbances. Sleep-related problems can be very troubling to the aging individual and are frequently the basis of visits to the physician and complaints to the nurse. Some of these problems result from changes that normally occur with aging; others may be caused or aggravated by acute or chronic health problems. Nurses must understand normal sleep patterns and be able to identify common age-related changes in sleep patterns and common sleep disorders in order to assess, plan, and intervene appropriately and effectively.

Normal Sleep and Rest

Periods of sleep and wakefulness occur in regular and somewhat predictable cycles. Most humans develop a pattern that repeats approximately every 24 hours. This cycle occurs in response to the day-night cycle of the sun and is referred to as **circadian** (from the Latin word meaning "about a day") or **diurnal** (from the Latin word meaning "daily") rhythm. Within this cycle, individuals develop their own unique patterns for waking and sleeping.

The usual times that people go to bed and rise differ widely among individuals. Some go to sleep at 10 PM and rise at 6 AM; others go to sleep at midnight and rise at 8 AM. These sleep-wake patterns can be disturbed by shift work, time-zone changes, illness, emotional stress, medications, and numerous other factors. The amount of sleep needed also varies widely among individuals. Some individuals function normally with less than 6 hours of sleep, whereas others require 9 hours of sleep or more to feel rested. The average amount of sleep required for people ages 20 to 60 years of age is 7.5 hours per day.

Sleep is under the control of the central nervous system. Current research indicates that wakefulness is regulated by the neurotransmitter norepinephrine. Sleep appears to be controlled by release of serotonin within the brainstem. Sleep is not a uniform state of unconsciousness; rather it is divided into a series of cycles of lighter and deeper stages of sleep. Immediately before falling asleep, most adults experience a stage of increased relaxation and drowsiness that typically lasts from 10 to 30 minutes. This is followed by four to six complete sleep cycles lasting between 1 and 2 hours each. Each cycle consists of four non-rapid eye movement (REM) stages and one REM stage (Box 14-1, Fig. 14-1). As the night's sleep progresses, REM periods increase in length and non-REM periods decrease in length. If sleep is interrupted at any time, the individual goes back to stage 1 of non-REM sleep and begins a new cycle.

Sleep and Aging

Because sleep efficiency decreases as age increases, many elderly complain that they do not feel refreshed after sleep. Although the amount of time spent in bed may increase with age, the amount of time actually spent sleeping decreases. The average 70-year-old sleeps only 6 hours per night, which is 1.5 hours less than younger adults sleep. A decreased amount of time is spent sleeping, and the nature of the sleep changes. Elderly individuals experience less stage 4 non-REM sleep and less REM sleep. These changes result in less deep restorative and refreshing sleep. Circadian rhythm also appears to change with age, resulting in earlier bedtime and earlier rising. In addition, sleep interruption and nocturnal awakening are increasingly common because the elderly are more easily aroused by environmental noise or stimuli.

Sleep Disorders

The most commonly reported sleep disorder is **insomnia,** which is defined as difficulty falling asleep or remaining asleep or the belief that one is not getting enough sleep. Insomnia is not a disease in itself but is a symptom of some other underlying problem. Different types of insomnia are identified based on the phase of sleep affected: (1) sleep initiation problems—those related to falling asleep; (2) sleep maintenance problems—those related to staying asleep; or (3) terminal insomnia problems—those related to abnormally early awakening. Identification of the type of insomnia problem present can help nurses to identify the underlying cause or causes and result in the best interventions.

Insomnia can be caused by medical conditions, psychologic factors, medications, and behavioral or environmental factors. Medical conditions that cause pain,

BOX 14-1

Stages of Sleep

STAGE 1: NON–RAPID EYE MOVEMENT (REM) SLEEP

- Lightest level of sleep
- Lasts a few minutes
- Decreased physiologic activity beginning with a gradual fall in vital signs and metabolism
- Person easily aroused by sensory stimuli such as noise
- If person awakens, feels as though daydreaming

STAGE 2: NON-REM SLEEP

- Period of sound sleep
- Relaxation progresses
- Arousal still easy
- Lasts 10 to 20 minutes
- Body functions still slowing

STAGE 3: NON-REM SLEEP

- Initial stages of deep sleep
- Sleeper difficult to arouse and rarely moves
- Muscles completely relaxed
- Vital signs declining but remaining regular
- Lasts 15 to 30 minutes

STAGE 4: NON-REM SLEEP

- Deepest stage of sleep
- Very difficult to arouse sleeper
- If sleep loss has occurred, sleeper will spend considerable portion of night in this stage
- Restores and rests the body
- Vital signs significantly lower than during waking hours
- Lasts approximately 15 to 30 minutes
- Possible sleepwalking and enuresis

REM SLEEP

- Stage of vivid, full-color dreaming (less-vivid dreaming may occur in other stages)
- Usually begins every 50 to 90 minutes after sleep has begun
- Typified by autonomic response of rapidly moving eyes, fluctuating heart and respiratory rates and blood pressure
- Loss of skeletal muscle tone
- Responsible for mental restoration
- Sleeper most difficult to arouse
- Duration increasing with each cycle and averaging 20 minutes

From Potter PA, Perry AG: *Basic nursing: theory and practice,* ed 3, St Louis, 1995, Mosby.

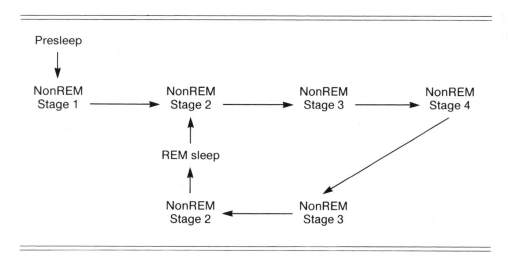

FIG. **14-1**   The adult sleep cycle. (From Potter PA, Perry AG: *Basic nursing: theory and practice,* ed 3, St Louis, 1995, Mosby.)

interfere with breathing, or cause frequent bladder or bowel elimination can contribute to frequent awakening. Common medical problems that may lead to insomnia include arthritis, bursitis, gastroesphageal reflux, chronic obstructive pulmonary disease, conges-tive heart failure, sleep apnea, prostatic problems, cystitis, and others. Nocturnal movement disorders, including restless leg syndrome (an irresistible urge to move the lower extremities) or nocturnal myoclonus (sudden repetitive jerking or kicking movements of the lower extremities), can also contribute to insomnia in the elderly.

Anxiety is likely to be related to difficulty falling asleep and interrupted sleep. Depression is most likely to be associated with early awakening but may also be related to hypersomnia (excessive sleepiness at a time of normal wakefulness). People with dementia often experience abnormal sleep cycles and are prone to waking and wandering during the night. Both prescription and over-the-counter medications are likely to affect sleep in the elderly (Table 14-1). Some medications make falling asleep more difficult, whereas others cause frequent awakening (Box 14-2). A few medications can result in hypersomnolent responses.

Behaviors that contribute to sleep problems include physical inactivity, poor sleep routines, late-night eating or exercise, the use of tobacco, and consumption of alcohol or caffeine. Environmental factors such as excessive noise, light, activity, or other distracting stimuli can also contribute to the problem. See Box 14-3 for a list of risk factors for problems related to sleep or rest in the elderly.

Occasional problems with insomnia are experienced by individuals of all ages, but these random, acute episodes are likely to result in chronic insomnia if not properly addressed. Chronic insomnia can result in daytime sleepiness, irritability, decreased ability to concentrate, and other problems related to sleep deprivation. Daytime sleepiness is often ignored or excused as a normal change of aging rather than a symptom of sleep deprivation.

TABLE 14-1

Characteristics of Medications Used to Promote Sleep

Classification	Examples	Precautions
Sedative/hypnotics	Zolpidem tartrate	May cause morning drowsiness, headache, "hangover," dizziness, or paradoxic excitement
Benzodiazepines	Flurazepam; diazepam; triazolam; lorazepam	Likely to cause daytime sedation and short-term memory impairment in the elderly, particularly with long-acting forms; associated with increased risk of falls; paradoxic excitement may occur; must be avoided in individuals with sleep apnea; legislation restricts use in nursing home settings
Antihistamines	Diphenhydramine	May result in agitation, confusion, orthostatic hypotension, urinary retention, and arrhythmias; can make the quality of sleep less restful; not preferred for the elderly
Antidepressants	Amitriptyline; desipramine; nortriptyline; trazodone	Potential side effects include urinary retention, constipation, orthostatic hypotension, and confusion; risk for cardiac arrhythmias, fatigue, headache, blood dyscrasias, altered blood glucose readings, nausea and, photosensitivity
Others	Chloral hydrate	Sedation with "hangover" effects; severe interaction with other sedatives; gastrointestinal toxicity

BOX 14-2

Drugs that Contribute to Sleep Disorders

- Caffeine
- Theophylline
- Alcohol
- Pseudoephedrine
- Corticosteroids
- Thyroxine
- Diuretics
- Neuroleptics
- Antidepressants
- Antihistamines (paradoxic reactions)
- Benzodiazepines (paradoxic reactions)

BOX 14-3

Risk Factors Related to Sleep or Rest Problems in the Elderly

- Pain
- Chronic respiratory or cardiovascular problems
- Frequent elimination
- Nocturnal movement disorders
- Anxiety, depression, or delirium
- Drugs likely to interfere with sleep
- Excessive environmental stimuli
- Excessive caffeine, alcohol, or tobacco use
- Sedentary lifestyle

NURSING PROCESS

SLEEP PATTERN DISTURBANCE

When assessing sleep patterns in the elderly, nurses must use a combination of objective and subjective data. Simply because an elderly individual's eyes are closed during nighttime checks does not mean that he or she is asleep. Nurses should watch closely for signs of fatigue and decreased participation in activities and should ask the elderly how they feel about the adequacy of their sleep and rest.

Assessment of Sleep and Rest

- Does the person feel rested after a night's sleep?
- What time does the person normally go to bed and rise?
- Is the person allowed to choose the time he or she goes to bed, or is it chosen by someone else?
- Does the person sleep continuously through the night or have interrupted sleep?
- Does the caregiver or bed partner report any abnormal breathing pattern, excessive snoring, or unusual movement during sleep?
- What causes the person to awaken? Pain? Noise? Other factors?
- Does the person have difficulty falling asleep?
- Does the person awaken early?
- Does the person nap or sleep during the day?
- Does the person ever fall asleep during activities?
- Has the person's behavior changed? Is he or she increasingly irritable, disoriented, or lethargic?
- Does the person appear to be tired?
- Do you observe any yawning or dark circles under the eyes?
- Does the person complain of feeling tired? When?

Nursing Diagnosis

Sleep pattern disturbance

Nursing Goals/Outcomes

The nursing goals for elderly individuals diagnosed with sleep pattern disturbance are (1) to verbalize an understanding of sleep changes associated with aging, (2) to verbalize appropriate interventions to promote sleep, and (3) to report feeling rested and refreshed on rising.

Nursing Interventions

The following interventions should take place in hospitals and extended-care facilities:

1. **Identify the factors that contribute to sleep dis-**
turbance. Nurses must identify the cause of sleep disturbance so that the most appropriate interventions can be selected. Various internal and external factors can interfere with sleep. Pain, whether it is chronic or acute, will interrupt or prevent sleep. The causes of pain must be identified and measures taken to make the elderly person as comfortable as possible. Medical conditions and the medications taken to treat them can affect sleep. Elderly persons with cardiovascular disease are likely to experience anginal pain during REM sleep that causes them to awaken. Ulcer patients secrete excessive amounts of acid during REM sleep, causing pain and awakening. Individuals with chronic obstructive pulmonary disease may experience dyspnea that is related to lying down during sleep. This may result in oxygen hunger and anxiety and may interfere with sleep. Anxiety and depression often result in early-morning rising and an inability to return to sleep once awakened. Medications for hypertension frequently cause altered sleep patterns. Environmental factors, including lighting, noise, and temperature change, should also be considered.

2. **Schedule nursing interventions to allow for adequate undisturbed sleep.** Nursing and medical interventions can interfere with sleep. Medication administration, dressing changes, or toileting can interrupt sleep. Although nurses do not have total control over the scheduling of medications and treatments, they should attempt to formulate a plan that causes the least interference with sleep. For example, if diuretics are given close to bedtime, urinary frequency may prevent the individual from getting continuous sleep. A schedule change that involves giving the diuretic early in the morning will decrease this problem. If a procedure is not essential for the well-being of an individual, it should not be scheduled during the night. Many treatments and medications are now specifically ordered "while awake" to eliminate any confusion or concern regarding interpretation of the order. The benefits to the patient must be weighed against the risks of sleep deprivation (see the following clinical situation box).

3. **Plan bedtimes and wake-up times to meet the individual's needs and desires rather than the institution's.** Although a regular bedtime schedule is advisable, this time should be chosen with input from the aging person. The fact that an elderly person resides in an institutional setting does not mean that sleep patterns established over a lifetime will change to fit the institution. The institution should allow for individual preferences. Many elderly persons find that they cannot sleep once they have gone to bed. They often lie awake

CLINICAL SITUATION

Mrs. Jones, age 79, had no problems participating in her activities of daily living until she was placed on an every-3-hours, day-and-night toileting schedule to prevent incontinence. After being awakened for five nights, she began to display an inability to dress and feed herself. The staff began to search for symptoms of illness or disease to account for this change but found none. Nursing notes indicated that Mrs. Jones was attending fewer activities, and she was observed napping in her room on several occasions. On the sixth night of toileting, Mrs. Jones remarked, "If you would just let me sleep I'd feel better."

The nurse put these pieces of information together and realized that although the toileting schedule reduced problems with incontinence, it caused other problems related to sleep. After a discussion with Mrs. Jones, her physician, and her family, it was determined that using incontinence briefs during the night would be the lesser of the evils. After three nights of uninterrupted sleep, Mrs. Jones began to dress and feed herself again and to participate in social activities instead of napping.

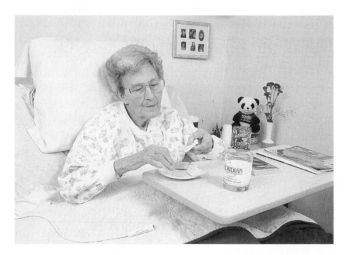

FIG. 14-2   A bedtime snack of milk, cheese, and crackers helps to promote sleep for this elderly woman. (From Sorrentino SA: *Mosby's textbook for nursing assistants*, ed 4, St Louis, 1996, Mosby.)

and become increasingly anxious. This anxiety further interferes with their ability to fall asleep. If the person is unable to sleep after 20 to 30 minutes, he or she should be encouraged to get up and quietly watch television, read, or listen to music. A lounge should be available so that this activity does not disturb the sleep of others. When the individual is tired, he or she should then return to bed. This supports the mental connection that bed is a place for sleep.

4. **Allow the individual to maintain rituals that help induce sleep.** Many elderly persons have rituals that help them sleep. These presleep rituals are highly individual and include hygiene activities, the use of special pillows, praying, and a variety of other activities. Nurses should discuss individual preferences and incorporate these into the plan of care.

5. **Assist in providing an environment that is conducive to sleep.** To prevent awakening roommates, use the minimum amount of light necessary and make as little noise as possible when checking patients or performing required treatments. Establish a schedule for routine rounds so that even if nightly sleep is interrupted, it will be at the same time each night. If possible, place individuals who have sleep difficulties in rooms away from noisy phones, work rooms, and other loud areas. Noise that goes unnoticed during the day, particularly conversation near the nurses' station and unanswered call systems, can disturb sleep at night. Provide lighting that allows for safety but does not interfere with sleep. Curtains and doors should be positioned to avoid undesired light. Some individuals can sleep only if there is a nightlight; others are disturbed by any light. Due to changes in circulation, many elderly individuals need an extra blanket for comfort at night. A warm, light blanket that does not feel "heavy" is preferred by many aging individuals.

6. **Provide comfort measures to promote sleep.** A comfortable environment promotes sleep. The bed should be clean, dry, and free of wrinkles. Top linens should be tightened or loosened to provide the greatest comfort. Sleepwear should be nonrestricting and of the type preferred by the individual. Oral hygiene should be encouraged or provided. The elderly should be encouraged to empty the bladder before going to bed in order to avoid the need to get up once they become sleepy. Nocturia occurs most commonly within a few hours of going to sleep. In addition, if the elderly person is left wet, sleep is disturbed for several hours. Awakening the person and changing wet clothes results in a return to normal sleep.

7. **Administer sleep medications (sedatives and hypnotics) as ordered.** Nurses should assess their patients or residents for desired effects and untoward effects of sleep medications. Because many medications that are used to promote sleep can cause orthostatic hypotension, individuals should be observed for dizziness, position changes should

NURSING CARE PLAN

SLEEP-REST

Mrs. Star, age 83, lives at Larkspur Court Residence Center. Her room is near the nurses' station. She is often observed to be awake during the night. She often does not want to get up for breakfast, stating, "I'm too tired." She yawns frequently during the day and takes frequent naps in her room. She complains, "I can't get comfortable, there is just too much noise around here."

NURSING DIAGNOSIS

Sleep Pattern Disturbance

DEFINING CHARACTERISTICS

- Observed periods of awakening at night
- Frequent yawning and napping
- Complaints of fatigue

GOAL/OUTCOME

Mrs. Star will report feeling adequately rested.

NURSING INTERVENTIONS

1. Identify specific factors that make sleep difficult for Mrs. Star.
2. Ask Mrs. Star if she can identify any changes that would help her sleep.
3. Consider a room change if possible.
4. Close her door to reduce extraneous noise.
5. Discourage daytime napping.
6. Encourage daytime physical activities.
7. Recommend that she avoid caffeine after dinner.
8. Teach relaxation techniques.
9. Provide comfort measures at bedtime.
10. Assess the need for further sleeping aids.

EVALUATION

Mrs. Star now states, "I really like my new room. It's much quieter so I don't have trouble sleeping at night. In fact, I've even started going to more activities now that I'm feeling more rested during the day." She is observed to be sleeping soundly when checked at night. Fewer daytime naps are documented in chart. You will continue the plan of care.

---

be made slowly, and assistance should be provided during ambulation in order to reduce the risk of falls or other injuries.

Medications to promote sleep should be a last resort because many sedative and hypnotic drugs can leave the elderly with lingering or "hangover" effects and can contribute to insomnia. These drugs can actually lead to disturbed sleep because they alter the nature and quality of sleep. Long-acting drugs can be retained in the body for an excessive amount of time, potentially leading to

confusion, disorientation, and daytime sleepiness. Medications that affect respiration should be used with extreme caution in the elderly. Low doses of drugs with short half-lives are best tolerated by the elderly.

8. **Provide nutritional supplements that aid sleep.** A light snack or beverage before bed is commonly requested (Fig. 14-2). Caffeinated beverages such as coffee should be discouraged because caffeine can interfere with sleep. Decaffeinated coffee, herbal tea, and milk are good choices. Milk is often

suggested because it contains tryptophan, which has sleep-inducing properties. Heavy meals put extra stress on the body and should be avoided near bedtime. Alcoholic beverages should also be discouraged because they may interfere with the normal sleep cycles and may lead to awakening due to diuresis.

9. **Promote emotional comfort by spending time listening to concerns.** Anxiety and depression interfere with sleep. A backrub or a few minutes of quiet conversation at bedtime may help relieve the concerns of the day and promote sleep in the elderly. Relaxation training or other stress management techniques may be appropriate for some individuals.

10. **Observe patients for patterns of fatigue or napping throughout the day.** Excessive napping or fatigue during the day can interfere with nighttime sleep. Nurses should assess for daytime behaviors that affect sleep. If individuals spend too much time napping, nurses should determine the reason. If boredom is the cause, diversional activities should be increased. If the individual is too fatigued or stimulated by the day's activities, then more frequent rest periods should be encouraged.

The following interventions should take place in the home:

1. **Use a journal to assess sleep and rest patterns.** Many elderly individuals who complain of sleep problems are unaware of their daily routines. Keeping a journal to record naps, bedtimes, periods of awakening, and time of rising in the morning often yields important information. If the individual cannot do this alone, a spouse or relative may assist. Any information that may be relevant (e.g., pain, nocturia) should be noted.

2. **Explain the importance of adequate activity and exercise throughout the day.** Adequate exercise and activity help promote good sleep. Excessive activity should be avoided within 2 hours of bedtime because such activity may raise body temperature and actually interfere with sleep.

3. **Assist the elderly in establishing an environment that promotes rest and sleep.** Nurses should verify that the conditions in the home promote rest and sleep. Verify that the elderly individual has an adequate bed and suitable covers. Make sure heating is adequate. If noise from neighbors or traffic is a problem, possible ways of dealing with this should be discussed.

4. **Discuss limiting fluid intake at night if nocturia is a problem.** If nocturia is interrupting sleep, the elderly should be encouraged to decrease fluid intake for 1 to 2 hours preceding bedtime. It is important that adequate fluid be consumed earlier in the day, however, to prevent fluid balance problems.

5. **Encourage the use of relaxation exercises, creative visualization, self-hypnosis, or other relaxation techniques.** Many techniques that promote relaxation can be used to help induce sleep. Numerous audiotapes and books are available to describe these techniques, many of which could benefit the elderly and are unlikely to cause the problems that are caused by medications.

6. **Use any appropriate interventions that are used in the institutional setting.**

A nursing care plan for sleep pattern disturbance is presented on p. 241.

SUMMARY

Changes related to sleep are a major concern for many elderly persons. Because sleep problems can result from normal age-related changes or other problems, concerns about sleep should not be taken lightly. A thorough assessment of sleep behaviors and appropriate interventions will help the elderly achieve the rest and sleep they require to function at the highest possible level.

READINGS AND REFERENCES

Becker PM, Jamieson AO, Brown WD: Insomnia. Use of a decision tree to assess and treat, *Postgrad Med* 93:66, 1993.

Brown University New Bureau Web site: *Hospital noise disrupts sleep for patients in the critical care setting*, www.brown.edu/Administration/News_Bureau/1996-97/96-063.html, 1997.

Gillin JC, Byerley WF: Drug therapy: the diagnosis and management of insomnia, *N Engl J Med* 322:239, 1990.

Hauri PJ, Esther MS: Insomnia, *Mayo Clin Proc* 65:869, 1990.

Knott L Web site: *Insomnia: a serious problem in the elderly*, www.docnet.org.uk/germed/apr96/insomnia.html, 1996.

Mayo Foundation for Medical Education and Research Web site: *Sleep disorders in the elderly*, www.mayo.edu/geriatrics-rst/Sleep.html, 1997.

National Institute on Aging Age Page Web site: *A good night's sleep*, www:mhsource.com/hy/age-sleep.html, 1990.

US Department of Health and Human Services: The dangers of sleeping pills, *Aging* 336:7, 1994.

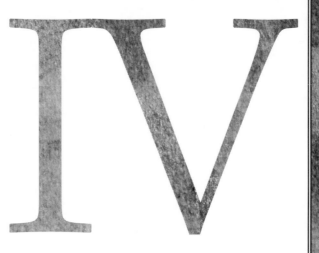

IV

PSYCHOSOCIAL CARE OF THE ELDERLY

chapter fifteen
15

COGNITION AND PERCEPTION

1. Describe normal sensory and cognitive functions.
2. Describe how sensory perception and cognition change with aging.
3. Discuss the effects of disease processes on perception and cognition.
4. Describe methods of assessing changes in perception and cognition.
5. Identify the elderly who are most at risk for experiencing perceptual or cognitive problems.
6. Identify selected nursing diagnoses related to cognitive and perceptual problems.
7. Describe nursing interventions that are appropriate for elderly individuals experiencing problems related to perception or cognition.
8. Discuss pain assessment and management as they relate to elderly individuals.

The cognitive-perceptual health pattern deals with the ways people gain information from the environment and the way they interpret and use this information. **Perception** includes the collection, interpretation, and recognition of stimuli, including pain. **Cognition** includes intelligence, memory, language, and decision making. Cognition and perception are intimately connected to the functioning of the central nervous system and the special senses of vision, hearing, touch, smell, and taste.

NORMAL COGNITIVE-PERCEPTUAL FUNCTIONING

The environment excites or stimulates the senses. The senses in turn pass these stimuli into the cerebral cortex where recognition (perception) and interpretation (cognition) occur. Specific regions of the cerebral cortex are responsible for detecting and processing the stimuli acquired by the various senses. Malfunction of the sensory organs or of the interpretation centers in the brain results in altered perception and cognition.

If the senses do not function appropriately, stimuli do not enter the brain and there is not enough information for accurate interpretation. Individuals with sensory deficits in one area may attempt to compensate for these deficits by gathering more information from those senses that function normally. People with hearing deficits often lipread or otherwise rely on visual cues. People with visual deficits rely more heavily on the senses of hearing and touch. People with multiple sensory deficits have great difficulty collecting information and often experience serious cognitive and perceptual problems. Adult hearing impairment has been associated with social isolation and depression. People with sensory deficits have a normal ability to think and learn, but for them the process is more difficult. The story of Helen Keller's life illustrates the difficulties experienced by a sensorially deprived person.

As discussed in Chapter 3, numerous sensory changes occur with aging. Common visual changes include farsightedness due to changes in the shape of the lens of the eye (presbyopia); decreased ability to respond to changes in light resulting in night blindness; and cataracts, which cloud the lens and result in blurred vision and sensitivity to glare (Fig. 15-1). Common auditory changes include loss of hearing acuity, particularly of higher-pitched sounds (presbycusis); loss of hearing due to decreased sound transmission (otosclerosis); and ringing in the ears (tinnitus), which can be caused by to Ménière's disease, age-related changes, or medications. Older adults are increasingly susceptible to misperception and therefore misinterpretation when one or more of these changes are present.

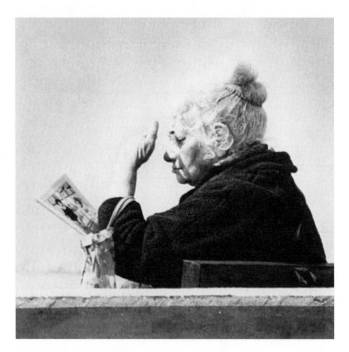

Fig. 15-1   Glare. (From Ebersole P, Hess P: *Toward healthy aging: human needs and nursing response*, ed 5, St Louis, 1998, Mosby.)

Cognition, or thought, takes place in the cerebral cortex of the brain. Cognitive development starts at the time of birth and perhaps even earlier. When the human brain is repeatedly exposed to stimuli, connections develop between nerve fibers of the cerebral cortex. Each time stimuli are introduced to the brain, they are associated (at an unconscious level) with the pool of facts, memories, and experiences that are stored there. Once these connections are firmly established, information is said to be "learned." Once learning has taken place, information or skills can be retrieved as needed. Memory enables people to retain and recall previously experienced sensations, ideas, concepts, impressions, and all information that has been previously learned. The human mind is extraordinary in its ability to learn and process extensive amounts of information. It is able to retrieve information on demand, correlate random pieces of information, make judgments, solve problems, and create ideas.

Cognition and Intelligence

People have different levels of cognitive ability. People often speak of intelligence quotients (IQs) when they try to describe cognitive ability. The IQ can be deceptive because there are different types of intelligence, and the standardized testing procedures do not measure all types of intelligence.

Fluid intelligence is the ability to perform tasks or make judgments based on unfamiliar stimuli. This is sometimes called the ability to "think on your feet." **Crystallized intelligence** (often called "wisdom") is the ability to perform tasks and make judgments based on the knowledge and experience acquired through a lifetime. Because young people have less knowledge and experience, they must rely more on fluid intelligence. With advanced age come an abundance of skills and knowledge that has been acquired over time, and crystallized intelligence is used more often.

Intelligence is often measured by means of tests. Although intelligence tests are commonly used, they have distinct limitations. Most written tests measure verbal and mathematic ability. A person who has had little formal education can have a high level of cognition and yet score poorly on standardized intelligence tests. Cognition is not the same as education. Cognition is the ability to think and reason. Many people have good cognitive skills but poor education.

Intelligence tests are normally timed. Because not all individuals process information at the same speed, two individuals with a similar pool of knowledge and skills may be judged very differently, simply because they respond at different speeds. Those with a rapid rate of information processing are typically judged to be more intelligent than those who take longer to process information, even if the end result is the same. This is probably reflective of our culture, which values speed.

Cognition and Language

Language is a product of cognitive function. In both spoken and written forms, language allows humans to communicate ideas and thoughts. Language develops early in life. By 2 years of age the average child has a vocabulary of several hundred words. Very specific areas of the brain are dedicated to language and change significantly as language skills improve.

Sensory and cognitive problems can result in poor language development or loss of language skills. Damage to the language centers of the brain can result in **aphasia,** a condition in which people are unable to understand or express themselves through language.

PERCEPTION-COGNITION AND AGING

Aging persons frequently experience sensory changes that interfere with the collection of information. Visual and hearing changes, changes in taste and smell, and changes in touch and sensation all interfere with the ability to collect accurate information from the environment (Fig. 15-2).

Many elderly people who are considered confused

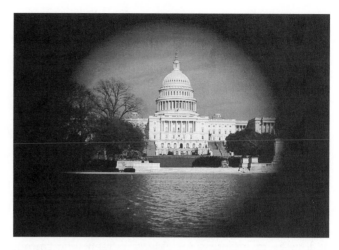

FIG. 15-2 *One type of altered vision that is common in the elderly: restricted peripheral visual field. (From Sorrentino SA: Mosby's textbook for nursing assistants, ed 4, St Louis, 1996, Mosby.)*

BOX 15-1

Possible Indicators of Hearing Loss

- Difficulty understanding women or children
- Trouble following a conversation if more than one person is talking
- Difficulty hearing over the phone
- Difficulty hearing because of background noise
- Complaints that other people are mumbling
- Increased volume of radio or television, particularly if those with normal hearing complain about the loud volume
- Straining to hear conversation at a normal volume

---

actually suffer from altered sensory perceptions. An elderly person who does not hear well (Box 15-1) or see well may walk into traffic or make mistakes about directions; these mistakes are not made because the individual is confused but rather because he or she does not have enough sensory information to make an appropriate decision. Multiple competing stimuli can also cause problems if the elderly are unable to focus on the important stimuli and disregard nonessential stimuli.

Intelligence does not automatically decrease with aging, nor does the ability to learn. Some people seem less intelligent as they age because of their tendency to be slower and more cautious in their responses. Rather than be embarrassed, they often take more time to be certain of the answer before they respond. This hesitancy or uncertainty may be mistaken for a lack of intelligence, which it is not.

Lack of formal schooling may make the elderly appear less intelligent. They may lack polish in their speech and have a more limited vocabulary than better-educated people. Many elderly who grew up in hard times ended their formal educations at a young age because they had to work to help support the family. When today's elderly entered the workforce, advanced education was not needed to earn a decent living. Many continued to read and learn and often exceeded what school would have provided. Often these elderly are intimidated by young, well-educated caregivers.

The speed at which information is processed and recalled changes with age. It is common for the elderly to take longer to recall a specific piece of information. Short-term memory is more likely to be affected than is long-term memory. An elderly person who cannot remember what he or she had for breakfast may very well be able to describe an event in great detail that occurred 50 years ago.

Some degree of forgetfulness or memory loss is common with aging. This problem can be very disturbing to the alert aging person. Many begin to fear that they are "losing their minds" or developing a serious problem. Careful assessment is needed to distinguish mild memory loss from an early indication of a more serious cognitive disorder.

There is no known reason why memory loss happens, but studies have shown that by 75 years of age even an alert elderly person may lose as much as 30% of memory. The more memories a person has developed throughout life, the more he or she will retain, so well-educated elderly tend to retain a higher level of function than less well-educated elderly. Even without formal education, many elderly persons are able to compensate for memory gaps by relying more on the large pool of experience gathered over a lifetime.

Healthy elderly people are able to learn new information no matter what their age. While the ability to acquire new information appears to decrease with age, it may be more a matter of a lack of desire to learn than the inability to acquire and retain the information. If a healthy elderly person wants to learn something, he or she is usually capable of doing so. Once information is learned, the alert elderly person can recall it as well as a younger person.

NURSING PROCESS
SENSORY-PERCEPTUAL ALTERATIONS

An elderly person can experience alterations in one or more of the senses. The extent of these alterations can range from very small changes to total loss of sensory function. The more serious the alteration, the greater the risks will be. Different nursing approaches are necessary for different types of sensory alteration.

Assessment of Sensory Changes

- Has the person mentioned any changes in the taste or smell of food?
- Can the person detect whether something is cold or warm?
- Can the person feel whether something is smooth or rough?
- Does the person have known vision problems (e.g., glaucoma, macular degeneration, cataracts, refractive errors)?
- Does the person see small details or shadows?
- Does the person frequently walk into or trip over objects?
- Can the person read? If not, why not? If yes, can he or she read newsprint or only large-print headlines?
- How close to the television does the person sit?
- Does the person wear eyeglasses? Single lens, bifocal, or trifocal?
- When was the person's vision last checked?
- Does the person respond when people speak to him or her at normal volumes?
- Can the person hear a whisper from someone behind or to the side of him or her who cannot be seen?
- Does the person turn the volume of the television or radio to a very loud level?
- Does the person turn his or her head to hear?
- Does the person wear a hearing aid?
- Does the person respond appropriately or inappropriately to questions?
- Can the person follow directions?

See Box 15-2 for a list of risk factors for problems related to cognition and perception in the elderly.

BOX 15-2
Risk Factors Related to Cognition and Perception in the Elderly

- Vision problems (total blindness, presbyopia, macular degeneration, cataracts, hemianopsia, detached retina, diabetes, glaucoma, significant refractive errors)
- Hearing problems (presbycusis, otosclerosis, conductive sensorineural deafness)
- Dementia (including Alzheimer's disease)
- Altered cerebral circulation (stroke, aneurysm, head injury)
- Drugs that affect the sensorium (alcohol, narcotic analgesics, tranquilizers, sedatives, hypnotics)
- Altered neurologic function resulting in decreased levels of consciousness
- Altered metabolic states (hypoglycemia, metabolic alkalosis)
- Environments with either inadequate or excessive sensory stimulation

Nursing Diagnoses

Sensory/perceptual alterations: visual, auditory, kinesthetic, gustatory, tactile, olfactory.

Nursing Goals/Outcomes

The nursing goals for elderly individuals with sensory-perceptual alterations are (1) to demonstrate improved ability to detect changes in the environment, (2) to interact appropriately with the environment, and (3) to demonstrate the ability to compensate for deficits by using prosthetic devices and alternative senses.

Nursing Interventions

The following nursing interventions should take place in hospitals or extended-care facilities:

1. **Ensure that all caregivers are aware of the person's sensory problems.** The Kardex should identify any vision or hearing problems and should be displayed in a prominent place on the patient's records. Nursing assistants and ancillary personnel should be made aware of sensory problems and appropriate methods of communication before attempting to provide care for an elderly individual with sensory deficits.

2. **Make appropriate sensory contact before beginning care.** If the aging person is hard of hearing, avoid startling him or her. Approach so that he or she can see you, or touch the individual gently on the hand before making more personal contact. If the person is visually impaired, speak up and introduce yourself when you enter the room. This lets the person know who is there, even if he or she cannot see a face clearly.

3. **Determine the best methods for communicating with the elderly.** Be patient and relaxed when working with the elderly (Fig. 15-3). When working with sensorially altered elderly persons, it is best to keep messages as simple as possible, use easily understood words, and speak clearly. It may be necessary to reword a statement if the first attempt is not understood. When explaining care or treatments, be careful to avoid information overload. When writing messages, ensure that the writing is clear and large enough to be seen easily.

   When dealing with hearing-impaired elderly, it is helpful to speak in a low tone of voice because hearing losses are usually in the higher frequencies of sound. Because many hearing-impaired people compensate by lipreading, it is best to stand in good light while facing the person and to speak slowly but not unnaturally so. Do not chew gum or eat while conversing. If one ear is better than the other, talking into the good ear may help. Background noise from television or radio should be kept to a minimum because it may distract the elderly or interfere with verbal communication.

   Use facial expressions, gestures, and other visual cues that are appropriate to the message. These cues can help the person understand what you are talking about. For example, when you want someone to follow you, hold out your hand and begin to walk. If it is time to groom the hair, show the person the brush and comb to help make the message clear.

   Persons with hearing impairments are not likely to understand messages spoken through the call signal speakers that are used in most care settings. In most facilities, even people with good hearing have problems with these devices. Caregivers should respond promptly and in person to calls from the sensorially impaired. More information regarding communication with the elderly is provided in Chapter 5.

4. **Modify the environment to reduce risks.** Lighting is important for the elderly. Because it takes the eye longer to adjust to bright light as we age, stairs and other hazardous areas should be designed to prevent glare. When an elderly person has a condition in which a portion of the visual field is lost (hemianopsia), the furniture should be arranged to maximize the person's ability to see (Fig. 15-4). Personal belongings should be placed toward the good side, and the person should be taught to turn his or her head and "sweep" the environment to pick up more visual cues.

5. **Verify that prostheses such as eyeglasses and hearing aids are functional.** Obtaining the proper corrective lenses is not a one-time requirement. As the eyes continue to change, a prescription that was once adequate may lose its effectiveness. Simply because a person wears eyeglasses does not mean that he or she can see clearly, particularly if he or

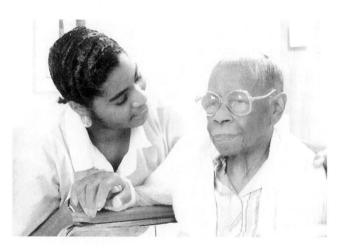

FIG. 15-3 Nurses can use touch to calm a person with Alzheimer's disease. (From Sorrentino SA: *Mosby's textbook for nursing assistants*, ed 4, St Louis, 1996, Mosby.)

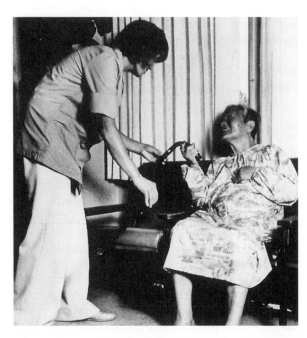

FIG. 15-4 Nurses should approach patients who have a left-sided hemiparesis from the right side. This elderly woman may not be able to see people to her left. (Courtesy of Ken Yamaguchi. In Castillo HM: *The nurse assistant in long-term care: a rehabilitative approach*, St Louis, 1992, Mosby.)

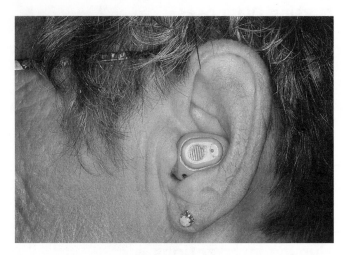

FIG. 15-5 A hearing aid inserted in the ear canal is barely visible. (From Elkin MK, Perry AG, Potter PA: *Nursing interventions and clinical skills*, St Louis, 1996, Mosby.)

she has had the eyeglasses for some time. Eye examinations should be performed regularly and prescriptions changed whenever required. Many aging individuals suffer from multiple refractive errors and require bifocals or trifocals to achieve adequate focus. Bifocals and trifocals can present problems because the wearers must move their heads to shift the line of vision to the proper section depending on what they wish to view. Some people find this so disturbing that they choose not to wear the correct prescription. Problems like these should be reported to the physician so that an acceptable solution can be found.

Eyeglasses must be cleaned before they are worn. Fingerprints and other debris can distort vision and make the glasses useless. To be of benefit, eyeglasses must also fit the person properly. Many glasses are too loose and slide down the nose; others are too snug and create uncomfortable pressure areas on the nose or ears. Often the elderly wear glasses with broken frames that are taped together. If the glasses do not help vision or are uncomfortable, the elderly are likely to avoid wearing them. Nurses should arrange a consultation with an eye specialist to get such problems corrected.

Hearing aids are worn by many elderly persons. These devices do not duplicate normal hearing and are not beneficial for everyone. Hearing aids can be built into eyeglasses or inserted into the ear canal.

Some of the older units hang over the external ear; newer models are almost invisible when worn (Fig. 15-5).

Many persons have difficulty adjusting to hearing aids and complain that they are bothersome. When first fitted with a hearing aid, the person may only be able to tolerate it for a few minutes a day. As they adjust to the device, the amount of time it is worn should be gradually increased. Elderly persons who are adjusting to wearing hearing aids often report that they make them nervous or jumpy to hear so many sounds. The elderly should be reassured that this is normal and that the jumpiness will go away as they become used to wearing the hearing aid. Many people who wear hearing aids report that the sounds they hear are "tinny" or "noisy," and that they hear feedback whistles or hums. These noises are usually caused by incorrect insertion or improper adjustment of the controls on the device.

Hearing aids require a certain amount of care and maintenance. Because they are fragile, care should be taken not to drop them. Most are made of plastic and should be kept away from very hot or very cold places. Before being inserted into the ear, hearing aids should be checked for cracks or rough edges that could injure the ear. The ear mold should be cleaned regularly. Special attention should be paid to the removal of cerumen, which may plug the canal and reduce the effectiveness of the device. Batteries should be checked and changed regularly because the hearing aid will not work properly without a good power source. To save the batteries, the hearing aid should be shut off when it is not in use. Batteries should be checked for corrosion and contacts should be cleaned, particularly if the device becomes wet. Storing unused batteries in the refrigerator can prolong their life. Old batteries should be discarded after a change so that they are not mistakenly saved and reused. This mistake can lead to confusion and frustration.

Caregivers who are not familiar with hearing aids should receive special training in how to place them in the ear canal properly. Hearing aids are useless unless they are worn properly. Nurses should always verify that a hearing aid has been applied to the correct ear. If the person wears two aids, they should be marked so that the correct device is placed in the correct ear. If the device still does not function properly, nurses may need to consult with an audiologist or speech therapist. If the elderly person is reluctant to wear the hearing aid, the nurse should do a thorough assessment to determine why he or she is refusing. A thorough re-evaluation of hearing may be necessary.

The following interventions should take place in the home:

1. **Modify the home environment to compensate for sensory changes.** Modifications in the home will help the elderly cope with sensory changes. Increasing the amount of light is the least expensive and most beneficial change. Lights should be positioned so that glare is avoided. Incandescent bulbs are better than fluorescent bulbs because they do not have a distracting flicker. Burned-out bulbs should be replaced promptly. It is even better if light bulbs are replaced when they begin to dim rather than waiting until they burn out.

Use of contrasting colors will help the elderly determine edges and borders. Contrasting strips should be applied to changes in elevation such as shower lips and steps. Contrasting door frames, dishes, pillows, personal care items, and toilet seats, will help the elderly distinguish these items more easily.

2. **Assist the sensorially impaired to develop techniques or acquire devices that will help compensate for losses.**

Hearing-impaired persons. Nurses should explain ways that hearing-impaired persons can improve communications. These include (1) telling others that they are hard of hearing, (2) focusing on the speaker and paying attention to what is being said, (3) facing the speaker or asking the speaker to face them, (4) asking the speaker to speak slowly and clearly but not to shout, and (5) asking the speaker to repeat when information is not clear.

Many special devices are available for hearing-impaired persons. Local telephone companies can provide special equipment such as amplifiers or video display terminals that will enable the elderly to maintain contact with others. Doorbells and mats that flash a light when someone is at the door are available. Alarm clocks that vibrate rather than ring can be purchased from specialty or department stores. Hearing-impaired individuals with adequate vision should be made aware of closed-caption television broadcasts, which provide a typed narration of news and many entertainment programs.

Visually impaired persons. Telephone dials can be modified with overlay rings that have large numbers to assist in dialing. Some newer telephones can be programmed with commonly used numbers so that the person needs to push only one button to dial. Handheld or floor-standing magnifying devices will help with reading or close work. Large-print books and magazines are available in most public libraries. Written materials can also be enlarged on photocopy machines to make reading easier. Books on audiotape are also available in stores and many libraries. Talking clocks that fit in a pocket are available.

3. **Use any appropriate interventions that are used in the institutional setting.**

NURSING PROCESS
ALTERED THOUGHT PROCESSES

Anything that damages or interferes with the normal functioning of the cerebral cortex can result in cognitive (i.e., thinking and judgment) problems. All changes in cognitive function must be given immediate attention. Prompt assessment of the type and severity of the disorder along with identification of the cause or causes will enable the caregiver to plan the most appropriate interventions for each individual. Cognitive function can be affected by sensory changes, physiologic factors, or emotional disorders. Cognitive problems can range from mild and reversible forms of disorientation to severe and irreversible forms of dementia (Table 15-1).

Sensory changes can result in behaviors that mimic cognitive problems but actually are not. The two should not be confused. Sensory misperception should be ruled out before further cognitive assessment is performed (see the following clinical situation box).

The term **confusion** is used to describe a wide range of behaviors. Both lay people and professionals use this term far too frequently—often incorrectly and inappropriately.

Confusion is defined as a mental state characterized by disorientation regarding time, place, or person that leads to bewilderment, perplexity, lack of orderly thought, and the inability to choose or act decisively

TABLE 15-1

Dementia: Types and Causes

Acute reversible dementia	Chronic irreversible dementia
Hypoxia	Alzheimer's disease
—Hypotension	Anoxia
—Anemias	Untreated acute dementia
—Ventilatory problems	Pick's disease
—Heart failure	Creutzfeldt-Jakob disease
Environmental changes	Alcoholism
	Untreated abnormal blood
Fluid and electrolyte imbalance	pressure
Metabolic disturbances	Hydrocephalus
—Acidosis	Heavy metal toxicity
—Hypoglycemia	Multiple cerebral infarction
—Hyperglycemia	
—Elevated blood urea nitrogen	
Drug toxicity	
Malnutrition	
Transient ischemic attacks	
Decreased sensory input	
Sensory overload	
Hypothyroidism	
Brain tumor	
Infection	
Subarachnoid hemorrhage	
Subdural hematoma	

From Wolanin MO: *Geriatr Nurs* 4:227, 1983.

and to perform activities of daily living. Confusion is categorized in different ways by different authorities, but one common system identifies three major forms: acute confusion, idiopathic confusion, and dementia.

Acute confusion, often called **delirium,** is characterized by disturbances in cognition, attention, memory, and perception. This type of confusion is usually caused by a physiologic process that affects the autonomic nervous system. Conditions that can cause delirium include uncontrolled pain, infection, metabolic disturbances, vitamin deficiencies, uremia, hypoxia, hypercalcemia, endocrine imbalance, myocardial infarction, constipation, drug toxicity, and drug withdrawal. Acute delirium has a sudden onset of hours or days. It is characterized by rapid mood swings, disorganized sleep cycles, changes in psychomotor activity (hypoactivity, hyperactivity, or both), tremors or spasmodic activity, rapid speech patterns, loss of attention, and a wide range of cognitive changes (Tables 15-2 and 15-3). Elderly individuals with underlying emotional instability can exhibit a full-blown psychotic episode with delusions and auditory or visual hallucinations. The severity of symptoms may vary throughout the day, and symptoms are often worse at night. Because the cause of dementia is usually physiologic, acute confusion does not respond well to behavioral approaches such as reorientation. Once the cause is identified and treated the symptoms generally disappear. Failure to identify and correct underlying physiologic problems can result in serious physical harm or even death.

Idiopathic confusion does not have an identifiable physiologic basis. It is most likely to occur when there is a stressful disturbance in lifestyle or life patterns such as occurs with the death of a loved one, depression, or relocation to a hospital or new living quarters. The onset of symptoms is likely to correlate to specific occurrences or situations, although this is not always the case. Idiopathic confusion tends to affect memory and the ability to concentrate. Affected elderly are often depressed. Common symptoms of idiopathic confusion include appetite changes, loss of interest in activities, changes in sleep patterns, agitation, feelings of worthlessness or guilt, fatigue, or other physiologic complaints. The ability to perform routine activities of daily living is not usually affected, but the willingness to perform these activities may be. Individuals experiencing this form of confusion usually respond well to reorientation interventions and to approaches that reduce stress levels. Symptoms may be reversible but may not disappear completely.

Dementia is a slow, insidious process that results in

TABLE 15-2

Differences Between Delirium and Dementia

Delirium	Dementia
• Rapid onset measured in hours or days • Reduced level of consciousness • Increased or decreased psychomotor activity • Altered sleep–wake patterns • Disorientation and perceptual disturbances • Memory impairment • Decreased attention span with disorganized thinking • Generally reversible if underlying problem is identified and treated; may recur with acute illness	• Usually a slow, insidious onset of symptoms over months or years • Initially no change in level of consciousness • Impaired memory with loss of abstract thinking, judgement, language skills (aphasia), motor skills (apraxia), and ability to recognize familiar people or objects (agnosia) • Generally not reversible

TABLE 15-3

Nursing Interventions for Delirium and Dementia

Delirium	Dementia
• Designed to treat underlying pathology and maintain physiologic integrity • Includes administration of fluids, nutrition, oxygen, antianxiety medications, etc. • Designed to control environmental stressors, to protect safety, and to promote comfort • Designed to control environmental stressors, to protect safety, and to promote comfort	• Designed to maintain or maximize level of function • Includes environment modification, activity-based therapies, communication strategies, etc.

progressive loss of cognitive function. Dementia is caused by damage to the cerebral cortex that is most commonly a result of disease conditions (e.g., Alzheimer's disease; see Box 15-3), multiple infarcts of the cerebrum secondary to stroke, or other brain pathology. Drug intoxication, Huntington's disease, Creutzfeldt-Jakob disease, Pick's disease, cerebral hypoxia, hyperthyroidism, subdural hematoma, and brain tumors are less common causes. Dementia is characterized by changes in memory, judgment, language, mathematic calculation, abstract reasoning, problem-solving ability, impulsive behavior, stupor, confusion, and disorientation. Changes related to dementia are progressive and believed to be irreversible. In the early stages, many cases of dementia are mistakenly considered a part of normal aging, which can result in delayed diagnosis and treatment. The stages of dementia are listed in Box 15-4. Many elderly who suffer from the early stages of dementia are able to recognize that something is wrong yet they do not know what it is. They may be rather creative in the types of excuses used to explain their problems. In the later stages, however, impaired cognitive function is dramatic and obvious to even a casual observer.

Common behaviors seen with advanced dementia include wandering, excessively emotional reactions **(catastrophic reactions),** combative behaviors, suspiciousness, and hallucinations or delusions. These agitated behaviors, which are often worse late in the day, are referred to as the **sundown syndrome** or **sundowning.** Affected persons often do not recognize even their closest family members and friends. These abnormal behaviors are frightening to the family and anyone who cares about the affected individual.

People suffering from dementia are at increased risk of injury and personal neglect. They are unable to recognize or understand hazards in the environment. Self-care deficits in eating, bathing, grooming, and toileting are common.

In the early stages of dementia, the family may be

BOX 15-3

Facts About Alzheimer's Disease

- Alzheimer's disease is not a normal part of aging. It is a progressive, degenerative, irreversible form of dementia.
- The disease was first identified in 1906 by Alois Alzheimer, a German neurologist.
- Most cases of Alzheimer's disease occur in people over 65 years of age, but it can occur at as early as 30 years of age.
- The incidence of the disease doubles approximately every 5 years from age 65 to 85.
- Alzheimer's disease affects both men and women of all religions, races, and socioeconomic backgrounds.
- The cause of the disease remains unknown, but genetic, chemical, viral, and environmental factors are suspected. Family history and the presence of the apolipoprotein E gene appear to indicate an increased risk for development of the disease.
- Alzheimer's disease causes gradual changes such as plaques and tangles in the nerve cells of the brain that can be detected on autopsy.
- Neurologic changes result in a loss of the ability to process information normally.

- The first signs of Alzheimer's disease are subtle changes in behavior. The disease affects each individual differently: The type and severity of symptoms as well as the order of their appearance will differ from person to person.
- People suffering from Alzheimer's disease lose the ability to think, remember, understand, and make decisions. Consequently, they are often unable to perform even the most basic activities of daily living. The ability to control basic body functions such as elimination is also lost.
- People with Alzheimer's disease suffer personality changes. They lose the ability to control moods and emotions, leading to unpredictable and often inappropriate behavior. Unusual behaviors include wandering, pacing, hiding things, swearing, disturbed sleep patterns, and repetitive actions.
- There is no known cure for Alzheimer's disease. A variety of medications are being tested for use with this disease, with varying degrees of success.

able to provide adequate care at home. With advanced stages, full-time supervision and total physical care are often required. Dementia is likely to result in institutional placement.

Dementia affects up to 10% of adults over 65 years of age who live in the community. Estimates of the incidence in those 85 years or older are as high as 50%. About half of the institutionalized elderly suffer from some form of dementia.

Assessment of Cognitive Changes

- Does the person mention any changes in memory?
- Does the person's family or significant others notice memory changes?
- Does the person have difficulty remembering recent or remote events?
- Can the person grasp new ideas, or does he or she have difficulty with this?
- Can the person make appropriate, informed decisions?
- Does the person find it difficult to learn new things?
- What helps the person learn new things?
- What is the person's dominant language?
- Does the person speak other languages?

BOX 15-4

Stages of Dementia

STAGE 1
 Forgetfulness
 Decreased judgment
 Loss of spontaneous emotional response
 Decreased ambition
 Decreased mental abilities, including verbal and mathematic skills

STAGE 2
 Increased level of forgetfulness
 Significantly impaired judgment
 Irritable behavior
 Agitation
 Confusion as to person, place, and time
 Episodes of incontinence

STAGE 3
 Inability to communicate
 Loss of contact with environment
 Total physical dependency
 Total incontinence

- What is the person's language/vocabulary level?
- What is the person's education level?
- How long is the person's attention span?
- Are there significant behavior changes, including hyperactivity (agitation, excitability, distractibility) or hypoactivity (lethargy, apathy, somnolence)?
- Is the person restless, uncooperative, belligerent, angry, withdrawn, or threatening?
- Has the person experienced any delusions or hallucinations?
- Are there particular times of day when behavior is most noticeably different
- Does the person have a history of stroke or other brain disease?
- Have there been any recent changes in medication or dosage?
- Are there any signs of infection (urinary tract infection, pneumonia)?
- What is the level of hydration?
- Is the person constipated?
- What is the person's oxygen saturation?
- What are the results of the Folstein Mini Mental State Examination (MMSE)? (See Chapter 8 for more details about this tool.)

See Box 15-2 for a list of risk factors for problems related to cognition and perception in the elderly.

Nursing Diagnosis

Altered thought processes

Nursing Goals/Outcomes

The nursing goals for elderly individuals with altered thought processes are to (1) remain free from injury, (2) assist in activities of daily living to the highest level possible, and (3) seek assistance when needed.

Nursing Interventions

The following nursing interventions should take place in hospitals or extended-care facilities:

1. **Assess behavior on admission and at regular intervals.** Correct identification of the type of cognitive loss is important so appropriate medical and nursing interventions can be planned and implemented. When a sudden change in behavior is observed in a person who has had normal cognition, a physiologic problem is usually suspected, diagnosed, and treated. For persons who already have a history of cognitive changes, however, it is more difficult to identify these changes. Progression from mild confusion to dementia is common but can be missed unless caregivers pay close attention to subtle changes in behavior.

2. **Provide assistive sensory devices.** Confusion is worse when there is inadequate or inaccurate sensory input. Make sure that eyeglasses, hearing aids, dentures, and uses other adaptive devices designed to maximize sensory perception are being worn when necessary.

3. **Orient the person to person, place, and time, and provide any other important situational information.** Call the person by the name they respond to best. Most often this is the first name, such as Mary, Jim, or Alice. Refer to calendars or clocks to orient to time of day, week, and month. Use calendars to show when key events such as birthdays, holidays, and special activities will occur. Remind the person where he or she is and describe daily events and procedures before they happen. If the person becomes combative, do not argue with him or her. Instead, focus on the feelings that the person exhibits by using reflective statements such as "I know that this isn't what you want to do right now, but it's dinnertime and the food is here."

4. **Provide a structured environment that ensures safety yet enables the person to keep active as long as possible.** Make sure the environment is free from hazards that could lead to falls. Individuals who get up frequently might benefit from wearing shoes even when in bed so they have better balance and footing when they get up.

   Some people suffering from dementia become less active; others demonstrate pacing or other repetitive movements. In order to maintain strength and joint mobility, inactive persons should be encouraged to perform some physical activity that they like each day. Specific activities should be identified and time should be structured into the care plan. Activity, occupational, and physical therapists can help develop a plan to meet individual needs (Box 15-5).

   Person who pace should be allowed to do so without restraint. Pacers should be encouraged to take rest periods during the day so that they do not exhaust themselves.

   Wanderers may need to be housed on a care unit with controlled exits that set off alarms when anyone passes through the door. Wandering can also be monitored by use of an electronic bracelet that sounds an alarm when the wearer tries to leave the unit or building. In home or hospital settings where these controls are not practical, bed or chair alarms (weight-sensitive pads that set off alarms when the person is off the pad) can be used to let nurses know that the person has gotten out of his or her bed or chair. Adequate lighting is important to reduce the likelihood of falls and to reduce fear induced by misperception of shadows.

5. **Provide continuity.** Too many new faces or

BOX 15-5

General Approaches for Dealing with Confused Elderly

- Provide a calm, safe, and structured environment with a controlled amount of stimuli.
- Use a calm, gentle, one-on-one approach.
- Speak normally and informally as though the person is not confused.
- Allow plenty of time; avoid hurrying.
- Determine the confused person's reality; avoid confrontation or forced reorientation to objective fact.
- Encourage reminiscence using family pictures, common activities, or objects.
- Provide familiar clothing and personal items from home.
- Redirect attention or use some other form of distraction to reduce anxiety due to disturbing thoughts.
- Provide safe, repetitive activities within individual capabilities (e.g., winding yarn, folding towels).
- Provide continuity of care with a limited group of caregivers.
- Develop and maintain daily routines for care and activities.
- Avoid sudden changes in routine, room, or caregivers.

---

changes are frightening and disturbing to the confused elderly. Whenever possible, care should be provided by a consistent group of caregivers who are able to develop a trust relation. The person should have access to familiar personal belongings such as pictures or a blanket or purse. These can provide comfort and help the person keep some contact with reality.

6. **Avoid use of physical and chemical restraints.** Keeping confused persons restrained in beds or chairs tends to increase their level of confusion. The use of physical and chemical restraints can be harmful and can actually make the behavior worse. Restraints are a form of imprisonment, and their use without a valid medical reason can be grounds for legal action. Restraints were traditionally used to "protect" people from falls or other injury. Too often, however, they were used so that nursing staff did not have to take time to adequately meet the elderly person's needs. Rather than protecting the elderly, restraints can actually cause harm and lead to physical deterioration. It may be more appropriate to keep the bed in low position or position a mattress on the floor next to the bed to reduce the risk of injury if the person does fall.

Current OBRA legislation recognizes the problems involved with restraint and currently restricts the use of chemical restraints to very specific situations. It is not appropriate to treat nonaggressive behavior with psychotropic medication. These individuals are more likely to respond to alternative therapies such as music, dance, exercise, art, or other forms of activity therapy. Verbal agitation is not typically responsive to medication. Under current guidelines, only constant yelling or screaming are a valid justification for antipsychotic medication. When psychotropic medications are used, they should be administered at the lowest dose and for the shortest possible time.

7. **Structure participation in activities of daily living.** If affected persons are able to perform any of their own physical care, they should be encouraged to do so, particularly in the early stages of dementia. This will help them maintain physical strength, and it also promotes self-esteem for those who are aware that they are losing functional ability. Routines should be kept simple. The care plan should be individualized for each person and followed consistently by all caregivers. Simple step-by-step directions should be provided. Choices should be kept to a minimum because they tend to increase anxiety and agitation. Clothing should be kept simple and should be modified to make dressing and undressing easy, thereby reducing frustration. Hair should be styled so that care is quick and easy. Shorter styles make shampooing and grooming easier and less time consuming. Mealtimes should be kept as pleasant as possible. Finger foods are more easily managed than those that require the use of silverware. Soup or beverages can be served in cups with handles that are easier to control. To prevent burns, careful attention should be paid to the temperature of hot beverages. Trays should be prepared before serving to minimize delay and frustration. Meat should be cut into easily digested pieces because the person may forget to chew before swallowing. Reminders to swallow are necessary in some cases. Toileting schedules can help reduce episodes of incontinence. Many confused elderly become increasingly agitated when they need to eliminate, even if they do not recognize the sensation.

8. **Structure the environment to minimize disruption; avoid sudden changes of room or environment.** Frequent change of staff, large numbers of strange people, excessive noise, and excessive

amounts of activity can be overly stimulating to those who suffer from dementia and should be kept to a minimum. Sudden changes of room, or even rearrangement of the furniture and belongings, can cause increased confusion, apprehension, and agitation. Whenever possible, room changes should be avoided. If it is necessary, the new room should be as similar to the old one as possible. Personal effects should not be moved unless necessary for safety.

9. **Develop a plan to deal with "acting out" behaviors.** Excessive stimulation and stress are likely to trigger catastrophic reactions or delusional behavior. Making decisions and responding to questions are stressful to those suffering from dementia and should be avoided. Certain actions on the part of nurses will help the person regain control. Distractions such as a walk or a cup of tea can be used to divert the person's attention. If this does not work, it may be necessary to take the person to his or her room or a quiet place free from the stimuli that caused the upset. Simple touch and reassurance, even sitting quietly with the person, may be enough to reestablish control.

   It is essential that nurses remain calm when confused individuals act out. It is not easy for nurses to deal with repeated irritating or hostile behaviors, but nurses must remember that anger, arguments, and explanations only confuse the person and make the situation worse. Even if nurses do not say anything negative to the person, body language may communicate a lack of acceptance. Frustration can be perceived by the elderly person despite their confusion. If nurses are unable to control their personal behavior, it may be necessary to leave the situation and seek support from other staff members in order to regain self-control.

10. **Use effective communication skills.** Use of effective communication techniques can promote positive interactions with the confused elderly. Smiles, eye contact, and gentle touch should be used. Express genuine interest and warmth. Listen to the confused person, even if the words do not make sense. Allow adequate time for the person to express him- or herself. When giving information, keep the messages short and simple, using words that are familiar to the person. Speak in a calm, natural tone of voice.

11. **Consult with family and the multidisciplinary team.** The family may be able to provide valuable information regarding the elderly person's likes, dislikes, routines, and fears. When they have been providing care in the home, families may also be able to provide suggestions for approaches that have worked in the past. Care of the confused elderly requires cooperation and coordination between various departments so continuity can be maintained. Regular "staffings" that include all relevant departments and disciplines provide an opportunity to review the person's current status and revise the plan of care.

The following interventions should take place in the home:

1. **Help the family accept the diagnosis.** The diagnosis of dementia is difficult for loved ones to accept. Allow opportunities for them to verbalize concerns and express their feelings of anger, frustration, or helplessness.

2. **Help the family adjust to the demands of providing care for a cognitively impaired elderly person.** Persons with severely altered thought processes cannot be left alone. It is difficult to devise a plan that enables the families to supervise the impaired elderly while also allowing them to continue with their own lives. Nurses can do several things to help families cope with this situation. Nurses can explain and demonstrate the types of behaviors, actions, and communication techniques that are likely to be effective. They can help families make modifications in the home environment that will provide optimum safety yet maintain some semblance of a normal home. Nurses can also recommend books and pamphlets that will provide families with more detailed and specific information. Several good books on the care of Alzheimer's victims are available in bookstores. The Alzheimer's Association has many good reference books and pamphlets, including a handbook titled *Home Care of the Alzheimer Patient.*

3. **Provide emotional support, and help the family identify coping strategies.** Coping with the day-to-day responsibilities of caring for a cognitively impaired elderly person is highly stressful. Regular visits to assess how the family is coping as well as time spent listening to concerns will help family members deal with their fears and anxieties.

4. **Identify community resources.** Support groups for the families of Alzheimer's disease or other dementia sufferers are available in many communities. Nurses should keep abreast of those that are available in each community so they can supply this information to concerned family members. Nurses should encourage family members to participate in these groups. Respite care programs are also available in many communities. These programs provide supervised care for a few hours—and even for days at a time—so that the family members can spend time doing the things they need or want to do without worrying about care responsibilities.

5. **Help families make arrangements for institutional placement, if necessary.** If the demands of caring for the impaired person become physically or psychologically excessive for the spouse or family, nursing home placement may be necessary. The family will often need assistance in making contact with these facilities or with a social worker who can help them with the planning. In addition to helping with the planning, nurses should provide emotional support to the family. The decision to move a loved one to a long-term care facility is exceedingly stressful, and the family is likely to experience feelings of helplessness or guilt.

6. **Encourage families to plan for "end-of-life" decisions.** The family will need to discuss issues such as a guardianship or health care decision maker. They should be encouraged to seek advice from the primary caregiver and a lawyer before severe mental deterioration occurs.

7. **Use any appropriate interventions that are used in the institutional setting.**

A nursing care plan for altered thought processes is presented on p. 259.

NURSING PROCESS

IMPAIRED VERBAL COMMUNICATION

The ability to communicate using words or language is a uniquely human skill. It is so much a part of our daily lives that we do not even consider the possibility of losing it. Yet many people are forced to live without the ability to speak or communicate using words. Individuals who experience cognitive or sensory changes frequently lose the ability to use words to communicate effectively.

Speech is the term used to refer to spoken language. Speech requires coordinated functioning of the brain, cranial nerves, pharynx, larynx, and lungs. The normal physiologic changes of aging affect the quality of speech. Normal speech in the elderly tends to be slower, softer, less fluent, less rhythmic, and breathier than in younger individuals, and it often has a tremulous quality. Speech is only a part of language.

Language is a broad term that includes all modes of spoken or symbolic communication. Language allows us to send and receive messages from other humans. We use language to convey our ideas and to make our wishes known to others. Without the ability to communicate, we are isolated from the world around us. Persons who lose the ability to use language or to speak are likely to experience problems. Elderly people with impaired verbal communication skills of-

ten become depressed, agitated, and frustrated, and they feel excluded from normal social interactions.

Language is a complex and not completely understood function of the brain. Both hemispheres of the cerebral cortex contribute to the process of encoding and decoding language, but two regions of the brain play key roles in language and speech: **Broca's area,** which is located in the posterior frontal lobe, and **Wernicke's area,** which is located in the posterior temporal lobe. If either of these areas is damaged by trauma or oxygen deprivation for prolonged periods of time from occlusion or hemorrhage, serious language problems can occur. The most common language problem seen in the elderly is called **aphasia** (or **dysphasia**).

Dysphasia should not be confused with dysphagia, which is difficulty swallowing. Stroke or head trauma can cause both problems. Speech pathologists are an excellent resource for information about speech problems and swallowing disorders.

Aphasia has been classified in several different ways. The most common classification includes **receptive aphasia,** in which the person has difficulty understanding language; **expressive aphasia,** in which the person is unable to express him- or herself using language; and **global aphasia,** in which the person loses the ability both to understand language and to express him- or herself using language. Each of these categories has several subclassifications.

Receptive aphasia is not the same as deafness. Communication problems in deaf people are caused by mechanical or neurologic defects that do not allow sounds to enter the nervous system. Persons suffering from receptive aphasia hear sounds normally but are unable to give these sounds meaning. In some cases this loss is complete; in others only specific language reception is lost. Some persons cannot understand spoken words but can understand written words. Others can repeat the spoken words but cannot give any meaning to them. Still others can understand single words but not sentences or word combinations.

Like receptive aphasia, expressive aphasia comes in more than one form. Broca's aphasia is a common form in which the person is able to understand verbal and written language but is unable to speak words fluently. The area of the brain that coordinates the muscles of speech is damaged. This form of aphasia is particularly frustrating because the person knows what he or she wants to say but cannot get the words out. In **Wernicke's aphasia,** the person is able to speak, but the words produced may be nonsensical or have little connection with reality (Table 15-4).

The term global aphasia is used when receptive and expressive language skills are lost. Persons suffering from global aphasia are profoundly affected. If any communication ability remains, it is in the form of a

---

NURSING CARE PLAN

COGNITIVE-PERCEPTUAL

Mr. Quick has a history of organic brain syndrome. He is not oriented to person, place, or time. He often cannot remember if he has eaten or what he should be doing at any given time. His behaviors are sometimes socially inappropriate; for example, he wanders into rooms and takes the belongings of other residents. He has a very short attention span and is unable to follow most directions. He likes to wander the halls and often laughs to himself. He will sometimes sit in the dayroom if the dayroom if the radio is playing and tap his foot to the music.

NURSING DIAGNOSIS

Altered thought processes

DEFINING CHARACTERISTICS

- Lack of orientation to person, place, and time
- Impaired ability to follow directions
- Short attention span
- Inappropriate social behaviors
- Inappropriate affect
- Repetitive behaviors

GOAL/OUTCOME

Mr. Quick will sustain no harm.

NURSING INTERVENTIONS

1. Address Mr. Quick by name.
2. Make eye contact before attempting to communicate.
3. Use pictures and familiar objects to orient him to his own room. Place a recognizable picture or other device at the door.
4. Provide a simple calendar or clock to help orient him to time.
5. Use simple language and short sentences.
6. Use concrete objects or other visual cues to explain things.
7. Allow adequate time for social interaction and communication.
8. Encourage participation in music therapy sessions.
9. Assess for changes in mental processes.
10. Notify the physician of significant changes in mental status.

EVALUATION

Mr. Quick is still not oriented to person, place or time. He continues to wander the halls on the unit when not distracted. He will sit still to fold and unfold towels or other repetitive tasks. He sings and claps along during music therapy sessions. You will continue the plan of care.

---

single sound that may be repeated with a variety of pitches, rhythms, and emphasis.

When an elderly person loses the ability to talk with others, he or she finds it difficult, if not impossible, to maintain normal roles and relationships. Even those who fully retain their intellectual function and understanding are viewed differently if they cannot speak clearly. Once the ability to communicate has been damaged, these elderly persons find that they are no longer treated as capable, competent adults but are instead treated as though they were deaf or retarded. Friends, family, and even health care professionals are increasingly likely to avoid people with impaired communication skills. This avoidance is rarely deliber-

---

TABLE 15-4

Comparison of Common Types of Aphasia

Broca's aphasia	Wernicke's aphasia
Lesion in frontal lobe	Lesion in temporal lobe
Expressive or motor	Receptive or sensory
Speech is slow, labored, hesitant, nonfluent, poorly articulated	Speech is rapid, fluent, normal in tone, clearly articulated, and long and rambling
Short sentences with little grammatic structure	May follow stereotyped patterns
	Nonsense or "jargon" speech indicates noncomprehension

---

ate; it occurs out of frustration or ignorance. Avoidance by others increases the likelihood of frustration, depression, social isolation, and loss of self-worth in the elderly.

Assessment

- Does the person have any sensory limitations? (see the assessment of sensory changes on p. 248).
- Has the person experienced any injury or surgery that altered the normal speech mechanisms?
- Does the person have a history of cerebrovascular injury or disease?

Nursing Diagnosis

Impaired verbal communication

Nursing Goals/Outcomes

The nursing goals for elderly individuals with impaired verbal communication are (1) to communicate needs with a minimum amount of frustration, (2) to demonstrate an increased ability to communicate needs and feelings, and (3) to express satisfaction with or acceptance of alternate methods of communication.

Nursing Interventions

The following interventions should take place in hospitals or extended-care facilities, and at home:

1. **Assess the elderly person's communication problems and abilities.** Communication problems and abilities differ from person to person. It is important that nurses understand the specific problems and capabilities of each person so that the plan of care can be individualized to best meet the individual's needs.
2. **Identify specific approaches that are effective for each person.** There are many techniques that can

facilitate communication. Nurses should try a variety of these to determine which are most effective. When working with a person who has impaired verbal communication, the following approaches are possible:

(1) face the person when speaking, and establish eye contact; (2) speak slowly, clearly, and in a low tone of voice; (3) speak in a normal tone of voice, and avoid shouting; (4) allow adequate time for communication (do not hurry the communication); (5) pace communication to avoid fatigue; (6) keep messages simple with one- or two-word phrases; and (7) use touch therapeutically.

3. **Document in the care plan the selected techniques that facilitate communication.** The specific approaches or techniques that are effective should be clearly documented in the plan of care so that all caregivers can use them consistently. This will reduce the frustration of both the affected person and the staff.
4. **Explain effective communication techniques to family members and friends.** Communication techniques should be explained to visitors, including family, friends, and clergy. This will promote positive interactions and enable both the affected person and his or her visitors to have a good experience. The more positive the interaction, the greater the likelihood of regular visits and interaction with the affected individual. This will enable the person to maintain somewhat more normal patterns of social interaction. It is wise to avoid large groups of visitors, which might interfere with the person's concentration and result in confusion, frustration, and fatigue.
5. **Teach the verbally impaired elderly methods for their communicating needs.** If the person is unable to communicate verbally, nurses should provide flash cards, pads, pencils, picture boards, or magic slates. If unable to use these, the person should be encouraged to use gestures. Open-ended statements such as "Show me what you would do with

---

NURSING CARE PLAN

COGNITIVE-PERCEPTUAL

Mr. White, age 68, suffers from Alzheimer's disease. He is able to understand simple commands and follow them. His speech is brief, hesitant, and garbled. It takes a long time for him to say anything. He often shakes his head and pauses when trying to think of words. He often repeats the phrase "Help me, help me." At times he becomes very frustrated when he cannot make his wishes known to his family or the staff. He spends much of his time alone in his room and has been observed crying after a particularly frustrating visit with his family.

NURSING DIAGNOSIS

Impaired verbal communication

DEFINING CHARACTERISTICS

*   Garbled speech
*   Inability to express ideas and feelings
*   Inability to find words
*   Inability to complete sentences

GOAL/OUTCOME

Mr. White will maintain the optimum level of interaction with family and staff.

NURSING INTERVENTIONS

1.   Ask *yes/no* questions whenever possible.
2.   Observe nonverbal communication.
3.   Use touch to communicate empathy.
4.   Speak slowly using short, simple sentences.
5.   Repeat, rephrase, and restate messages.
6.   Decrease environmental distractions.
7.   Establish eye contact before starting communication.
8.   Provide visual cues whenever possible.
9.   Use pictures of familiar items.
10. Allow ample time for responses.
11. Explain basic communication techniques to family.
12. Consult with speech therapist regarding other communication techniques that may benefit Mr. White.

EVALUATION

Mr. White follows some simple one- or two-word directions once his attention is obtained. He points to common objects on a picture board and occasionally leads caregivers to an object when told to "show me." Continues to have episodes of crying and pleas of "Help me." His family states that he "seems less upset" when they sit with him in a quiet area or when they look at a family picture album. You will continue the plan of care.

(the item in question)" may help the individual describe his or her needs.

6.   **Consult with a speech therapist/pathologist to determine the most effective communication strategies.** Speech therapists are specially trained to identify and treat communication disorders. Whenever possible, speech therapists should be consulted as soon as a communication problem is suspected. The recommendations should be incorporated into the plan of care and supported by all caregivers.

A nursing care plan for impaired verbal communication is presented above.

NURSING PROCESS

PAIN

Some stimuli, such as pain, have their origin within the body. Either physiologic damage or psychologic distress can result in the sensation we call pain.

Pain is a subjective perception. It is what the person tells you it is. Everyone experiences the sensation we call pain in a unique way. Because no two people mean exactly the same thing when they say they have pain, nurses must attempt to detect and determine the severity of another person's pain through careful assessment.

Nurses cannot see pain or measure pain with a meter, but they can detect its presence by careful listening and observation. Much information regarding the severity, quality, and location of pain can be gained from listening to how the person describes his or her pain, observing the individual's level of activity, and watching body language for subtle cues such as grimacing, guarding of a body part, or drawing away when a body part is touched. Various visual pain scales (Fig. 15-6) can help determine the severity of pain.

Response to pain differs from person to person. Culture, sex, spiritual beliefs, and age all play a role in what a person considers painful and how he or she responds to it. Some people believe that pain and suffering are punishments or ways to atone for wrongs they have done in their lives. Others believe that pain is a test of their faith.

Some cultures teach that a person should be stoic or uncomplaining or that pain should be hidden and tolerated with a minimum amount of intervention. Other cultures teach that it is acceptable to express pain by crying, moaning, and yelling. These individuals expect relief from the pain as quickly as possible. Nurses coming from one cultural perspective may be totally puzzled when confronted by patients from another. Nurses who think that a person who is quiet cannot be in pain will often fail to look for pain in quiet patients. Nurses who are silent sufferers will often become upset with the dramatic behavior of more demonstrative people.

The elderly are at increased risk for pain because of the higher incidence of disease conditions with aging. Some elderly have a decreased ability to sense pain, whereas others are highly sensitive to painful stimuli. There is no proof that pain decreases with aging. Pain influences the way the elderly feel about themselves and how they interact with others. Chronic or unrelieved pain can lead to behavior changes. Elderly persons who demonstrate anger, depression, or isolation from others should be evaluated for pain.

Many elderly deny pain because they fear they will be avoided or lose their independence. They live with pain because they think that it is a normal part of growing old. It is not. Pain is an indicator that something is wrong in the body. It does not have to be tolerated simply because the sufferer is old.

Determining the presence of pain in confused elderly persons is even more difficult. If pain is not recognized and assessed, serious harm may result. Failure to recognize pain can cause delays in the treatment of serious medical conditions and delays in response to a change in condition.

Confused elderly have difficulty interpreting painful stimuli, identifying its location, and communicating the nature of their distress to caregivers. They do not always respond to pain in the typical ways that nurses expect. Changes in body language, vital signs, and level of confusion are possible indicators of pain. The presence of pain is likely to result in agitation; increased pulse, respiratory rate, and blood pressure; and an increased level of confusion.

Assessment of Pain

- Does the person complain of pain?
- Is the pain constant or intermittent?
- Where is the pain?
- Is the pain generalized or localized?
- How would the person describe the pain (e.g., is it burning, stabbing, radiating, gnawing)?
- How long has the person had the pain?
- Does the pain interfere with activities of daily living?

Which Face Shows How Much Hurt You Have Now?

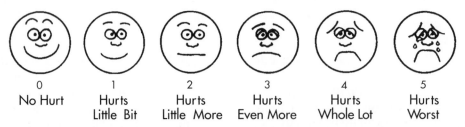

| 0 | 1 | 2 | 3 | 4 | 5 |
| No Hurt | Hurts Little Bit | Hurts Little More | Hurts Even More | Hurts Whole Lot | Hurts Worst |

FIG. 15-6 FACES Pain Rating Scale. (From Wong DL: *Whaley and Wong's essentials of pediatric nursing*, ed 5, St Louis, 1997, Mosby.)

- Does the pain interfere with sleep?
- What helps the person control the pain?
- Does the person take any medication for the pain?
- What medication does the person take and how often?

Nursing Diagnoses

Pain, chronic pain

Nursing Goals/Outcomes

The nursing goals for acute or chronic pain are (1) to report an improved comfort level or decrease in pain, (2) to verbalize the ability to cope with pain, and (3) to demonstrate techniques that provide relief from pain.

Nursing Interventions

The following nursing interventions should take place in hospitals or extended-care facilities:

1. **Thoroughly assess the nature and severity of the pain.** All pain is not the same. It is easy to miss significant changes in an elderly person's condition, particularly someone who suffers from chronic pain. A thorough assessment should be done to determine whether current pain is similar to previous pain or is different in degree, location, or severity (Table 15-5). If the person is cognitively impaired or noncommunicative, it is particularly important to watch nonverbal cues. Many times a close family member who knows the person's normal responses can help nurses interpret the person's behavior.

2. **Provide comfort measures.** Many times simple

TABLE 15-5

PQRST Method for Pain Assessment

Component	Assessment Questions	Examples
Provocation or Palliation	What activities or circumstances precede or cause the pain? Did the pain occur suddenly or gradually? What makes the pain better or worse?	Pain only occurs when stomach is empty. Pain occurs after exercise. Pain builds from mild to severe. Pain decreases with rest.
Quality	What does the pain feel like? Try to elicit client's own words.	Dull, aching, sharp, burning, crushing, stabbing, tearing, cramping, throbbing, grinding.
Region, Radiation or Referral	Where is the pain located? Can the client touch the specific area? Does it remain localized to a small area or does it involve a larger area of the body? Is pain present in one or more areas of the body? Does the pain begin in one area and then move to another area? If so where does the pain move to?	Pain localized in temporal region of skull. Entire abdomen hurts. Pain in pelvic area and region of the scapula. Pain starts in chest and radiates down left arm.
Severity	How severe is the pain on a scale of 1 to 10? Which illustration best represents pain (use a picture board ranging from a happy face to a face with a frown and tears).	Pain reported at level 7.
Timing	When did the pain start? How long does the pain last? Is the pain continuous or intermittent? Does the pain only occur at certain times of the day?	Pain first noted at 7 AM. Pain has been present for 6 hours. Pain "comes and goes." Pain only noticed during evening.
Additional questions	Has the patient experienced any pain like this in the past? Is the current pain similar or different than previous episodes? Did the client take any medication for pain? Was the medication effective at relieving pain? How effective? How long was it effective?	History of intermittent headaches. Current headache much more severe than ever experienced previously. Acetaminophen reduces but does not eliminate the discomfort for 2 to 3 hours.

comfort measures (e.g., repositioning, giving a backrub, or toileting) can reduce pain. Fear and anxiety can increase pain. Listening to the elderly and providing emotional support often help reduce pain.

3. **Avoid actions that increase pain.** Simple actions like jarring the bed or moving an individual too rapidly can increase pain. Because movement may increase pain, care should be used when moving, transferring, or otherwise touching persons in pain. Often a simple touch, an explanation of what to expect, or acknowledgment of the pain shows that the nurse is sensitive to the feelings of the elderly person.

4. **Anticipate situations likely to cause pain.** Because confused persons are unable to report pain accurately, nurses need to anticipate activities or procedures that are likely to cause pain and institute measures to prevent or reduce it.

5. **Teach nonpharmacologic approaches to pain control.** Many nonpharmacologic approaches are available for pain control. Biofeedback, meditation, hypnosis, and imagery are all useful in pain control. These techniques are often not attempted with older adults because caregivers feel that they will not accept or understand the techniques. Many elderly are not only capable of learning these techniques, but they are pleased to have some control in the relief of pain.

6. **Administer medications as ordered.** Studies have shown that nurses tend to underestimate rather than overestimate pain in others. This leads to more suffering than is needed. Nurses are often afraid that administering medication will lead to addiction or dependence. In fact, timely administration of medication before pain becomes severe actually decreases the total amount of medication used. The type and dosage of medication used to control pain in the elderly are highly individualized and may differ from those used with younger adults.

The following interventions should take place in the home:

1. **Help the elderly and their families develop a plan to cope with pain.** Pain, particularly the chronic pain endured by many elderly persons, can be physically and psychologically exhausting for the affected person and his or her loved ones. Nurses should help those living at home to develop a plan built on the interventions that are most effective for them. The elderly and their families should be shown how to incorporate these pain-relief measures into daily activities so that pain is kept to a minimum and the person is able to lead as normal a lifestyle as possible.

2. **Use any appropriate interventions that are used in the institutional setting.**

SUMMARY

Perceptual changes are among the most common problems experienced by the elderly. Altered vision and hearing present multiple concerns related to safety and lifestyle. Pain, while not a routine problem of aging, can interfere with the elderly person's ability to lead a fulfilling life. Nurses must be alert to changes in these areas and identify ways to support as normal a lifestyle as possible. Providing care for elderly individuals who are experiencing severe cognitive changes, particularly those with dementia, challenges the skills and capabilities of nurses, families, and all health care providers. Ongoing assessment of perceptual and cognitive functioning is necessary to detect subtle but potentially dangerous changes. Prompt recognition of problems and careful selection of appropriate interventions will allow the aging person to maintain the highest level of function possible.

READINGS AND REFERENCES

Anderson LN, Clarke JT: De-escalating verbal aggression in primary care settings, *Nurse Pract* 21:95, 1996.

Andresen GP: How to assess the older mind, *RN* 55:34, 1992.

Anti-Ontong D: Patient management consultation: cognitive and affective assessment of the geriatric patient, *Med Surg Nurs* 2:70, 1993.

Arguelles T, Lowenstein DA: Cognitive tests and test translations: research says si to development of culturally appropriate cognitive assessment tools, *Generations* 21:25, 1997.

Balneaves L: Tune in to your client, *Can Nurse* 90:37, 1994.

Carr P: Clues, *Home Healthcare Nurse* 10:60, 1992.

Cognitive and functional impairment, *Am Fam Physician* 51:633, 1995.

Cooper JW: Managing disruptive behavioral symptoms: today's do's and don'ts, *Nursing Home* 43:54, 1994.

Drachman DA, Swearer JM: Screening for dementia: cognitive assessment screening test (CAST), *Am Fam Physician* 54:1957, 1996.

Evans C, et al: Caring for the confused geriatric surgical patient, *Geriatr Nurs* 14:237, 1993.

Evans L: Sundown syndrome in institutionalized elderly, *J Am Geriatr Soc* 35:101, 1987.

Forrest J: Assessment of acute and chronic pain in older adults, *J Gerontol Nurs* 21:15, 1995.

Fromm CG, Metzler DJ: Preparing your older patient for surgery, *RN* 56:38, 1993.

Green PM, Gildemeister JE: Memory aging research and memory support in the elderly, *J Neurosci Nurs* 26:241, 1994.

Halls GR, Wakefield B: Acute confusion in the elderly: what to do when the clouds roll in, *Nursing 96,* 26:32, 1996

Hunt L: Aging and the visual system, *Insight* 18:6, 1993.

Jubeck ME: Are you sensitive to the cognitive needs of the elderly? *Geriatr Nurs* 13:217, 1992.

Kolanowski AM: Clinical importance of environmental lighting to the elderly, *J Gerontol Nurs* 18:10, 1992.

Kuhlman G, DeBoer G, Wilson HS: *Applying the nursing process for clients with organic mental syndromes and disorders.* In

Wilson HS, Kneisl CR, editors: *Psychiatric nursing,* ed 4, Redwood City, Calif, 1992, Addison-Wesley.

Level of cognitive dysfunction should indicate the need for long-term care, *Brown University Long-Term Care Quality Letter* 6:1, 1994.

Linblade DD, McDonald M: Removing communication barriers for the hearing-impaired elderly, *Med Surg Nurs* 4:379, 1995.

Marchello B, Boczko G, Shelkey M: Progressive dementia: strategies to manage new problem behaviors, *Geriatrics* 50:40, 1995.

McConnell EA: Myths and facts about pain in the elderly, *Nursing 93* 23:83, 1993.

Mentes JC: A nursing protocol to assess causes of delirium: identifying delirium in nursing home residents, *J Gerontol Nurs* 21:26, 1995.

Miller J, et al: Assessment of discomfort in elderly confused patients: a preliminary study, *J Neurosci Nurs* 28:175, 1996.

National Institute on Aging-Age Page Web site: *Aging and your eyes,* www.aoa.dhhs.gov/aoa/pages/agepages/eyes.html, 1995.

National Institute on Aging-Age Page Web site: *Hearing and older people,* www.aoa.dhhs.gov/aoa/pages/agepages/hearing.html, 1995.

National Institute on Aging-Age Page Web site: *Forgetfulness: it's not always what you think,* www.mhsource.com/hy/ageforget.html, 1996.

Roses AD: Apolipoprotein E genotyping in the differential diagnosis, not prediction, of Alzheimer's disease, *Ann Neurol* 38:6, 1995.

Shelton DL: Report gives facts on mental health needs of elderly, *American Medical News* 38:12, 1995.

Sullivan-Marks EM: Delirium and physical restraint in the hospitalized elderly, *Image* 26:295, 1994.

SELF-PERCEPTION AND SELF-CONCEPT

LEARNING OBJECTIVES

1. Discuss the concepts of self-perception and self-concept.
2. Describe how self-perception and self-concept change with aging.
3. Discuss the effects of disease processes on self-perception and self-concept.
4. Describe methods of assessing changes in self-perception and self-concept.
5. Identify the elderly who are most at risk for experiencing problems related to self-perception and self-concept.
6. Identify selected nursing diagnoses related to self-perception or self-concept problems.
7. Describe nursing interventions that are appropriate for elderly individuals experiencing problems related to self-perception and self-concept.

NORMAL SELF-PERCEPTION AND SELF-CONCEPT

The attitudes and perceptions people have about themselves and their abilities and self-worth make up what is often called our self-identity. People form their self-identities from their values, life experiences, and interactions with others. People with good self-worth and high self-esteem share certain characteristics. They have strong personal values and feel that they have the ability to control their lives. They have had positive life experiences and have received positive feedback from others. People with poor self-worth and low self-esteem are just the opposite. They tend to have weak personal values and feel that they have little control over their lives. They have had primarily negative life experiences and have received negative feedback from others.

We form our self-identities by comparing ourselves and our experiences to some ideal. This can be an internal ideal drawn from our personal values or an external ideal drawn from the society around us. Many people experience problems with self-worth because they always measure themselves against external standards. Contemporary standards are communicated again and again by advertising and the media. People who are young, thin, rich, successful, and attractive are idealized. Anyone who does not meet these superficial and artificial standards is somehow judged to be "inferior" and is thus viewed negatively by our society. Few people are able to meet all of the idealized criteria. This results in a large number of people in contemporary society who suffer from negative self-esteem.

In trying to meet external standards, people are likely to lose themselves and their internal values. The more we look to the external forces, the less likely we are to have high self-esteem. The more we look internally for our self-worth, the more satisfied we will be in the long run. Shakespeare summed it up nicely in *Hamlet:* "This above all: to thine own self be true/And it must follow, as the night the day, thou canst not then be false to any man."

It is easy to say that people should draw on internal ideals to maintain self-esteem, but this is difficult in light of external pressures and feedback. In today's society, people usually have more negative experiences than positive ones. Therefore, problems relating to self-perception and self-esteem are common in people of all ages. Problems relating to self-esteem are particularly common among the poor, the infirm, and the elderly.

Feedback from others affects our perception of ourselves. People who have caring friends and families tend to have higher levels of self-identity and self-esteem. Strong families and friends provide support for each other. They help each other keep things in perspective by providing positive feedback and buffering each other from an often negative world. A good family and good friends play an important part in building and maintaining our self-esteem.

Persons who lack supportive family and friends are likely to have a poor perception of self and low self-esteem. Those who come from dysfunctional families or are separated from loved ones run a high risk of poor self-perception and low self-esteem. These people are more likely to suffer from negative feedback because they lack the necessary support to provide balance.

A real or perceived ability to make choices plays an important role in self-perception and self-esteem. People who feel capable of controlling what happens perceive things far differently from those who perceive no control over their lives.

Our sense of self-control starts with our bodies. Adults are used to having control of their bodies and bodily functions. Control of the movement of body parts and of elimination are so basic we do not even think of them—at least not until we lose control of them for some reason. Consider how you would feel if tomorrow you woke up and could not move or could not control your bladder or bowels. Would your sense of self-worth and self-esteem change?

Adults are also used to having control and making choices regarding their activities. Choices regarding activities of daily living (e.g., hygiene practices, amount and type of clothing, amount and type of food, amount and type of exercise and sleep) are determined by and are reflections of an adult's self-perception and level of self-esteem.

Loss of control results in depression, powerlessness, helplessness, hopelessness, fear, and anxiety. Loss of control destroys self-esteem.

Problems related to self-perception and self-esteem are not as obvious as are physical problems. By their very nature, self-perception and self-concept are subjective. Many people find it difficult to talk about their feelings, frequently finding themselves unable or unwilling to put their feelings into words. More often our perceptions of self-worth and self-esteem are exhibited to others through behavior. Significant behaviors include the amount of attention paid to personal hygiene and grooming, the type and frequency of emotions exhibited, body posture, the amount and type of eye contact, and voice and speech patterns. People with very high self-esteem appear to be very much in control of themselves and their lives. They are usually well-groomed, maintain an erect body posture, make eye contact with others, speak clearly in a normal tone of voice, and exhibit emotions appropriate to a given situation.

People with very low self-esteem often appear disinterested and out of control. They often appear unkempt or disheveled. They may slump or slouch, and there seems to be little purpose to their movement. Eye contact is infrequent. The amount of communication with others is reduced, is negative in nature, and is often mumbled or abrupt. Emotions can vary from expressions of sadness to full-blown anger.

Most people's self-esteem and behavior fall between these two extremes. As long as behavior falls within the accepted range of normal, people tend to disregard or overlook what is going on inside other people. Only when behaviors move outside of the normal range do we seriously attempt to understand what is happening inside the person to cause those behaviors.

SELF-PERCEPTION/SELF-CONCEPT AND AGING

Erickson has identified the major task of late life as maintenance of ego integrity (the sense of self-worth) versus despair. Attitudes toward aging, the level of self-esteem throughout life, the extent of physical change due to aging and illness, the presence or absence of emotional support systems, and the ability to maintain a degree of control will have an impact on whether aging adults will be successful in accomplishing this task.

Aging individuals must come to grips with their own perception of aging. It is difficult to see oneself getting old. Many elderly persons express dismay with the realization and can even identify a particular moment when they perceived themselves as "old." One older woman recently attended her 50th high school reunion. She reported having a good time but wondered what *she* was doing with all of these "old people." A subtle but real change in her self-perception occurred after that incident. Before then, she did not feel old; afterward, she was more aware of her age.

Poor self-concept, depression, and other negative feelings are common among the elderly. Elderly persons who have had a poor self-concept throughout their lives are not likely to gain self-esteem with aging. Even those who had a healthy level of self-esteem during their younger days are likely to experience problems during aging. This is due in part to today's societal attitudes.

Ageism is prevalent in our youth-oriented society, which far too often portrays the elderly as physically and mentally inept, nonproductive, and dependent.

Considering these negative images of aging, it is easy to understand why many people do all within their power to avoid the physical signs of aging. In an attempt to maintain their sense of self-worth, aging persons with adequate financial resources may try cosmetic surgery, hair dye, and hair transplants. It is difficult for some younger people to understand how radically the changes of age or illness can destroy self-image and self-esteem in the elderly. Many younger persons feel that these cosmetic measures look absurd, and they mock the elderly, which further lowers the aging person's self-worth. It will be interesting to see what these insensitive people do as they age.

Elderly people who accept the negative societal perceptions are likely to suffer more than those elderly who refuse to accept these stereotypes. Unfortunately, those who start with the poorest self-concept are the ones who are most likely to accept the negatives and are particularly vulnerable to loss of self-worth. Physical, social, and economic changes that occur with aging result in changes in the way elderly persons perceive themselves and their bodies. The greater the amount of change, the more likely the person is to experience problems related to self-concept. Small changes in appearance or function (e.g., wrinkles or aches and pains) nibble at the edges of self-worth. Serious illnesses (particularly those that result in obvious disfigurement or major loss of function, such as strokes) take a large bite out of the aging person's perception of self.

Frequent and significant losses (including decreasing physical health; decreasing mental quickness; loss of significant others; loss of pride in appearance, roles, or possessions; and loss of independence) threaten the perception of control that is important to most adults. These losses can result in a variety of problems, which often increase in severity if unchecked.

Institutional placement further damages self-worth by stripping the elderly of many of the personal belongings that make up the visible part of their identity. It is a rare facility that is able to accommodate more than a small amount of clothing and a few mementos of a lifetime. A lifetime of 80 years is often reduced to a small closet and bedside stand.

While losses of physical and functional abilities are damaging to self-worth, loss of the emotional support of loved ones is even more devastating. Death is an increasingly common visitor to the elderly. This does not make it less frightening; rather it is a reminder of one's own mortality. The friends and loved ones who made life worthwhile slip away, one by one. The positive messages that a person is worthwhile, lovable, and loved become less frequent, and the reasons for living disappear. Losses due to death or separation from friends and family can leave the elderly without those sources of positive feedback that nourish self-worth.

We cannot prevent loss due to death, but loss due to separation is another matter. The breakdown of the extended family and geographic mobility are increasingly isolating the elderly. Elderly persons who are separated from their families and significant others are at increased risk for experiencing diminished self-worth. Separation is increasingly associated with placement in an institutional setting. The elderly often feel rejected and isolated when nursing home placement is necessary. It is a natural response for the elderly to feel they have been "put away" because they have little value or worth. These individuals often feel unimportant, unloved, and unwanted. Even if this is completely untrue, the perception greatly decreases their sense of self-worth. If family and friends visit often and show positive concern, self-esteem can be maintained. Too often, however, this is not the case. It is in institutional settings—where nobody really knows or cares about the "inner" person—that many elderly lose their remaining sense of self-esteem and self-worth.

SELF-PERCEPTION AND SELF-CONCEPT ALTERATIONS

When the elderly have a poor self-concept, fears and anxieties increase. As control over one's life decreases, self-esteem plummets even lower, and the elderly fall victim to feelings of hopelessness and powerlessness, which lead to depression. Depression leads to isolation from others, further decreasing the sense of self-worth.

Assessment of Self-Perception and Self-Concept

- Does the person verbalize fears or concerns?
- Are these fears of a known or an unknown source?
- Does the person verbalize loss of control over his or her life?
- Has the person recently experienced significant losses?
- Has the person recently moved or been separated from significant others?
- What is the person's general appearance and posture?
- Does the person make or avoid eye contact?
- Does the person verbalize concerns regarding changes in his or her appearance?
- Does the person make negative comments regarding him- or herself?
- Does the person avoid looking in the mirror or at altered body parts?
- Does the person question his or her worth?
- Does the person verbalize feelings of failure?

BOX 16-1

Risk Factors Related to Self-Perception and Self-Concept in the Elderly

- Conditions that result in change of body appearance (surgical removal of body parts, burns, obesity, skin lesions, chemotherapy, disfiguring endocrine disorders such as acromegaly or Cushing's disease)
- Inability to control bodily functions
- Significant losses (of significant others, possessions, social roles, financial status)
- Recent relocation (particularly if involuntarily)
- Chronic pain

- Does the person verbalize hopelessness or despair?
- Does the person spend most of his or her time alone, or does he or she interact with others?
- Does the person accept directions from caregivers passively, or does the person express the desire to make his or her own decisions?
- Does the person exhibit aggression, anger, or demanding behaviors?
- Are there any signs of autonomic nervous system stimulation (e.g., increased pulse or respiratory rate, elevated blood pressure, diaphoresis)?
- Does the person manifest any behaviors typical of emotional upset (pacing, hand wringing, crying, repetitive motions, tics, aggressiveness)?
- Are there changes in vocal quality (e.g., quivering)?
- Does the person complain of headaches?
- Does the person have difficulty focusing on activities, remembering things, or making decisions?
- Has the person experienced changes in eating or sleeping patterns?
- Has the person started to give away treasured possessions?
- Does the person verbalize the desire to end his or her life?

See Box 16-1 for a list of risk factors for altered self-perception and self-concept in the elderly.

NURSING PROCESS

BODY IMAGE DISTURBANCE

People experiencing body image disturbance are likely to refuse to look at or touch the affected body parts. In severe disturbances, the individual may deny that the change has occurred and act as though nothing has happened. Many persons who suffer with this problem are unwilling to discuss their concerns with others for fear that they will be rejected or made to feel "different." If they are willing to verbalize their concerns, they may speak of themselves in a disembodied way, as though the deformity or change is not really happening to them. They may speak of themselves very negatively or with a great deal of disgust that they are no longer what they once were. They may become preoccupied with their body function and excessively concerned about every minor change. They may need reassurance that nothing else will happen to them. Many persons with altered body image will refuse to participate in their own care and resist any plans for rehabilitation. They are likely to verbalize feelings of worthlessness and powerlessness.

Nursing Diagnosis

Body image disturbance

Nursing Goals/Outcomes

The nursing goals for elderly individuals with body image disturbances are (1) to verbalize concerns regarding changes in body appearance or function, (2) to identify their personal strengths, (3) to acknowledge and look at the actual changes in body appearance, (4) to verbalize willingness to modify lifestyle to accommodate physical changes, and (5) to demonstrate readiness to participate in therapy and use necessary assistive devices.

Nursing Interventions

The following interventions should take place in hospitals, extended-care facilities, and at home:

1. **Assess the elderly individual's perceptions of self, including strengths and support systems.** Even with serious impairment, the elderly can have strengths that will help them cope with change. Nurses will need to identify the unique strengths of each person so that these can be drawn on when planning care.
2. **Establish a trusting relationship.** To help the elderly work through and accept physical changes or deformities, nurses must demonstrate acceptance both verbally and nonverbally. Actively listening to concerns and planning care to include opportunities for the patient to verbalize his or her feelings help to build trust.
3. **Provide care in a nonjudgmental manner.** Because nurses are the people most likely to actually see any deformity, it is particularly important that they show no sign of revulsion or disgust when providing care. Nurses must take particular care not to show even *subtle* body language or facial expressions that could be perceived by the elderly as a sign of nonacceptance.
4. **Encourage the person to look at and touch affected body areas.** Nurses are so used to seeing physical deformities (e.g., stomas and amputations) that they may not be aware of just how frightening these are to the affected person. Many people need time and encouragement to even look at the affected body part. Some will depersonalize the change and refer to "it" as though the deformity was something apart from themselves. Looking at and touching the deformity will help the person accept reality. Until he or she is able to do this, the individual will not be ready for teaching or self-care.
5. **Focus on abilities, not disabilities.** In order to become motivated, a person must feel that he or she is capable of doing the activity. Many elderly persons—even those with severe deformities—are capable of doing *something*. Focusing on what can be done instead of on what cannot be done promotes feelings of self-worth.
6. **Assist in selecting clothing and/or dressing the elderly in a manner that de-emphasizes body changes.** Clothing that draws attention away from obvious deformities helps maintain body image. Sweaters, lap robes, and properly fitted clothing can be used to make deformities less obvious.
7. **Ensure that the person is carefully groomed.** Soiled clothing should be changed promptly. The face and hands should always be kept clean and free from food or other debris. Little things like neatly combed or styled hair, a shave, or the application of a tasteful amount of makeup can make the person feel better about his or her appearance. How a person looks makes a difference in how he or she feels. An elderly person should never be made to look "cute." The elderly should always be groomed appropriately for their age.
8. **Coordinate rehabilitative care with other departments.** Physical therapy, occupational therapy, speech therapy, pharmacy, and other departments may be involved in the care of individuals who have experienced significant changes in body function. Nurses spend the most time with these individuals and are most aware of the total effect of various therapies. Nurses should coordinate these activities in the care plan to ensure that all the groups are working toward the same goals. It is also important for nurses to monitor their patients' responses to the therapy and their ability to tolerate the effort required in therapy.

NURSING PROCESS
SELF-ESTEEM DISTURBANCE

There are many reasons why the elderly are at risk of losing self-esteem. Those who have low self-esteem are likely to display certain characteristic behaviors.

Body language of persons with low self-esteem is similar to that of depressed individuals. They are often observed with the head slumped on the chest or shoulder; the facial expression is one of sadness; and they usually avoid eye contact. These individuals are likely to speak of themselves in negative terms. Statements such as "Don't waste your time on me" or "I can't do anything right" are indicative of low self-esteem. The speech of individuals with low self-esteem is full of statements of sadness, loss, depression, anxiety, and anger. They can see very little that is positive about their lives and tend to focus on negative experiences. People with low self-esteem pay little attention to hygiene or grooming. They tend to be very passive, letting caregivers control all facets of their lives. They may demonstrate extreme dependence on others, even if they are capable of doing things for themselves. They are unlikely to initiate activities, and if they do they are likely to leave activities unfinished. They are resistant to positive feedback and may argue or become angry with anyone attempting to give it. Elderly persons with low self-esteem are likely to avoid social contact; if forced to be in contact with others, they tend to avoid interaction and stay at the edges of the group or activity.

Assessment

See the assessment for self-perception and self-concept on p. 269.

Nursing Diagnosis

Self-esteem disturbance

Nursing Goals/Outcomes

The nursing goals for elderly individuals with self-esteem disturbances are to (1) identify personal strengths, (2) express feelings and concerns, and (3) practice behaviors that promote self-confidence.

Nursing Interventions

The following nursing interventions should take place in hospitals, extended-care facilities, and at home:

1. **Explore feelings and concerns.** To plan effective interventions to improve feelings of self-worth, nurses must be aware of the unique concerns and feelings of each elderly individual.
2. **Demonstrate acceptance of older adults as people with value and self-worth by responding to concerns, encouraging them to make choices, following through with their requests, and including them in care planning.** Taking time to actually listen and respond to the needs communicated by the elderly is the best way of demonstrating accep-

tance. Too often the nurses "listen" and then do something completely different from what the elderly person requested. This is a subtle way of indicating that the person does not matter. If nurses are unable to comply with the aging person's requests, an explanation should be given so that the individual understands the reasons.

3. **Encourage participation in self-care activities.** Participation in self-care activities allows the elderly to retain a sense of self-worth. Even small acts like washing their own faces or eating a piece of toast can help make the elderly feel some control over their person (Fig. 16-1).
4. **Provide opportunities for reminiscence. Reminiscence,** sometimes called "life review," is a phenomenon that is especially important to the elderly. Nurses tend to focus on the present. Because there is so much to do, we do not take time to listen to old stories. We are so busy making sure that the elderly are oriented to the present that we tend to forget about their past. Some nurses think that talking about all of the "old stuff" is downright boring. Nurses even make the mistake of thinking that participating in these often sentimental and nostalgic conversations is inappropriate, unnecessary, and not a part of nursing care at all. These errors can result in nurses missing important information regarding the mental health and self-esteem of the aging person.

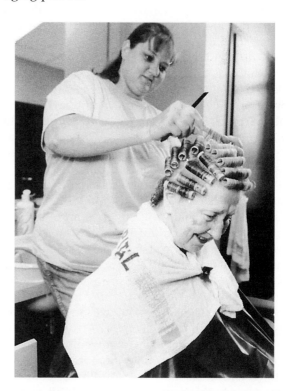

FIG. **16-1** Having her hair done by a visiting beautician, this long-term resident is actively participating in her own care and is able to retain her sense of self-worth. (Courtesy of Barnes Extended Care, St Louis.)

272 PSYCHOSOCIAL CARE OF THE ELDERLY

All people, particularly the elderly, need to feel that their existence has made a difference. As death approaches, the elderly need to feel that their lives have had purpose and meaning. Absence of self-worth leads to despair and hopelessness. Erickson stressed the importance of seeing value in the life stories of the elderly.

People of all ages reminisce (i.e., think back to earlier times in their lives). This process helps people work through previous problems and recognize previous successes. It helps resolve conflicts and enables the elderly to cope with the present and future and to go on with life and living. Life review is not just looking back at the "good old times"; rather it is a process of determining that one's life has had value and merit. It is a way to meet the challenges of the present, and it is a way to prepare for death.

Elderly individuals who have completed a life review—either on their own or with assistance—seem to have a certain serenity. They accept that although not perfect, their lives have been worthwhile. Some find areas of discontent that they are still able to correct: they can still find lost friends, finish incomplete personal business, and make amends. Life review is a healthy process. It is a normal and necessary way that all individuals, particularly the elderly, can maintain mental health.

Reminiscing can be done individually or in groups. Elderly persons who reminisce alone (as many do) are often highly critical of themselves, feeling that they did not "make the right choices" and "do the right things." By reminiscing with others, the true value and merit of life often become clearer. Group sharing tends to be less intense than one-on-one communication. In addition, the memories of one person often trigger similar recollections among other group members. Different perspectives on situations can help the elderly see themselves and their responses in a different light.

When working with a group of elderly persons, nurses should ensure that the group is not too large or some individuals will not have an opportunity to participate. Five to eight people can effectively participate in a group at one time. It is essential that nurses remain open and actively listen to all participants. Various devices can be used to stimulate reminiscences. Items such as picture albums, old movies, magazines, newspapers, or songs can be used to start the conversation. Activities such as writing poems, assembling picture albums, making collages, or writing an autobiography may be helpful. Open statements such as "Tell me about when you came to this country" can be helpful as well.

5. **Encourage the family to participate in reminiscence by providing pictures or items that bring** **back memories of happy times.** Families should be encouraged to take the opportunity to share in the memories of their elderly members. Many families find boxes of old pictures among the elderly person's belongings. Sometimes the people and events are familiar, other times they include many unknown and unfamiliar individuals. A review of these pictures often helps trigger memories in the elderly and enables them to show a side of themselves that their adult children and grandchildren never knew anything about. Pictures of a smiling young couple kissing, dancing, taking their children to the park, or taking part in any number of other activities can help the elderly person remember better times. It can also help the family realize that, like themselves, their parents were really young once—facing the same dreams and challenges. This knowledge can help them grow closer and more aware of the continuity of family and can provide an opening for older people and their families to share feelings that they might otherwise feel uncomfortable addressing (Fig. 16-2).

6. **Encourage families to communicate positive feelings to the elderly person.** Too often at funerals grief-stricken family members are heard to say "I wish I had told my mother (or father) how much she (or he) meant to me." The best way to prevent these regrets is to say and do these things when the

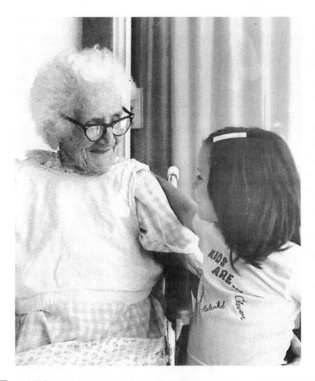

FIG. 16-2 Bringing young and old together is an important part of the self-esteem of the elderly. (Courtesy of the American Society on Aging.)

elderly person is still alive. It means a lot to all of us to hear that we are appreciated and loved. It means even more to the elderly, who may be questioning whether their lives had any meaning. Young family members are often hesitant to say positive things face to face because they assume that the older person "knows" how they feel or because they just feel awkward saying them. It's interesting to observe how many people have no trouble saying something negative but have trouble putting something positive into words. It is no wonder that so many people, particularly the elderly, have an altered sense of self-worth.

The greeting card industry has capitalized on this characteristic by mass producing cards to help people convey feelings they cannot verbalize. Many elderly persons treasure greeting cards they receive from family because this is the closest they get to true communication of feelings from family members. Sometimes families need to be reminded and encouraged to meet the need for positive support. Anything nurses can do to help families recognize the importance of positive communication will help the elderly.

NURSING PROCESS

FEAR

Fear is a feeling of dread or apprehension regarding an identified source. Fear is not unique to the elderly; but as functional abilities decrease, fears may become more obvious. The most common fears identified in the elderly include fears of change and disruption in their lives or routines, crime and victimization, loss of loved ones, disease, injury, pain and suffering, loss of independence, financial destitution, and loneliness. Interestingly, death was not the most feared item; in fact, many elderly people express less fear of death than do younger persons. They may state that they fear the unknown, but not death itself. Many even view death as a release from fears and an opportunity to rejoin loved ones.

Fear is closely related to anxiety. Individuals with known fears usually also experience anxiety, although anxiety can occur without a known fear. People respond to fear in different ways. Some might verbalize feelings of helplessness, others might withdraw from contact with other people, and still others might respond aggressively. Aggressive responses to fear are often misinterpreted by caregivers as anger. Fear can also result in physiologic symptoms due to stimulation of the sympathetic nervous system. Such symptoms include dilated pupils, dry mouth, trembling, elevated blood pressure, increased pulse and respiratory rate, palpitations, diaphoresis, diarrhea,

and urinary frequency. Physiologic stimulation due to high-level anxiety can be dangerous to aging individuals who are already compromised by endocrine, respiratory, cardiovascular, or neurologic disease.

Assessment

See the assessment for self-perception and self-concept on p. 269.

Nursing Diagnosis

Fear

Nursing Goals/Outcomes

The nursing goals for fearful individuals are (1) to identify specific fears, (2) to identify coping strategies that were helpful in the past and use these when fears arise, and (3) to use strategies that help control fear.

Nursing Interventions

The following interventions should take place in hospitals, extended-care facilities, and at home:

1. **Provide opportunities for the elderly to express their fears.** Fear is debilitating. It stops people from being able to take positive actions. Identifying fears is the first step in dealing with them. If the elderly demonstrate signs of fear during care, nurses should stop the activity and give the individual the opportunity to express his or her fears. These fears should then be taken into account when planning a strategy to reduce or eliminate them. Nurses should be careful not to minimize or deny the person's fears. Avoid using clichés such as "Don't worry, we know what we're doing," because such statements convey the idea that the person's feelings do not count.

2. **Remove or reduce the most common sources of fear.** Each of us fears different things. Fear of falling and fear of loud noises are common from the time of birth. Falling is a very real fear to elderly persons who require assistance in transfers, particularly transfers that involve hydraulic devices. This fear can be reduced by ensuring that there is adequate help and by providing ongoing reassurance during the transfer.

3. **Provide explanations for all care procedures.** Fear of the unknown is common at all ages. Many activities and treatments that are familiar to nurses are extremely strange and frightening to the elderly, who may fear that the procedure will cause bodily harm or pain. Nurses should be careful to explain why the procedure must be done, what will happen, and what the person can do to help. Explana-

tions will not always remove the fear, but they usually do reduce it.

NURSING PROCESS

ANXIETY

Anxiety is an unsettled or uneasy feeling caused by a vague or unidentified threat. Anxiety can be mild, moderate, or severe; in extreme cases, it can reach the level of panic. Anxiety can be acute or chronic. Anxiety is more prevalent among the elderly than among any other age group, with studies revealing that as many as 10% of the elderly report chronic, often debilitating, forms of anxiety. Mild anxiety can actually be good for people, even the elderly. A little anxiety keeps people vigilant for potential hazards. A little anxiety provides the motivation for positive actions such as seeking health care. Those who have never experienced anxiety would have little reason to plan ahead or take precautions in life. However, persistent or high-level anxiety can interfere with a person's ability to perceive situations accurately and to respond to them appropriately. In addition to behavioral changes of anxiety, stimulation of the sympathetic nervous system can result, with physiologic changes identical to those seen with fear.

Assessment

See the assessment of self-perception and self-concept on p. 269.

Nursing Diagnosis

Anxiety

Nursing Goals/Outcomes

The nursing goals for elderly individuals diagnosed with anxiety are to (1) identify methods that help reduce anxiety and (2) experience fewer episodes of anxiety.

Nursing Interventions

The following nursing interventions should take place in hospitals, extended-care facilities, and at home:
1. **Encourage the elderly to verbalize their thoughts and feelings.** Once thoughts and feelings are put into words, individuals are often more able to recognize the causes of their anxiety. Once the causes are recognized, strategies can be designed to help the person cope with anxiety. Other people (e.g., nurses) can frequently see patterns in the verbalized thoughts and feelings of anxious people. This perspective is more objective and often helps the

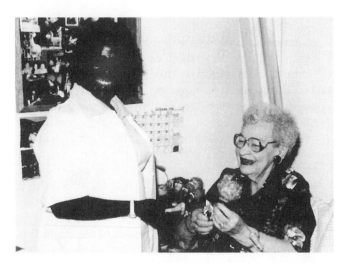

Fig. 16-3 A nurse admiring the creative work of a resident. Crafts may help lessen anxiety in older adults. (From Castillo HM: *The nurse assistant in long-term care: a rehabilitative approach*, St Louis, 1992, Mosby.)

person gain a better understanding of him- or herself. Allowing the elderly person to verbalize anger and irritation or to cry may enable them to calm down.
2. **Provide a quiet environment and reduce excessive stimulation.** Excessive noise or activity usually increases anxiety. A quiet room with minimal contact and stimulation may help calm the elderly. Reassurance with gentle touch and empathetic communication may also help. Stimulating beverages such as coffee should be avoided.
3. **Provide distraction or diversion.** Moderate anxiety may decrease if the individual becomes involved in another activity that he or she finds pleasant. Quiet activities such as listening to music, watching television, or working on a craft are soothing to many elderly persons (Fig. 16-3).

NURSING PROCESS

HOPELESSNESS

Hopelessness is a subjective state in which people feel unable to solve problems or establish goals. They *feel* that they have no alternatives or choices, even when they actually can control what occurs. Hopeless persons express feelings of complete apathy in response to problems. They are often heard making statements such as "What's the use in trying; nothing will go right anyway" or "Nothing ever goes right for me." Because hopeless persons cannot see any possible solutions, they tend to be passive and uninterested. They find it difficult if not impossible to solve problems or make decisions. The body language of hopeless individuals is that of despondency. In most cases, these persons display few emotions (although some respond with anger). Self-destructive behaviors are common among hopeless elderly. Failure to eat, to take prescribed medication, or to follow-up with medical care are often signs of hopelessness. In extreme cases, hopeless individuals may become suicidal. The suicide rate in elderly is higher than that in any other age group, and the numbers appear to be rising. Any elderly person who demonstrates severe signs of hopelessness should be watched closely. Hopeless elderly persons who abuse alcohol or other depressant medications are at higher-than-average risk for suicide.

Assessment

See the assessment of self-perception and self-concept on p. 269.

Nursing Diagnosis

Hopelessness

Nursing Goal/Outcome

The nursing goal for elderly individuals diagnosed with hopelessness is to identify activities or interventions that promote hopefulness.

Nursing Interventions

The following interventions should take place in hospitals, extended-care facilities, and at home:

1. **Visit the elderly frequently and spend time exploring the factors that contribute to feelings of hopelessness.** It is necessary to spend time with the elderly to develop enough trust for them to share their concerns. Regular visits that are not related to direct physical care show that nurses are concerned with the person. It is important to get the person to verbalize their feelings. Unless nurses know their specific concerns, it is impossible to design approaches that will help a particular aging individual. Hopelessness is often related to other nursing diagnoses, particularly spiritual despair, grief, and depression.

2. **Assess the potential for self-destructive behaviors or suicide.** Frequent verbalization in the elderly of the wish to harm themselves or to commit suicide must be taken seriously. The depressed elderly and those who have recently experienced significant loss are at highest risk for suicidal thought. Elderly persons who live alone are more likely to try to take their own lives. Some commit suicide passively by refusing to eat, by refusing medical care, or by failing to comply with medical treatments such as taking medications. Other elderly persons choose a very active form of suicide such as drug overdose, shooting, or hanging. The very frail elderly are

---

BOX 16-2

Suicide and the Elderly

- At least 6000 people 65 years of age or older commit suicide each year.
- White men are the most likely group to commit suicide.
- Medical illness is a major contributing factor to suicide.
- Social isolation, serious depression, and a history of self-destructive behaviors increase the risk for suicide.
- Life events such as loss of a loved one, uncontrollable pain, and major life changes such as retirement increase the risk of suicide.

BOX 16-3

Interventions Related to Suicide

ASSESS FOR SIGNS OF DEPRESSION
—Changes in appetite or sleep patterns
—Unexplained fatigue
—Apathy or loss of interest in life
—Trouble concentrating or indecisiveness
—Social withdrawal from family and/or friends
—Loss of interest in normal activities or hobbies
—Loss of interest in personal appearance
—Crying for no apparent reason

ASSESS FOR OTHER BEHAVIOR CHANGES
—Giving away treasured possessions
—Talking about death or suicide
—Taking unusual or unnecessary risks
—Increased consumption of alcohol or drugs
—Failure to follow through with prescribed medication or diet
—Purchase of a weapon

DEMONSTRATE INTEREST AND BECOME INVOLVED WITH THE PERSON
—Take clues of suicide seriously; do not ignore them.
—Ask the person if he or she is considering suicide.
—Avoid judgmental statements.
—Offer hope and help the person seek alternatives.
—Promote a safe environment by removing easy suicide methods.
—Seek help from persons or agencies that specialize in suicide prevention.

more likely to attempt passive forms; the stronger person is more likely to choose an actively destructive method (Boxes 16-2 and 16-3).

NURSING PROCESS

POWERLESSNESS

Powerlessness occurs when the elderly feel they have lost control of what happens to them. Such feelings may result from the loss of control of physical functions or body parts or from loss of a body part. Powerlessness is common with hospitalization or placement in an extended-care facility. Nurses often contribute to feelings of powerlessness by taking over or taking charge of the elderly. Doing too much for a person is perhaps more damaging than doing too little. By their very competence, caregivers can intimidate the elderly and destroy any initiative for them to even attempt self-care. Individual dignity and control are too often sacrificed to efficiency. This is particularly true of the elderly who require more time to accomplish tasks. It is easier for the staff to do something for the elderly than to wait for them to do it.

Life in an institutional setting tends to be regimented and restrictive. In an attempt to meet the needs of many people, it is easy to lose track of the uniqueness of the individuals. The needs of the institution often take priority over the desires of the individual. If the importance of the elderly is not recognized by caregivers, the institution will completely control the lives of each individual.

Persons who are acquiescent and relinquish control of their lives to others without question are often viewed as the "good" or adjusted residents. Those who protest and demand their own way are viewed as the "bad" or maladjusted residents (Fig. 16-4). These are mistaken notions. Persons who give up control are more at risk of low self-esteem, hopelessness, powerlessness, and social isolation than are those who manipulate, argue, or complain in order to maintain some control over their lives.

Assessment

See the assessment of self-perception and self-concept on p. 269.

Nursing Diagnosis

Powerlessness

Nursing Goals/Outcomes

The nursing goals for elderly individuals diagnosed with powerlessness are (1) to identify actions in which they can exert control and (2) to make decisions and have input in the plan of care.

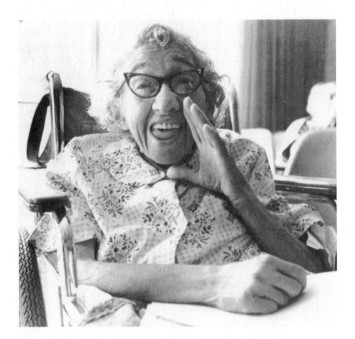

FIG. 16-4 Assertiveness. (Photograph by Marianne Gontartz. Courtesy of the American Society on Aging.)

Nursing Interventions

The following interventions should take place in hospitals, extended-care facilities, and at home:

1. **Allow the elderly to make choices whenever possible.** Even in institutional settings, choices should be made by the elderly as often as possible. Menus can be planned to include options such as sandwiches for people who do not like the menu items. A variety of suitable clothing can be displayed before dressing so that individuals can select the articles they desire. Enough activities should be available so that the person can find one that interests him or her.

2. **Encourage the elderly to do as much as possible for themselves.** When people perform their own care, they feel more in control. Such control of simple things can help maintain a sense of being able to influence what happens.

3. **Adapt the environment to encourage independent activity.** Nurses should evaluate the environment, taking into consideration the strengths and the limitations of the elderly. Many elderly lose their sense of power because things in the environment are outside of their control. When the elderly must always ask for things or call on nurses for help, the nurses control the situation. Modifying the environment so that all necessary or desired items (e.g., walkers) are close at hand gives control back to the elderly. Elevated toilets can reduce the need to call for assistance. Providing snacks and beverages in a readily accessible place such as a lounge provides control.

4. **Explain the reasons for any changes in the plan**

NURSING CARE PLAN

SELF-PERCEPTION/SELF-CONCEPT

Mrs. Green, age 90, was living independently until recently, when she suffered a fall that resulted in a broken hip. Her family is unable to provide the ongoing care she requires because they too are getting old and they live in a different state. Mrs. Green is a new resident of Golden Grove Nursing Home. She is very passive and allows the staff to do everything for her despite the fact that she is capable of doing many things for herself. She does not express any feelings or preferences about her care, meals, or anything else. When asked about her perceptions she says, "It doesn't matter. You'll do whatever you want anyway." She prefers to remain in her room.

NURSING DIAGNOSIS

Powerlessness

DEFINING CHARACTERISTICS

- Passive behavior
- Apathetic responses
- Verbalization of lack of control
- Nonparticipation in care

GOALS/OUTCOMES

Mrs. Green will participate in decision making regarding her care and identify actions within her control.

NURSING INTERVENTIONS

1. Visit daily for 10 to 15 minutes to allow Mrs. Green to verbalize her feelings and concerns.
2. Respect Mrs. Green's right to private space. Allow her to choose what belongings she wants and where she wants them.
3. Actively include her in care planning, present her with options, and then follow through with her choices.
4. Explain the reasons for any changes that must be made.
5. Keep the call signal handy and respond promptly when called.
6. Meet her requests promptly.
7. Encourage participation in personal care.
8. Assist her in identifying areas in which she can retain control.

EVALUATION

The nursing assistant reports that Mrs. Green is demonstrating more assertive behaviors such as insisting on choosing her own clothing and stating preferences about meals. She has been heard saying "I will do that later when I am ready!" You will continue the plan of care.

of care. At times the plan of care may need to be changed. When this is necessary, the elderly should be informed as soon as the change is known. The reasons for the change should be explained so the person understands that the change occurred because of certain circumstances and not simply because the nurses are assuming control of the patient's right to make choices.

5. **Avoid being overprotective or directive.** Nurses and other caregivers often do not allow the elderly to use their abilities. In the name of concern and caring, caregivers do too much for the elderly. This can lead to one of two possible outcomes: either the elderly person becomes angry and tells the caregiver to leave him or her alone, or the elderly person gives up and lets the caregiver do everything. In the first case, the person may not get help when he or she really needs it. In the latter, the person is likely to experience a rapid loss of ability. The best approach is a balanced one in which caregivers sup-

port and encourage the elderly to perform as much for themselves as is safely possible. Unless the situation is harmful, nurses may have to learn to accept less than perfection and avoid redoing what the person has done for him- or herself. Redoing what has already been done can strip away the elderly person's dignity and make him or her feel impotent and childlike. Therefore, help should be provided only when it is needed and only to the extent it is needed.

6. **Respect the elderly's right to refuse.** The ultimate power held by patients is the right to refuse care. Elderly persons who are in control of their mental faculties retain this right, and nurses cannot force them to do anything against their wishes. When a person refuses food, care, or medication, nurses should first determine the reasons for the refusal. Once the reasons are known, nurses should develop a plan to reduce or remove the objections. Unless the reasons for refusal are known, any approaches are likely to be unsuccessful. Often a good explanation of the importance of the treatment or medication can overcome objections and relieve conflict. In other cases, minor modifications such as changing the method or timing of medications will work. For some individuals, consultation with the dietitian, physician, or other specialist is needed to solve the problem. If alert older persons continue to refuse care despite attempts to gain acceptance, nurses should accept the refusal. This does not mean that further attempts to gain compliance cannot or should not be made in the future. When a person refuses some or all parts of his or her care, nurses should document all of the facts of the situation as well as all interventions that were tried.

If the elderly are unable to make judgments because of impaired cognitive function, a different situation exists. In these cases, the families or guardians should be actively involved in planning care.

These individuals may be able to suggest ways to get the person to cooperate. Persons who hold legal guardianship can speak for patients in determining what should be done. Nurses should also discuss these concerns and problems with the physician. Many times changes in the medical plan can eliminate problems.

A nursing care plan for powerlessness is presented on p. 277.

SUMMARY

Both age- and disease-related changes affect the elderly's image of themselves; societal values and life experiences also play a role. Self-concept is closely related to the elderly person's values, beliefs, roles, and relationships. When the elderly suffer losses in any important area of life, self-concept is threatened. If these individuals are able to maintain a sense of self-worth and personal value, few problems occur. If they feel that they are of little value, serious problems, including fear, anxiety, hopelessness, and powerlessness, will result. These disturbances can significantly affect the elderly's response to care. Nurses should pay close attention to what older adults have to say about themselves. Measures should be taken to provide emotional support, enhance personal control, and promote self-esteem in the elderly.

READINGS AND REFERENCES
Carpenito LJ: *Nursing Diagnosis: application to clinical practice,* ed 6, Philadelphia, 1995, JB Lippincott.
Genevay B: See me! Hear me! Know who I am! An experience of being assessed, *Generations* 21:16, 1997.
Janelli LM: Are there body image differences between older men and women? *West J Nurs Res* 15:327, 1993.
Porter EJ: Non-equilibrium systems theory: some applications for gerontological nursing pressure, *J Gerontol Nurs* 212:24, 1995.

chapter seventeen
17

ROLES AND RELATIONSHIPS

LEARNING OBJECTIVES

1. Describe normal roles and relationships.
2. Describe how patterns of roles and relationships change with aging.
3. Discuss the effects of disease processes on the ability to maintain roles and relationships.
4. Describe methods of assessing changes in roles and relationships.
5. Identify the elderly who are most at risk for experiencing problems related to changes in roles and relationships.
6. Identify selected nursing diagnoses related to role or relationship problems.
7. Describe nursing interventions that are appropriate for elderly individuals experiencing problems related to changing roles and relationships.

NORMAL ROLES AND RELATIONSHIPS

A **role** is a socially accepted behavior pattern. People tend to establish their identities and to describe themselves based on the roles they play in life. Man, woman, husband, wife, adult, senior citizen, parent, child, son, daughter, student, teacher, doctor, nurse, worker, and housewife are some common roles. People play many roles over a lifetime and often must attempt to play several roles simultaneously.

Roles are identified, defined, and given value by the society in which a person lives. Each member of society learns the status of various roles and learns to expect certain behaviors, symbols, and relationships that are acceptable for each role. The behaviors, symbols, and relationship patterns can differ widely, depending on the values and norms of the society in which the individual lives. The value assigned by society indicates the status of each role. Those in high-status roles generally possess more privileges and receive more rewards. For example, modern society gives bosses higher status than employees, teachers higher status than students, employed persons higher status than unemployed persons, and younger, more productive members of society higher status than older, retired members.

Relationships are connections formed by the dynamic interaction of individuals who play interrelated roles. Most people develop a wide range of relationships within their families, at work, and during day-to-day social activities. The way individuals occupying each role interact with each other describes their relationships. Relationships can be short or long-term, personal or impersonal, intimate or superficial. Relationships change over time and are affected by the role changes of the people involved.

Each culture and subculture set standards for designated roles and relationships. People in various roles or relationships are expected to behave in accord with accepted standards, which include things like the amount and type of clothing or jewelry that are appropriate. Standards specify the type of housing, the means of transportation, and even the type and amount of food consumed. Standards specify how individuals in the culture relate to each other in social and work situations. For example, the role perception for a middle-class American businessman is that he is expected to wear a suit and tie with minimum jewelry, live in an apartment or house in the suburbs, drive a conventional car, eat healthy meals, show up for work on time, and show respect to the boss. If this businessman showed up late for work wearing jeans and a sweatshirt, wearing an earring and riding a motorcycle, and eating a hamburger and telling the boss not to "bug" him, most people would be shocked. Yet this behavior is not considered atypical for a college student—even one who is studying to be a businessman.

A simple, or **homogeneous**, society is one in which all members share a common historical and cultural experience. There is little confusion or conflict in a homogeneous social system because the symbols, behaviors, and relationships are perceived in the same way by all members of the society. Everyone knows the accepted roles and how people in each role are expected to relate to each other. Therefore, there is little question and few problems with regard to role or relationship expectations.

A more complex, or **heterogeneous**, society is one in which the members of many diverse subcultures with different historic and cultural experiences must interact. These subcultures may have their origin in race, religion, ethnic heritage, or age. Because subcultures do not share the same experiences, their symbols, behaviors, roles, and relationships are not perceived in the same way by all members of the larger society. Roles and role expectations are not always clear, and this lack of shared perceptions frequently leads to misunderstandings, confusion, and conflict.

American culture is very heterogeneous and is becoming even more so. Problems are likely to occur when people with different role and relationship perceptions are required to interact with each other. The greater the differences in role perceptions, role symbols, and role relationships, the greater the likelihood of cross-cultural misunderstandings will be. This explains the confusion or stress many people experience when they interact with individuals of different ages or from different cultural backgrounds. It also explains why a person who was raised in a specific culture is more comfortable with similar individuals and finds it difficult to establish close relationships with people from different cultural backgrounds. It also explains why people of different ages may have difficulty understanding each other. The diversity of the population contributes to the prevalence of role and relationship problems in contemporary American society.

However, this is not the only role or relationship issue people face. In addition to the interpersonal conflict or confusion seen in modern society, individuals can also experience *internal* role conflict and confusion. Problems occur when the demands of multiple roles and relationships must be met at the same time, particularly when the expectations of one role conflict with those of another. For example: women today are often expected to be wife, mother, and employee. They are expected to keep the home, prepare meals, supervise the children, be active in school or community programs, be social and sexual companions to their spouses, and be productive workers who are capable of doing everything while working with everyone, and always arriving on time with smiles on their faces. Unless she is superwoman, she is bound to fall short of someone's expectations.

Most people occupy multiple roles and develop a variety of relationships throughout their lives. People think of themselves and establish their identities in terms of their roles and relationships. If you ask people to describe themselves, you will typically receive a list of roles or relationships (e.g., mother, engineer, supervisor) rather than a list of personal characteristics.

Because people form their self-image based on their roles and relationships, they are likely to have difficulty accepting changes in either. Our identity and sense of self are threatened when roles are lost and the associated relationships change. The longer the role was held and the more intense the relationships, the greater the grief will be. When a person's role changes, the symbols and indicators of role and status also change. Loss of symbols or status is often as painful as the loss of the role. People may grieve a change of role or loss of relationship as much as they grieve the loss of a loved one.

ROLES, RELATIONSHIPS, AND AGING

As previously discussed, societies establish and define the boundaries of various roles. Individuals are judged by how well they understand and comply with their assigned roles. "Old person" is a role that has many connotations and expected behaviors. The ageists in contemporary American society would define the role of the elderly as helpless, infirm, cranky, and useless. Some elderly accept this stereotype and act the part. However, more and more elderly are continuing in productive roles and maintaining successful relationships well into their eighties and nineties.

The longer a person occupies a particular role, the more familiar and consequently more comfortable he or she becomes with it. The more comfortable people are in their roles and relationships, the harder it is to adjust to changes.

The elderly must adjust to many predictable role and relationship changes associated with aging. The elderly must adjust to retirement, altered relationships with adult children, changes in housing, loss of valued possessions, loss of friends due to relocation or death, and loss of a spouse to death, loss of health, and loss of independence. All of these changes and losses are potentially very traumatic to the elderly.

Many elderly resent the fact that society forces them to retire. Age 65, which was once the typical retirement age, no longer is. This is partially due to financial reasons; but it is also because many elderly people do not want to retire because they feel that they would lose too much of their identity if they did. They say, "I don't know what I would do if I couldn't work." Elderly persons who do retire may adjust well or poorly, depending on the adequacy of their other roles to keep them satisfied. Generally, the more roles and relationships a person develops at younger ages, the better his or her ability to adjust will be when some of those roles and relationships are lost.

When an occupational role no longer exists, the individual often grieves its loss. Many people look forward to retirement but once retired find that they miss both the status that role gave them and the interaction with other people. They often resent the fact that they are no longer viewed as productive, contributing members of society. They are no longer lawyers, plumbers, nurses, or teachers; they are just retired people.

To maintain a connection with those who are still employed, many retired elderly continue to think of themselves as a part of their occupation. A nurse remains a nurse for life, a plumber remains a plumber, and so on. Even if they have not worked in the occupation for years, most elderly persons continue to identify with their previous occupational roles. This may be particularly obvious in elderly professionals (e.g., physicians, lawyers, professors, ministers) who never stop using their titles. Many expect to retain the same status level and respect as was paid to them when they were actively employed and are highly insulted if this respect is not forthcoming.

There are some roles from which a person cannot "retire." Homemaker is one such role. Elderly persons who have spent the largest part of their lives managing a home—doing the cooking, cleaning, sewing, and other duties required of a homemaker—may feel lost when they are forced by circumstances of ill health or finances to give up the home. Many elderly homemakers (primarily women) have few other roles and feel a great sense of loss when institutionalized. Those who took the time to develop hobbies or social interests and relationships outside of the home tend to adapt better than do those who had no interests other than their homes.

The elderly do not give up the role of parent just because their children are adults. The role of parent is usually identified as being self-sufficient and in control. Role conflict and altered family relationships are likely to occur when older adults attempt to continue to direct their children's behavior long after the children are adults or when the parents lose the ability to function independently and are forced to become dependent on their children. Successful adjustment to

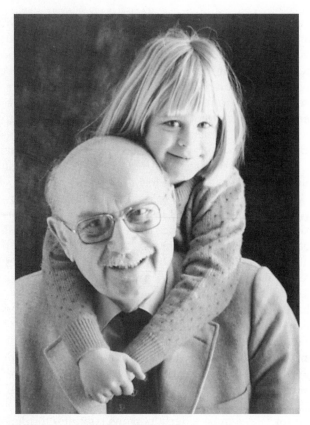

FIG. 17-1 Grandparenting. (Courtesy of the American Society on Aging.)

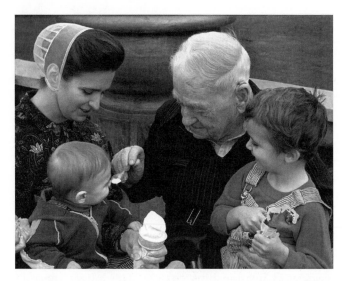

FIG. 17-2 Grandfather helping with the responsibilities of feeding baby. (Courtesy of Rod Schmall, West Linn, Ore.)

changes in the parenting role is very difficult and requires a great deal of patience, tact, and accommodation on the part of all family members. Families who have a history of altered parenting or poorly developed family relationships are likely to have serious problems leading to abuse or isolation of the elderly person from his or her family.

In addition to being the parent of adult children, many older adults are grandparents. The role of grandparent is often described as being much more pleasant than that of being a parent. As one grandmother said "I can have all of the fun and enjoyment of children without the responsibility." Another grandmother replied, "Yes, it's nice when they come to visit, but it's nice when you can send them home."

Grandparenting allows older adults to share their wisdom and experiences with a new, young generation. Because grandparents are often under less daily stress and are not the primary disciplinarians of the children, they are usually more relaxed and have more time to spend on "nonessential" activities such as conversation and play (Fig. 17-1). It is common for retired grandparents with time on their hands to entertain children with stories or teach them skills, hobbies, or games that the grandparents learned as children. When positive interactions take place between grand-

parents and grandchildren a close bond is often formed that benefits both parties (Fig. 17-2). Mobility and the resulting separation of family members often make it difficult for this relationship to develop. Both parties are usually worse off for not knowing the other.

Many elderly persons have occupied the role of spouse for 30, 40, or 50 or more years. With the death of a partner, these persons are deprived of a significant role and relationship. Marriage is one of the most personal and intimate relationships. A successful long-term marriage requires a great deal of effort, the loss of this intensely personal relationship triggers a high level of emotional distress. Many widowed elderly experience severe grief and social isolation as a result of the loss. They describe themselves as feeling as though half of them was missing, of feeling half-alive. Many widows and widowers find their grief to be so overwhelming that they cannot even continue to perform normal activities of daily living.

The loss of friends due to relocation or death also results in changed social roles and relationships. Many activities require more than one person to be fun. Many elderly have formed friendships or social groups over the years. As more and more of the members move away or die, the elderly person is likely to become more and more socially isolated. Elderly persons who outlive their families and friends often feel that their lives are without purpose.

Many elderly change housing arrangements out of choice or necessity. The house may be too big, too expensive, or too difficult to maintain. This is particularly true when the health of one or both occupants fails or when a widow is unable to keep up the home after loss of the spouse. Moves to smaller accommodations frequently necessitate the sale or distribution of personal possessions accumulated over a lifetime. This loss of possessions makes the process of moving even more traumatic for the elderly. In some ways they are "giving away" their lives.

Loss of health and independence are probably the most traumatic losses because they involve changes in the very essence of who people are. When the elderly lose health and independence, they lose control over their own destiny. They are at the mercy of others (either family or strangers) for care and sustenance.

Assessment of Roles and Relationships

- What is the person's marital status (i.e., single, married, widowed, divorced)?
- If the person has lost a spouse or significant other, how long ago did this occur?
- Does the person live alone or with others?
- If the person lives with others, who are they and how are they related? What is the family structure?
- How does the person describe relationships within the family?
- What family interactions have you or others observed?
- Does the person belong to any social groups?
- Does the person have close relationships with friends?
- Is the individual employed? What are the relationships at work?
- Has the person retired from work? How long ago? What are his or her feelings regarding retirement? What does the person do to occupy his or her time?
- Does the person feel a part of the community or neighborhood?
- If in a long-term care setting, has the person established relationships with other residents?
- Has the person recently relocated? From home to an acute-care setting? From home to an extended-care facility? From one unit or room to another?
- Does the person spend a great deal of time alone?
- Does the person speak excessively with others or remain silent?
- Does the person exhibit signs of withdrawal, anger, depression, sorrow, fear, or shock?
- Has the person verbalized concerns regarding losses of persons, jobs, or abilities?
- Have the person's sleep or eating patterns changed?
- Has the person's ability to concentrate changed?

See Box 17-1 for a list of risk factors for problems related to changes in roles and relationships in the elderly.

BOX 17-1

Risk Factors Related to Changes in Roles and Relationships in the Elderly

- Recent loss of a spouse, child, close friend, significant other, or cherished pet
- Recent loss of lifelong or valuable roles
- Recent major adjustment in his or her living situation
- Inability to perform familiar roles owing to loss of functional abilities

---

NURSING PROCESS
DYSFUNCTIONAL GRIEVING

Grief is a strong emotion. It is a combination of sorrow, loss, and confusion that comes when someone or something of value is lost. This reaction could come in response to the loss of a person, role, relationship, health, or independence.

Grief affects thoughts, emotions, and behavior and creates a wide range of physical sensations. The normal grief response follows a somewhat predictable pattern, although the exact amount of time any given individual will need to work through a loss will differ (Table 17-1).

Grief is normal after the loss of a significant role or relationship. Grieving leads to dysfunction when the person has an exaggerated or prolonged period of grief. Continued sadness, anger, or denial are indicative of poorly resolved grief. Many times grief is so severe that it prevents the person from normal functioning (Box 17-2). Elderly persons experiencing dysfunctional grief may completely shut themselves off from normal support systems, lose interest in all activities, and even fail to perform the basic activities of daily living.

Assessment

See the assessment of roles and relationships on this page.

Nursing Diagnosis

Dysfunctional grieving

Nursing Goals/Outcomes

The nursing goals for elderly individuals with dysfunctional grieving are (1) to verbalize their grief; (2) to use available support systems; and (3) to participate in activities of daily living.

TABLE 17-1

Stages of Grieving

SHOCK AND NUMBNESS (FIRST 2 WEEKS)

Feelings: Disbelief, denial, anger, and guilt

Behaviors: Crying, searching, sighing, loss of appetite, sleep disturbance, limited concentration, muscle weakness, inability to make decisions, emotional outbursts

SEARCHING AND YEARNING (2 WEEKS TO 4 MONTHS)

Feelings: Despair, apathy, depression, anger, guilt, hopelessness, self-doubt

Behaviors: Restlessness, poor memory, impatience, lack of concentration, crying, social isolation, loss of energy

DISORIENTATION (4 TO 7 MONTHS)

Feelings: Depression, guilt, disorganization

Behaviors: Resistance to seeking help or reaching out to others, trying to live as if nothing happened, restlessness, irritability

REORGANIZATION (UP TO 18 TO 24 MONTHS)

Feelings: Sense of release, sense of obsession with loss decreases, renewed hope and optimism

Behaviors: Renewed energy, reorganization of eating and sleeping habits, improved judgement, renewed interest in activities and goals for the future

Modified from Davidson G: *The mourning process,* Web site: http://www.netmediapro.com/add/grieving.htm#gro5

BOX 17-2

Normal Loss/Grief Reactions

PHYSICAL
Persistent fatigue
Tightness in chest
Muscle weakness
Shortness of breath
Susceptibility to minor illnesses
Hypersensitivity to noise
Dry mouth
Headaches
Grinding teeth
Tension
Nausea
Hyperacidity
Dizziness

EMOTIONAL
Anger
Anxiety
Ambivalence
Depression
Fear
Irritability
Loneliness
Numbness
Panic

Sadness
Guilt
Shock
Helplessness
Apathy

COGNITIVE
Confusion
Forgetfulness
Disorientation
Disbelief
Preoccupation
Decreased attention
Inability to concentrate

BEHAVIORAL
Absent mindedness
Crying
Decreased motivation
Restlessness
Social isolation
Inconsistency
Irritability
Diminished productivity
Sleep disturbances
Appetite disturbances

Nursing Interventions

The following nursing interventions should take place in hospitals, extended-care facilities, and at home:

1. **Establish a trusting relationship to encourage verbalization of feelings regarding the change or loss.** Before sharing their true feelings, the elderly must develop trust in their nurses. Trust comes only when they believe that the nurses truly care about them as unique human beings and that the nurses will be understanding and sensitive to their feelings. It takes time and effort to develop trust.

   Trust cannot be forced. It may take days, weeks, or even months for a grieving person to share his or her deepest feelings. Although trust cannot be forced, nurses can take actions to promote its development. These actions are summarized in Box 17-3.

2. **Assess the source and acknowledge the reality of the grief.** Grief is very much like pain. It is a complex and personal emotion. Because most people find it difficult to deal with grief, they avoid grieving persons and avoid discussing anything that approaches the source of the grief. These behaviors leave the problem unresolved. To help with grief, it is essential that the grieving person identify and confront the loss. Nurses can help by spending time with grieving individuals and by allowing them the opportunity to verbalize their grief. Once able to verbalize and acknowledge their grief, nurses can use problem-solving methods to help the elderly develop coping strategies.

3. **Encourage the elderly to participate in activities of daily living.** Grieving individuals are often totally preoccupied with their loss. Although this preoccupation is understandable, it is incompatible with normal living. The more grieving people are able to maintain contact with day-to-day activities, the sooner they will be able to go on with life. Nurses can help by providing structure to the day. A plan of care that allows for preferences while setting limits helps provide this structure. A daily schedule that is well planned and predictable often enables the grieving elderly to regain some control and to cope with the changes. Encouragement and positive feedback for participation in daily activities help motivate positive behaviors.

4. **Identify sources of support.** Although nurses can provide some support to grieving elderly persons, many others can also help. Family, friends, spiritual advisers, counselors, therapists, and support groups are all valuable sources.

   Many pamphlets, books, and other materials are available to help people who are experiencing grief. Many are available in libraries, physician's offices, or other locations where the elderly congregate.

NURSING PROCESS

SOCIAL ISOLATION AND IMPAIRED SOCIAL INTERACTION

Social isolation, the sense of being alone, is a common problem among the elderly. Those experiencing social isolation are likely to be uncommunicative and withdrawn and to have few visitors or other social interactions. Social isolation is a result of many factors and can be unintentional or intentional. The more people are separated from family and friends, the greater the likelihood of social isolation will be.

Most social isolation is unintentional. Separation due to death is a common and unavoidable part of aging. Many elderly people simply outlive their families and friends. These people are likely to become isolated unless they establish new social outlets. Separation due to relocation is also common. Today it is unusual for family members to remain in a single community. Young family members move to find job opportunities; elderly family members move to retirement communities.

Decreased physical mobility and limited finances can result in social isolation. Physical changes can restrict an elderly person's ability to move about and make social contacts. Financial limitations can lead to separation from others because of the lack of adequate money to buy appropriate clothing or transportation to social activities.

Intentional isolation is less common and is most likely to occur when the elderly fear not being accepted by others. Those who suffer from grief may be too upset or absorbed in their own problems to interact with others. Elderly persons experiencing changes in body image from such procedures as amputation or colostomy are also likely to isolate themselves from others. Elderly persons who have cognitive or perceptual problems may isolate themselves because they do not understand what is going on around them.

BOX 17-3

Actions that Promote Trust

- Spend time with the person.
- Actively listen to what the person says.
- Address the person by name.
- Smile.
- Use a warm, friendly voice.
- Make appropriate eye contact.
- Respond to questions honestly.
- Provide consistency of care.
- Respect confidentiality.
- Follow through on commitments.

Assessment

See the assessment of roles and relationships on p. 283.

Nursing Diagnosis

Impaired social interaction

Nursing Goals/Outcomes

The nursing goals for elderly individuals with impaired social interaction are (1) to demonstrate increased participation in social activities and (2) to identify actions or resources that will help reduce social isolation.

Nursing Interventions

The following nursing interventions should take place in hospitals, extended-care facilities, and at home:

1. **Assess the reason or reasons for the social isolation.** Because many factors can lead to social isolation, nurses should identify those that affect each individual. Interventions should be directed at specific problems.
2. **Promote social contact and interaction.** Telephone calls and mail can be used to maintain contact with family and friends. Phones should be readily available and located so that the elderly can have privacy yet comfort when using them (Fig. 17-3). Phones can be equipped with amplifiers for those who are hard of hearing. Mail should be delivered promptly. Visually impaired elderly should be offered help in reading mail.

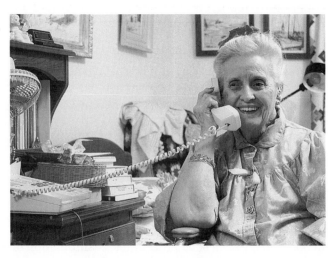

FIG. 17-3   A resident maintaining social contact by using the telephone. (From Sorrentino SA: *Mosby's textbook for nursing assistants*, ed 4, St Louis, 1996, Mosby.)

Social rooms and lounges should be available for the elderly to use for visits. If the individual is confined to bed, privacy to conduct visits in the room should be given.

Information about all activities in a facility should be well communicated to the elderly residents. Nurses should offer encouragement to those who are reluctant to participate in activities.

Careful planning is needed to prevent social isolation in elderly individuals with restricted physical mobility. Nursing care should be scheduled so there is adequate time for social interaction. The care plan should provide for any assistance required to enable participation in social activities.

3. **Spend one-on-one time with the isolated person.** Those who cannot or will not participate in social interaction will need extra attention from the nursing staff. One-on-one interaction, even for brief intervals during the day, will help these persons maintain some social contact. Over time, nurses can attempt to motivate these individuals to try other forms of social contact.
4. **Initiate referrals.** Many times the social worker, chaplain, or activities department can help socially isolated elderly persons to identify acceptable social activities.

NURSING PROCESS

ALTERATION IN FAMILY PROCESSES

Normal changes in family processes were discussed in Chapter 1. Whenever elderly persons or their families verbalize concern or confusion related to a change in roles or relationships, family dynamics should be assessed. Alterations in family processes can occur at any age but are most common when an aging family member becomes dependent.

Assessment

See the assessment of roles and relationships on p. 283.

Nursing Diagnosis

Altered family processes

Nursing Goals/Outcomes

The nursing goals for elderly individuals with altered family processes are (1) to express their feelings regarding changes in roles and relationships and (2) to work with family members to develop strategies for coping with changing roles and relationships.

Nursing Interventions

The following nursing interventions should take place in hospitals, extended-care facilities, and at home:

1. **Assess interactions between the elderly and their families.** Nurses should spend time sitting in when family members visit their aging relatives. Nurses should be alert for signs of destructive emotions such as anger or frustration. If these are evident, a rest time or coffee break should be suggested to reduce the tension and allow the family members a chance to calm down. When they have been separated, nurses can try to explore their feelings individually and suggest coping strategies.

2. **Encourage all family members to verbalize their feelings.** It is best to explore the feelings of family members independently. Many people, both old and young, are afraid to express their real feelings in the presence of other involved parties. Nurses should spend time with the elderly and each individual family member in private settings. During this time, it is important to convey to all concerned family members that all feelings, including those of anger and frustration, are acceptable and will be held in confidence. Expressing the negative emotions that are triggered by the stress of coping with changing roles and relationships is not easy for most people and will take time. Once feelings are identified, then positive coping strategies can be developed.

3. **Assist family members in identifying personal and family strengths.** Each person and each family have weaknesses and strengths. The key to maintaining or repairing family dynamics is identification of the strengths. Love, concern, and shared spiritual values can be used as a basis for positive relationships.

4. **Encourage family members to visit regularly.** When an aging family member is hospitalized or resides in an institutional setting, the family may feel useless or unnecessary. Some family members feel that their presence is not desired by the nursing staff. Nurses should recognize that family members are able to relate to the elderly in unique and special ways. Rather than make the family uncomfortable, the nursing staff should do everything possible to make them feel welcome and at ease. Greeting family members by name helps forge bonds of mutual caring. Responding promptly to requests and showing small considerations (e.g., offering the family members a cup of coffee) can go a long way in making them feel valued.

5. **Encourage the family members to assist in elder care.** Family members are often able and willing to help the nursing staff care for aging loved ones. Assisting with care provides the family with the opportunity to show their concern for the aging person. Assisting with care should not be expected or demanded, but it should be encouraged if the family appears willing. The amount of involvement will differ from family to family. Some family members may desire to perform a great deal of the care, even bathing and feeding. Others are more comfortable helping with less technical things such as hair grooming or shaving. Nurses can help families by providing all necessary equipment, by teaching families safe and effective ways to perform tasks, and by providing positive comments for a job well done.

6. **Assist families in identifying factors that are interfering with normal interactions.** Normal physiologic changes, illness, disability, side effects of medication, decreased finances, and other events can affect the behavior of the elderly and interfere with normal family interactions. Nurses should do a thorough assessment to determine the factors at play in any given situation. Once the causative factors are identified, nurses can work with the elderly and their families to develop a plan that eliminates or reduces the problems and thereby facilitates more normal interactions.

7. **Explore community resources.** If the family dynamics are severely altered, nurses may be unable to meet the family's needs. Special assistance in the form of support groups, geriatric social workers, or geropsychiatric clinics are available in many communities. Nurses should be aware of the resources available in a specific community and make information about these resources available to all family members.

A nursing care plan for social isolation is presented on p. 288.

SUMMARY

People play many roles and have many integral relationships over a lifetime. When aging results in loss of these roles and changes in relationships, grief is a normal response. However, if the grief response is severe, the elderly person may lose all interest in life. Grieving people are often unwilling to participate even in normal daily care or activities. To break through this grief, nurses must attempt to build a trusting relationship in which the elderly person can work through the loss and grief. Hopefully, this will enable the person to find new meaning in life and to build new relationships.

The elderly may become isolated from social inter-

NURSING CARE PLAN

SOCIAL INTERACTION

Mrs. Hixton is an alert, generally healthy 77-year-old widow who lives alone in the home she and her husband shared until his death from cancer last year. Her daughter lives several hundred miles away and calls occasionally. The home hospice nurse who visited regularly during her husband's illness stopped by as part of her routine follow-up and found that Mrs. Hixton spends most of her time in the house with the shades drawn and only goes out to buy groceries and other necessary items. She drives to church weekly but does not speak to other church members. She speaks hesitantly to the nurse and makes little eye contact during the conversation. With tears in her eyes she states that "Nobody cares about me anymore; they all have somebody, but I have nobody."

NURSING DIAGNOSIS:

Social isolation

DEFINING CHARACTERISTICS

- Feelings of rejection and being alone
- Absence of supportive family or friends
- Withdrawal from contact with others
- Sad, dull affect
- Lack of eye contact
- Preoccupation with own thoughts

GOALS/OUTCOMES

Mrs. Hixton will demonstrate increased participation in social activities and identify actions or resources that will help reduce social isolation.

INTERVENTIONS

1. Allow Mrs. Hixton time to verbalize feelings of sadness or depression relating to loss of her spouse.
2. Encourage her to develop a list of family members and friends with whom she previously socialized.
3. Encourage her to make contact with her daughter by phone on a weekly basis.
4. Identify social activities that were previously of interest.
5. Encourage participation in a grief counseling group.
6. Consult with minister regarding visitations.

EVALUATION

Mrs. Hixton hesitantly expressed willingness to attend one session of grief counseling. During this session she sat quietly and listened to others explain what they were going through. At the next home visit she told the nurse "I think I'll go to another session. There was another woman there who's having the same problems I am. She offered to have coffee with me." You will continue the plan of care.

action. Social isolation may result from ineffective methods of coping with grief or from impaired family dynamics.

Roles and relationships are maintained through communication with others. If the ability to communicate with others is impaired (as is the case with many of the common disorders of aging such as stroke or dementia), the ability to maintain relationships is af-

fected. Elderly persons with impaired communication are likely to feel isolated from family and friends and from normal social interactions (see the following critical thinking box).

Nurses who work with the elderly should understand the effects of changes in roles and relationships. An understanding of the significance of these losses will enable nurses to more effectively assess the be-

CRITICAL THINKING • ROLES

Identify five roles you currently have. Write these on separate slips of paper and turn them over on a table. Pick up one slip at random and look at it. Now throw it away. You have just lost that role. What impact does it have on your life? How does it change your relationships with others? How do you think others will now perceive you? How do you feel about the loss? How is your self-image affected?

Now repeat this over and over again until all of the slips are gone, asking yourself the same questions. When all of the slips are gone, what do you have left?

havior of the elderly and to plan interventions that will be of benefit.

READINGS AND REFERENCES

Clements M: What we say about aging, *Parade* Dec 12, 1993.

Davis S: The enduring power of friendship, *Am Health* 15:60, 1996.

Elder's "favorite" story can provide insights, *Brown University Long-Term Care Quality Letter* 5:S2, 1993.

Field D, et al: The influence of health on family contacts and family feelings in advanced old age: a longitudinal study, *J Gerontol* 48:P18, 1993.

Glass TA, et al: Change in productive activity in late adulthood: McArthur studies of successful aging, *J Gerontol* 50:S65, 1995.

Gratton B, Haber C: Three phases in the history of American grandparents: authority, burden, companion, *Generations* 20:7, 1996.

Kane RA: From generation to generation: thoughts on legacy, *Generations* 20:5, 1996.

Maynard J: The grandest lessons: we may not always approve of their approach to childrearing, but grandparents have a lot to offer our children, *Parenting* 10:75, 1996.

McGowen JB: Successful aging linked to productive activity, *J Commun Health Nurs* 12:252, 1995.

Taxel L: Bridging the generations, *Nat Health* 23:80, 1993.

Tobin SS: Cherished possessions: the meaning of things, *Generations* 20:46, 1996.

Venkatraman MM: A cross-cultural study of the subjective well-being of married elderly persons in the United States and India, *J Gerontol* 50:S35, 1995.

Ventura M: Confessions of an eternal romantic: passion and enduring love often seem at odds. So why do we keep striving to capture both in the same relationship? *Psychol Today* 30:34, 1997.

Weissbourd B: The grandparent bond, *Parents Magazine* 72:113, 1997.

chapter eighteen

COPING AND STRESS

1. Explain the concepts of stress and coping.
2. Identify the physical, emotional, and behavioral signs of stress.
3. Describe methods for reducing stress.
4. Discuss changes in stress and coping that occur with aging.
5. Identify the elderly who are most at risk for experiencing stress-related problems.
6. Discuss methods of coping with stress and depression.
7. Identify selected nursing diagnoses related to stress-related problems.
8. Describe nursing interventions that are appropriate for elderly individuals who are experiencing problems related to stress and coping.

NORMAL STRESS AND COPING

Stress is a normal part of life. No one lives without it. Stress occurs whenever a person is faced with a real or perceived threat or experiences a significant or life-altering change. Stressors include *external physical threats* such as extreme heat or cold, noise, or physical trauma; *internal* or *psychological threats* such as thoughts and feelings; and *external social threats* such as job pressures or changeable social relationships. Stress often results from a combination of these factors. The more stressors a person faces, the greater his or her level of stress will be. Stress occurs whether the threat or change is positive or negative.

Each of us faces a steady stream of life events with which we must cope. Some are temporary or minor events such as taking a test or giving a speech that may cause mild distress for a short period of time. Major life events such as the death of a spouse, serious injury, birth of a child, or marriage are likely to cause significant stress that lasts for a longer period of time. People experiencing high levels of stress feel exhausted, anxious, and vulnerable.

Different experiences are stressful to different people. Individual perceptions play an important role in determining what constitutes a stressor. Muscle pain, for example, is a stressor to most people but not to an athlete who views it as a measure of training. Public speaking is highly stressful to most people, but not to a politician who does it every day.

Various rating scales have been developed to quantify the amount of stress caused by common social and psychologic occurrences in the lives of elderly people (Table 18-1). In these rating scales, various events are based on the proportional amount of distress involved. These scales are useful general guides when one attempts to measure the amount of stress caused by a particular event. Stress is cumulative, and a combination of several smaller stressors can have the same effects as a major stressor. The more stressors a person faces at a time, the greater the likelihood will be of physical, cognitive, and behavioral changes.

When confronted with stressful events, the body undergoes predictable physiologic responses that prepare the body to withstand the threat and maintain homeostasis. The general adaptation syndrome, developed by Dr. Hans Selye, describes the collective responses of the body to stress. According to this theory, stress activates both the sympathetic and parasympathetic components of the autonomic nervous system, initiating a series of physiologic responses.

The general alarm reaction, often called the *fight-or-flight response,* occurs first. In this stage, the body undergoes a predictable range of responses or physiologic changes that are designed to overcome the threat. If these physiologic responses are effective, the body enters a stage of resistance during which it returns to normal functioning. If the responses are not effective, the body depletes its energy reserves and enters the stage of exhaustion. In the most severe cases, this exhaustion can result in death.

Physical Signs of Stress
Cardiovascular signs

People experiencing stress often report that their hearts are "racing" and "pounding." When the sympathetic nervous system is activated by stress, the heart rate and amount of blood ejected from the heart during each contraction increase. These changes allow more blood and oxygen to reach the body tissue, thereby preparing it for action. The peripheral blood vessels constrict so that more blood reaches the brain and the heart. This increases blood pressure and often leaves the hands and feet feeling cold and clammy. The blood glucose level increases to provide increased energy for the muscles.

Respiratory signs

The respiratory rate increases and the bronchial passages dilate during stress to allow increased oxygen exchange. Under severe stress, the respiratory rate may become too rapid, resulting in hyperventilation. Hyperventilation can result in a tingling sensation in the extremities, faintness, dizziness, and even convulsions if the acid-base balance is seriously altered.

Musculoskeletal signs

Muscle tension in the back, neck, and head increases with stress. Tension headaches, teeth grinding, and backaches are among the most common complaints.

Gastrointestinal signs

Peristalsis decreases with stress, as does the production of digestive enzymes. These changes result in loss of appetite, nausea, abdominal distention, and vomiting. Some individuals complain of heartburn or develop gastric or duodenal ulcers. Decreased peristalsis usually results in excess intestinal gas and constipation, but diarrhea is also quite common with stress.

TABLE 18-1

Stokes/Gordon Stress Scale–Selected Items

Rank	Event or situation	Weight
1	Death of a son or daughter (unexpected)	100
2	Decreasing eyesight	99
2	Death of a grandchild	99
3	Death of spouse (unexpected)	97
4	Loss of ability to get around	96
4	Death of son or daughter (expected, anticipated)	96
5	Fear of your home being invaded or robbed	93
5	Constant or recurring pain or discomfort	93
6	Illness or injury of close relative	92
7	Death of spouse (expected, anticipated)	90
7	Moving in with children or other family	90
7	Moving to an institution	90
8	Minor or major car accident	89
8	Needing to rely on cane, wheelchair, walker, or hearing aid	89
8	Change in ability to perform personal care	89
10	Loneliness or aloneness	87
11	Having an unexpected debt	86
11	Your own hospitalization (unplanned)	86
12	Decreasing hearing	85
13	Fear of abuse from others	84
13	Being judged legally incompetent	84
13	Not feeling needed or having a purpose in life	84
14	Decreasing mental abilities	84
15	Giving up long-cherished possessions	82
15	Wishing parts of your life had been different	82
16	Using your savings for living expenses	80
17	Change in behavior of a family member	79
18	Taking a relative or friend into your home to live	78
19	Concern about elimination	77
19	Illness in public places	77
20	Feeling of remaining time being short	76
20	Giving up or losing driver's license	76
20	Change in sleeping habits	76
21	Difficulty using public transportation	75
23	Uncertainty about the future	73

continued

TABLE 18-1—cont'd

Stokes/Gordon Stress Scale–Selected Items

Rank	Event or situation	Weight
25	Fear of your own or your spouse's driving	71
27	Concern for completing required forms	69
27	Death of a loved pet	69
29	Reaching a milestone year	67
32	Outstanding personal achievement	64
33	Retirement	63
35	Change in your sexual activity	59

Adapted from Stokes SA, Gordon SE, *User's manual, SGSS*, Pleasantville, NY: Pace University, Lienhard School of Nursing, 861 Bedford Rd, Pleasantville, NY 10570, 1988.

Urinary signs

Autonomic nervous stimulation results in decreased urine production but increased urinary frequency.

Cognitive changes

In addition to physiologic changes, stress affects the way we think, feel, and act. Although some stress is normal and necessary, high stress levels can be physically and mentally exhausting.

Mild stress results in an increased state of alertness. Individuals experiencing mild stress are able to pay attention to details, to learn, and to solve problems. With increased stress levels these abilities decrease rapidly.

Persons experiencing severe stress are likely to miss obvious details and might forget even the most basic information. Problem-solving ability is severely affected. Under stress, people are likely to develop "tunnel vision," in which they become narrowly focused on one aspect of a problem and ignore other important facts. These individuals are likely to act irrationally or impulsively and make poor choices. Some become incapable of making any decisions at all. Some research even indicates that stress can cause physiologic changes in the the brain that have an adverse effect on memory.

Emotional changes

People experiencing high levels of stress are likely to complain of fatigue, tension, and anxiety. They often report a sense of foreboding or a feeling that something is wrong. They may appear distracted, irritable, short-tempered, or even angry. People living with

Symptoms of Depression as Listed in DSM-IV

- Changes in appetite and weight
- Disturbed sleep
- Motor agitation or retardation
- Fatigue and loss of energy
- Depressed or irritable mood
- Loss of interest or pleasure in usual activities
- Feelings of worthlessness, self-reproach, or excessive guilt
- Suicidal thinking or attempts
- Difficulty with thinking or concentration

DSM-IV—Diagnostic and Statistical Manual of Mental Disorders, ed 4, Washington DC, 1994, American Psychiatric Association.

high-level stress often verbalize feelings of poor self-worth or low self-esteem. They may appear to be so wrapped up in their own problems that they have little capability for or interest in interacting with others. When stress becomes severe, people may experience signs of clinical depression or even verbalize suicidal thoughts.

Depression, which is a major problem among the elderly, is not easily identified or diagnosed. Depression is often missed because it occurs in conjunction with the numerous physical and social changes that occur with aging.

Depression is more than the "down moods" that everyone experiences. Depression is a whole-body syndrome that causes physiologic, emotional and cognitive changes in the elderly. The notion of "mental illness" is unsettling to many elderly people, who feel that seeking help for "mental problems" is a sign of a weakness that they should be able to overcome alone. Elderly persons are more likely to seek attention for physical symptoms than they are for feeling depressed. Symptoms such as chronic pain, appetite loss, sleeplessness, loss of interest, and even dementia-like behavior are often attributed to other problems, and the underlying depression is missed. This is unfortunate because 60% to 80% of the identified cases of depression can be treated using psychotherapy, medication, or a combination of both.

Depression is not a normal part of aging. In fact, studies have shown that most elderly people are satisfied with their lives. It appears that working through the stressors of a lifetime has enabled many elderly people to develop a high level of self-knowledge and strong coping skills. Depression appears to be most common when the elderly are under physiologic stress. It is also likely to occur when the elderly perceive that they have lost control of a situation, that

Goals of Treatment for Depression

- Decreased symptoms of depression
- Reduced risk of relapse and recurrence
- Improved quality of life
- Improved medical health status

they lack the support of significant others, or that their normal coping mechanisms have been overwhelmed by the number or severity of stressors (Boxes 18-1 and 18-2).

Behavioral changes

People attempt to cope with stress in different ways. Some avoid all interactions or tasks that might increase their stress level, whereas others take on additional duties in an attempt to block out the source of their distress. In either case, performance is likely to suffer. People under stress tend to be disorganized, make more errors, and leave tasks incomplete. They may appear and even sound muddled.

The thoughts, statements, and actions of stressed people often jump around in a scattered or disconnected manner. They may pace, hum, or perform other ritualistic actions such as finger drumming, key jangling, or toe tapping. Temper tantrums, shouting, and other aggressive behaviors can occur without warning.

Stress and Illness

Stress and illness are closely linked. Research has shown that both mental and physical illness result in stress and that stress increases the risk of both mental and physical illness. A physically ill person is less able to cope with additional physical or psychologic stressors, which take energy away from the already depleted reserves and decrease the ability to cope. Stress can interfere with the ability to learn, function, and follow through with the plan of care. Decreasing the number of stressors or in other ways decreasing the stress level can prevent illness or improve a person's ability to cope with existing illnesses.

People differ in their abilities to cope with stress. Those who do not learn to cope effectively with normal day-to-day stressors cannot function normally when the stress level is high and are at risk for becoming physically or mentally ill. Those who do learn good coping strategies can maintain their ability to function despite high-level stress. Many different coping or defense mechanisms are used as part of day-to-day living (Box 18-3). People who are able to cope

---

BOX 18-3

Common Coping or Defense Mechanisms

- *Repression*—The removal of anxiety-producing thoughts or experiences from conscious awareness
- *Denial*—Refusing to acknowledge some painful aspect of external reality that is obvious to others
- *Rationalization*—Creating an acceptable reason for unacceptable thoughts or actions
- *Intellectualization*—Making generalizations to avoid disturbing thoughts or feelings
- *Displacement*—transferring emotions about a situation or person onto another
- *Suppression*—Avoiding thinking about distressing situations
- *Projection*—Attributing one's own feeling to another
- *Sublimation*—Channeling negative energy into socially acceptable behaviors
- *Substitution*—Keeping so busy with activities that there is no time to think about stressors

---

effectively usually use several of these mechanisms, which are neither good nor bad. Coping mechanisms only become dysfunctional when they are used excessively or inappropriately as a way of avoiding dealing with the stressors.

Stress Reduction and Coping Strategies

There are two basic categories of coping style: problem-focused strategies and emotion-focused strategies. Problem-focused coping strategies attempt to change or eliminate the stressful event or threat. Emotion-focused strategies attempt to change the person's response to the stressful event or threat. The type of strategy used depends on the personal significance of the event and the perceived ability to alter the outcomes.

One effective way of reducing stress is to avoid or escape the stressor(s). When an event has little personal significance or when there is little likelihood of having an impact on the outcome of an event, avoidance may be the best choice. When people know that certain events are likely to increase their stress level, the best alternative may be to avoid these situations whenever possible. It is often simpler and wiser to avoid stress than to endure it. When facing a major stressor, it is wise to eliminate as many smaller stressors as possible so that energy is available to cope with the major problem.

When stressors cannot be avoided, when their personal significance is high, or when the person believes he or she can affect the outcome, other methods can be used. Confrontational, cognitive, and problem-solving methods are very effective means of dealing with these types of stressful situations.

In order to use a problem-solving method, one must first identify and examine his or her stressors. Once the stressors are identified, their importance to the individual can be determined. Only then can alternative actions to reduce the stress be explored. For example, the individual can continue to face the stressor (e.g., an annoying coworker) and live with the consequences **(confrontational)**, change jobs **(escape)**, decrease contact with an annoying person **(avoidance)**, or consciously work to change his or her attitude toward the annoying person **(emotional distancing)**. The choice made is based on a deliberate decision. The mere fact that the person retains control and makes a choice helps reduce the stress level.

Many people need to be taught how to use the problem-solving method for coping with stress in their lives. Learning to use this process with small or minor stressors can help people learn to cope with major stressors. Some find that physical activity helps them cope with stress. Exercise may reduce excessive levels of stress-related hormones and may allow the body to regain homeostasis. The particular physical activity chosen should be one that the stressed individual enjoys and participates in willingly. Physical activity should be carried out in moderation, not to a level of exhaustion where it becomes another form of stress.

Relaxation techniques can be used to help people cope with stress. The most common forms of relaxation technique include progressive relaxation, meditation, imaging, biofeedback, and self-hypnosis.

In addition to these techniques, the support of friends and family benefits most people. Talking through problems and stresses can facilitate problem solving. If the level of stress is too severe for routine stress-reduction techniques, professional help from counselors, ministers, or mental health professionals may be necessary.

COPING AND STRESS WITH AGING

Stress is as much a fact of life for the elderly as for the younger population. However, the amount and types of stressors do seem to change with aging (see Table 18-1). Many negative life events have been identified as producing stress in the elderly, but there are fewer positive life events that produce stress as we age. Many of the stressors of the elderly involve losses.

Loss of a spouse or child, home, vision, and driver's license can result in the loss of a purpose in life and may place a severe strain on the coping abilities of the elderly. Too many or too frequent stressors can overwhelm the elderly, particularly those already under physiologic stress due to physical illness.

The ability to cope with stress differs widely among the elderly. Generally, those who have learned good coping strategies and have used them through a lifetime will continue to do so into old age. Those who did not learn at a younger age how to cope with stress will continue to experience problems.

Because of the unchanging nature of so many of the stressors seen with aging, the elderly are more likely to emotionally distance themselves from situations they cannot change. They are increasingly likely to seek support in spiritual or philosophic beliefs that help them cope with these uncontrollable situations.

NURSING PROCESS

INEFFECTIVE COPING

Assessment of Coping and Stress Tolerance

- Does the person verbalize feelings of tension, stress, frustration, or depression?
- Does the person complain of changes in eating habits?
- Does the person complain of changes in bladder or bowel elimination patterns?
- Is the person experiencing changes in sleep patterns?
- Does the person have difficulty making decisions or solving problems?
- Does the person appear agitated, aggressive, angry, or hostile?
- Is the person depressed or withdrawn?
- Does the person smoke or consume alcohol excessively?
- Has the person experienced an increased frequency of illness or accidents?

See Box 18-4 for a list of risk factors for problems related to coping or stress in the elderly.

Nursing Diagnosis

Ineffective individual coping. Ineffective coping occurs when a person is unable to solve problems or adapt to the stressors in his or her life. Individuals experiencing ineffective coping frequently verbalize feelings of anxiety, anger, or depression and can often

---

BOX 18-4

Risk Factors Related to Coping or Stress Tolerance in the Elderly

- Recent social, physical, emotional, or financial losses
- Physical illness
- Major life changes

BOX 18-5

Alcohol-Related Problems in the Elderly

- The incidence of alcohol-related problems in community-dwelling elderly ranges from 1% to 6%. In those hospitalized for medical problems the incidence increases to 7% to 22%. In those hospitalized in mental health or psychiatric units the incidence increases even more (to 28% to 44%).
- Alcohol related problems often go undetected in the elderly because symptoms are often mistaken for dementia or medical problems. For example, gastrointestinal problems are more likely to be correlated to antiinflammatory medications than to alcohol consumption.
- Alcohol use in the elderly contributes to liver disease, dementia, peripheral neuropathy, insomnia, poor nutrition, incontinence, depression, inadequate self-care, and medication reactions. Use of alcohol increases the risk of falls, hip fractures, and other accidents.
- Elderly men are more likely to use alcohol to cope with financial problems, whereas elderly women are more likely to use alcohol to cope with death or loss of relationships.

---

be heard to use phrases such as "I just can't cope anymore." In addition, they may complain of changes in physical function that occur as a result of stress. Loss of appetite, nausea, "sour stomach," altered bowel or bladder elimination patterns, and sleep disturbances are common complaints. Elderly persons who are having problems coping often appear to be agitated. This agitation can interfere with the ability to make even simple decisions, solve problems, and participate in self-care activities. In severe cases, the person may appear angry and hostile or may withdraw from contact with others. If these individuals live independently, they may abuse tobacco, alcohol, or drugs in an attempt to cope with their stress (Box 18-5, Fig. 18-1).

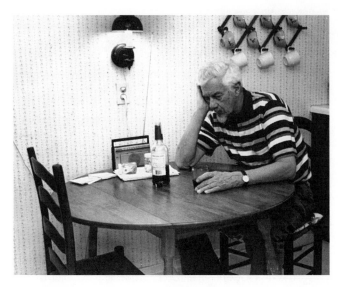

FIG. 18-1 Loneliness and hopelessness can be manifestations of alcohol abuse. (Courtesy of Ursula Ruhl, St Louis.)

Nursing Goals/Outcomes

The nursing goals for elderly individuals with ineffective coping are (1) to communicate feelings of stress; (2) to identify personal strengths and effective methods of coping; and (3) to participate in decision making.

Nursing Interventions

The following nursing interventions should take place in hospitals or extended-care facilities:

1. **Maintain continuity of care to develop a stable, trusting relationship.** Before elderly persons will verbalize their concerns, they must develop trust in their caregiver(s). This trust is best gained by keeping the number of caregivers to a minimum. A plan of care should be developed with the individual. To reduce stress, this plan should be followed with minimal changes.

2. **Encourage the elderly to verbalize their feelings.** Verbalization provides the elderly with an opportunity to express their concerns and solve problems. Merely putting feelings into words often reduces the stress that comes from holding back anxious thoughts. Nurses should be careful to remain nonjudgmental and should allow the elderly to express a full range of feelings, including fear, anger, hostility, and grief.

3. **Ensure that the elderly receive adequate nutrition, rest, and pain relief.** Persons who are hungry, fatigued, or in pain are likely to have difficulty coping with other stressors. Nurses should plan care in order to minimize these basic physical stressors.

4. **Assist the elderly in identifying personal strengths and previously successful coping strategies.** Most elderly people have used a variety of coping strategies throughout their lives. Unless the elderly suffer from chronic mental illness, they have probably managed to cope rather successfully to have reached old age. The coping behaviors that were used throughout life can act as a basis for coping with current situations.

5. **Explain a variety of stress-reduction techniques.** A variety of stress-reduction techniques can be used to help aging persons reduce stress. **Progressive relaxation** is a simple technique that can be used by the elderly. To learn to relax, the person is first taught to identify the difference between muscle tension and relaxation. Once he or she can identify the different sensations, the person is taught to alternately tighten and relax muscles, starting at the feet and working upward through the body. This is done until the entire body is relaxed. With practice, this technique can be done quickly, effectively, and at will.

    Self-hypnosis takes relaxation a step further and allows individuals to actually place themselves in a trance-like state. This technique is more complex and more difficult to learn than other relaxation techniques. Commercial audiotapes are available to teach self-hypnosis.

    Imaging is another relaxation technique in which individuals are taught to think of a calm, peaceful setting. This can be whatever setting the individual finds most relaxing. The person should visualize this setting and try to picture it in great detail, taking pleasure from each aspect of the environment. He or she should then imagine being in this environment, relaxing and enjoying the experience.

    Meditation is a somewhat more difficult—but highly beneficial—relaxation technique. Time and effort are required to learn to meditate effectively. In order to meditate, individuals must learn to shut out external stimuli and focus on calming their thoughts. To gain this internal focus, most meditators use a **mantra,** which is a word or sound that is repeated over and over again. To facilitate meditation, the individual should be provided with a quiet place where distractions can be minimized and should be assisted into a position that promotes comfort and relaxation.

6. **Encourage the elderly to participate in activities.** Physical and diversional activities can reduce stress by focusing excess nervous energy in productive ways, but persons experiencing stress may be reluctant to participate. These individuals should be encouraged but never forced to attend these activities because forcing will only increase stress.

7. **Consult with mental health specialists, ministers, or counselors.** There are many techniques that can help the elderly cope with stress. If the problem is severe or if nurses are unable to help the elderly cope with stress, it is wise to consult with a specialist.

The following interventions should take place in the home:

1. **Encourage the family to provide emotional support to the elderly.** It is often difficult for the elderly (or anyone else) to cope with stress alone. Families should be encouraged to spend time with the elderly, listening and providing emotional support. If the family dynamics are disturbed and the family is a source of stress, it may be necessary to reduce family contact and help the elderly person identify other sources of emotional support such as friends, ministers, or others.

2. **Identify community resources that can provide support to the elderly and their families.** Many elderly persons and their families have difficulty coping on their own. Most communities have mental health clinics or senior citizen help lines to assist in times of stress.

3. **Use any appropriate interventions that are used in the institutional setting.**

NURSING PROCESS
RELOCATION STRESS SYNDROME

Relocation stress syndrome describes the physiologic or psychologic stress that occurs when a person is transferred from one environment to another. Relocation stress is a common problem with aging and can occur with many types of relocation:

- From a private home to the home of a family member
- From home to an apartment or other shared living arrangement
- From one area of the city to another
- From home to a hospital
- From home to a long-term care facility
- From home to a hospital then to a long-term care facility
- From one unit in the hospital or long-term care facility to another unit in the same facility
- From one room to another in a hospital or long-term care facility

Elderly persons who are required to change residence are likely to experience losses, fears, and concerns that increase stress. Loss of independence, loss of personal possessions, loss of friends and neighbors, fear of the unknown, and concern about the future all increase stress. Stress is greatest when many losses or changes have occurred, when these changes occur in rapid succession, when the changes are unexpected, and when the individual has had little or no say in the decision-making process.

Elderly persons experiencing relocation stress syndrome exhibit emotional, behavioral, and physical signs of stress. Most newly relocated elderly persons experience feelings of powerlessness, helplessness, and insecurity. They often verbalize an unwillingness to relocate or dissatisfaction with the new living arrangements. They are likely to express feelings of grief, anger, apprehension, anxiety, loneliness, depression, and confusion. To cope with these feelings, the elderly may demonstrate a variety of behaviors.

Some attempt to maintain control of the situation by demanding attention and verbalizing many needs. They may be more dependent on caregivers than their physical condition justifies. Others attempt to cope with the stress by becoming hostile or angry. They often deny the necessity of the change and refuse necessary assistance or care. Still others cope by withdrawing and isolating themselves from contact with staff, other residents, and even family. These behaviors are usually a result of lack of trust or feelings of powerlessness in the new setting.

In addition to behavioral changes, the recently relocated elderly are likely to experience physical signs of stress. Changes in eating habits, weight loss, gastrointestinal changes, changes in elimination patterns, and changes in sleep patterns are commonly seen in newly relocated elderly persons.

See the assessment for coping and stress tolerance on p. 295.

Nursing Diagnosis

Relocation stress syndrome

Nursing Goals/Outcomes

The nursing goals for elderly individuals with relocation stress syndrome are (1) to recognize the reasons for the move or change; (2) to identify ways to maintain control and decision-making powers in the new environment; (3) to verbalize concerns about new living arrangements; and (4) to identify methods for coping with change.

Nursing Interventions

The following nursing interventions should take place in hospitals or extended-care facilities:

1. **Encourage verbalization of feelings, fears, and concerns about the move or change.** When a person holds in all fears and concerns, his or her stress

NURSING CARE PLAN

COPING-STRESS

Mrs. Mack, an 81-year-old woman, recently moved into Brookline Care Center. You observe that she looks sad. She spends most of her time alone, sitting in her room looking out the window. She repeatedly asks, "Why did they have to do this to me? I was happy where I was. I just wanted to stay there until I died." She makes many demands of the staff and asks many questions. She complains that she has difficulty sleeping in strange surroundings with other people so close by.

Her chart reveals that she has a variety of health problems, including heart trouble and a history of high blood pressure. Until recently, she lived independently in her own apartment and required minimal help with getting to doctor's appointments and grocery shopping. Recently she had become more forgetful, and her daughters were increasingly concerned about her safety and well-being living alone. Both daughters agreed that a care center would be most appropriate and they found one near one of their homes that was reasonable in cost and that had a vacancy. They made arrangements for the move and notified the landlord before discussing the plans with Mrs. Mack. The daughters moved a few of her personal belongings with her, but many were sold or given to family members.

NURSING DIAGNOSIS

Relocation stress syndrome

DEFINING CHARACTERISTICS

- Sad affect
- Apprehension
- Verbalization of concern about move
- Increased dependency
- Increased demands and verbalization of needs
- Change in sleeping patterns

GOALS/OUTCOMES

Mrs. Mack will verbalize an understanding of the reasons for her move, identify concerns about her new environment, and identify ways to cope with the change.

NURSING INTERVENTIONS

1. Encourage Mrs. Mack to verbalize her feelings about the move.
2. Allow expressions of anger or frustration about the family's actions.
3. Encourage Mrs. Mack to discuss her feelings with her family.
4. Explain the reasons that necessitated the move.
5. Involve Mrs. Mack in decision making and care planning.
6. Maintain stable care assignments to build trust.
7. Encourage a positive attitude about change.
8. Offer opportunities to participate in social activities.
9. Encourage her family to bring in more valued personal belongings.
10. Consult a social worker or minister as appropriate to facilitate positive family interactions.

EVALUATION

Mrs. Mack's family has brought additional family pictures, some favorite pillows, and a lap robe that had been stored in a closet. They also purchased a small color television with a special earphone for listening in bed. Mrs. Mack states "I still don't like it here, but I know that my family thinks it is best for me. They are trying to make it better I guess." You will continue the plan of care.

level remains high. Allowing the elderly to discuss their concerns openly and freely initiates the problem-solving process. Anger is common when the elderly disagree with the move. This anger should be accepted as a normal and even healthy response.

2. **Discuss the reasons for the move or change.** Nurses and families should be open and honest about the reasons for a move or change. Any questions the individual has should be answered as completely and honestly as possible. Attempting to shield the elderly from the often harsh reality is likely to result in anger and loss of trust.

3. **Include the elderly in care planning.** Whenever possible, active participation of the elderly in care planning should be encouraged. This allows the elderly to maintain some degree of control over decisions that affect their lives. Whenever possible, choices should be offered and the individual's preferences should be respected.

4. **Encourage a positive attitude about the move or change.** Nurses should help the elderly identify the benefits that will come with the change and should avoid making personal or negative comments about the move.

5. **Maintain continuity of care to enhance feelings of trust.** When an aging person is newly relocated, the number of persons providing care should be kept to a minimum and care should be given in a consistent manner. The individual's preferences should be respected and his or her needs met promptly. This will help build a sense of trust and decrease the stress that results from rapid or unpredictable changes.

6. **Encourage the use of familiar objects and belongings.** The elderly should be encouraged to bring as many prized personal possessions as space allows. Personal belongings enhance the sense of belonging. Seeing and using familiar items makes a new environment seem more familiar and reduces stress. Personal possessions should be positioned or displayed so that the person can easily reach or see them. Because most people feel that their personal belongings are extensions of themselves, these belongings should always be treated with care and respect by caregivers.

Relocation to a new environment can be confusing and even disorienting to the elderly. Selected equipment such as calendars, clocks, night-lights, and personal belongings will help the elderly make a smoother adjustment to a new environment.

The following interventions should take place in the home:

1. **Allow the elderly to participate in decision making and planning for the change.** It is important to include the elderly in decisions that will have a significant impact on their lives. When a major change (e.g., a change in residence) is necessary, the elderly person, his or her family, and possibly a social worker should make decisions together. The person should know the reasons for the change and the available options. When choices are available, the preferences of the individual should be respected. Enabling the elderly to retain control of the choices reduces the sense of powerlessness and thus stress.

2. **Anticipate fears and concerns, and allow adequate time to implement the change, when possible.** Nurses should help the elderly and their families anticipate and plan for the change. In cases in which a change in environment occurs because of a medical emergency, planning is not possible. In many cases, however, there is adequate time to prepare the elderly for a change. This time should be used to allow the individual to accept the fact that a change of environment is necessary. In addition, the individual can sort through personal belongings and distribute or discard them as desired. Scheduled visits to the new environment before the actual move allow the person to become more familiar with the physical structure and people.

3. **Use any appropriate interventions that are used in the institutional setting.**

A nursing care plan for relocation stress syndrome is presented on p. 298.

SUMMARY

Stress is a fact of life. Although the stressors may change throughout life, stress affects people of all ages. The major stressors of aging relate to losses. Loss of ability, loss of loved ones, loss of home, and many other losses are stressful to the elderly, affecting physical and emotional status. Stress can result in behavioral changes. Excessive levels of stress are harmful. Each individual uses a variety of coping mechanisms to deal with stress. The effectiveness or ineffectiveness of these coping strategies is of concern to nurses. Interventions that reduce stress and support positive coping mechanisms can be beneficial.

READINGS AND REFERENCES

Web site: *If you're over 65 and feeling depressed,* www. mhsource.com/hy/over-65.html, 1990.

Aldwin CM, et al: Age differences in stress, coping, and appraisal: finding from the normative age study, *J Gerontol* 51:P179, 1996.

Barnhouse AH, Brugler CJ, Harkulich JT: Relocation stress syndrome, *Nurs Diagn* 3:166, 1992.

Brugler CJ, Titus M, Nypaver JM: Relocation stress syndrome: a patient and staff approach, *J Nurs Admin* 23:45, 1993.

Donlon BC: Clinical outlook: behavioral slowing—how nurses can help patients to adapt, *J Gerontol Nurs* 20:46, 1994.

Gingerich BS, Ondeck DA: Aging, *J Home Health Care Nurs* 6:1, 1994.

Goldman R: Mind over matter: anti-stress tips for anti-aging, *Total Health* 19:1997.

Jenike MA Web site: *Neuropsychiatric assessment and treatment of geriatric depression,* www.mhsource.com/edu/psytimes/p950529.html, 1995.

Johnson TE, Lithgow GJ, Murakami S: Hypothesis: interventions that increase the response to stress offer the potential for effective life prolongation and increased health, *J Gerontol* 51:B392, 1996.

Kurlowicz LH: Depression in hospitalized medically ill elders: evolution of the concept, *Arch Psychiatr Nurs* 8:124, 1994.

Manion PS, Rantz MJ: Relocation stress syndrome: a comprehensive plan for long-term care admissions, *Geriatr Nurs* 16:108, 1995.

McDougall GJ: Older adults' metamemory: coping, depression, and self-efficacy, *Appl Nurs Res* 6:28, 1993.

Moneyham L, Scott CB: Anticipatory coping in the elderly, *J Gerontol Nurs* 21:23, 1995.

National Institute on Aging Age Page Web site: *Depression: a serious but treatable illness,* www.mhsource.com/hy/age-dep.html, 1992.

Nypaver JM, Titus M, Brugler CJ: Patient transfer to rehabilitation: just another move? *Rehabil Nurs* 21:94, 1996.

Pearlin LI, Skaff MM: Stress and the life course: a paradigmatic alliance, *Gerontologist* 36:239, 1996.

Rossen EK, Buschmann MT: Mental illness in late life: the neurobiology of depression, *Arch Psychiatr Nurs* 9:130, 1995.

Solomon R: Coping with stress: a physicians guide to mental health in aging, *Geriatrics* 51:46, 1996.

Solomon R: Successful aging: how to help your older patients cope with change, *Geriatrics* 29:41, 1994.

Valente SM: Recognizing depression in elderly patients, *Am J Nurs* 94:18 1994.

Wang WL, Anderson FR, Mentes JC: Home healthcare nurses knowledge and attitudes toward suicide, *Home Health Care Nurse* 13:64, 1995.

Woodward W, Thobaben M: Helping the elderly cope with mental changes, *J Home Health Care Pract* 6:15, 1994.

VALUES AND BELIEFS

LEARNING OBJECTIVES

1. Discuss the impact of personal values and beliefs on everyday life.
2. Identify values and beliefs commonly found in today's elderly population.
3. Discuss how beliefs and values impact the health practices of the elderly.
4. Explain the relationship of values and beliefs to health practices.
5. Compare the spiritual practices of major religions as they relate to death.
6. Describe methods of assessing beliefs and values.
7. Identify the elderly who are most at risk for experiencing problems related to values and beliefs.
8. Identify selected nursing diagnoses related to values or beliefs.
9. Describe nursing interventions appropriate for elderly individuals who are experiencing problems related to values or beliefs.

Most elderly persons have established a pattern of values, goals, and beliefs that guide their decisions and choices. These values and beliefs have their origins in the individual's religion, philosophy, family, culture, and society.

Values and beliefs are essential to the human spirit. They are the intangibles that set humans apart from other animals. Values and beliefs affect all aspects of our lives and play an important role in promoting health and coping with illness. Values and beliefs influence how we live and how we die.

Values influence the decisions we make throughout life. They are the "rights and wrongs," the "thou shalts" and "thou shalt nots" that everyone uses to steer their way through the myriad choices made during a lifetime. The choices of spouse, living arrangements, dress, eating patterns, and patterns of health maintenance are all influenced by our personal value system.

The personal value system is developed early in childhood. Many experts believe that most of our values are well established by the time we reach 10 years of age. The idea that the values that guide our lives for 80 or 90 years are established so early is significant and the implications for parents, schools, and society are tremendous.

Values are based on the beliefs that are stressed by the family, culture, church, school, and media while a person is growing up. The beliefs that were reinforced while we were young will most likely have the greatest influence on our personal value system.

Because people develop their values based on a unique combination of time, place, and experiences, no two people have exactly the same beliefs and values. People of similar ages, cultural backgrounds, and experiences are likely to share similar beliefs and values. People of different ages, cultural backgrounds, and experiences are likely to hold different beliefs and values.

People who formed their values during the Great Depression, for example, see the world quite differently than do those born during World War II or during the Baby Boom of the 1950s. People raised with strict moral or religious values are very likely to feel differently than people raised without the benefit of moral or religious training. People raised in traditional nuclear families are likely to have different values than people raised in other family structures. People raised before the advent of television are very likely to have different values than those raised with television. People growing up when war was viewed as a patriotic duty have different values than those raised during a time when any war was viewed as immoral.

People see the world through their own value and belief structure and use this as a filter by which they judge other people and events. Each of us has a great deal of difficulty understanding people whose values are different from our own.

It is human nature for each person to feel that his or her personal beliefs and values are somehow superior to those of others. People with belief and value patterns similar to our own are likely to be viewed positively, and interactions with these people are likely to be of a friendly nature. People with beliefs and values that are different from our own are likely to be viewed negatively, and interactions with these people may be difficult or even antagonistic.

Misunderstanding and conflict often occur when people with two different or contradictory sets of values interact. Statements such as "He just doesn't understand me" or "I just don't understand them" usually indicate a conflict in beliefs or values. Think of the number of times you have heard parents say this about their children and vice versa. Think of the number of times a member of one ethnic or religious group says it about another. Think of the times nurses say this about a patient of a different age, race, or background.

Understanding the values and beliefs of others is not easy, yet the willingness to try to understand or empathize is an important part of nursing care. In order to be effective, nurses must be willing to really listen to each person they care for and avoid judging the other person by their own values. It is difficult to withhold judgments based on personal values and to approach others with understanding. Nonjudgmental interaction requires a high level of patience and excellent communication skills.

Values and beliefs are not easily changed. This is true for ourselves and others. The most effective way to change beliefs and values is through education, which can be gained through reading, academic study, and interaction with individuals of diverse backgrounds. Patient teaching and positive interactions can help people change their beliefs. Increasing their personal knowledge about the beliefs and values of the more common cultural, religious, and social groups can help nurses change beliefs. Open-mindedness and understanding of the wide range of beliefs and values existing in an increasingly diverse world enable nurses to work effectively with a wide variety of people.

COMMON VALUES AND BELIEFS OF THE ELDERLY

Although the elderly population is no more homogenized than are younger age groups, they are likely to share some beliefs and values. People 60 years of age or older developed their value systems in a world that was very different from today. Many of the beliefs and values that are very important to the elderly have no significance to younger persons. This is difficult for the elderly to understand and it is difficult for younger family members or caregivers to appreciate. The value and belief patterns of the elderly are likely to challenge the understanding of predominantly younger nurses. Nurses must be careful to determine what beliefs and values are at work before making judgments or planning interventions. Unless the underlying belief or value is correctly identified, nurses are likely to choose ineffective interventions that lead to frustration or anger for all involved.

Economic Values

Many of today's elderly were strongly affected by the depression of the 1930s. They were "taught the value of a dollar" and to "waste not, want not." Financial independence is important to these individuals, and they may experience intense feelings of shame if forced to "accept charity." They may save or hoard items, even items that present health hazards, because they value saving rather than wasting. Many elderly people are dismayed when nurses or family members throw away food or medical supplies and may attempt to retrieve these items, particularly when they are left alone. They may store an excessive number of personal belongings and clutter up their homes until they become a safety hazard. The elderly may refuse to see a doctor or wait until they are seriously ill because they are concerned about the costs. They may refuse to buy medication, take less than the prescribed amount of medication, or fail to discard old prescriptions because of cost concerns.

Intrapersonal Values

Many elderly were raised valuing respect and obedience to elders. They often cannot understand why their families do not automatically accept what they say and follow their directions. As discussed in Chapter 17, interactions within the family can present many challenges. The more divergent the values of the various family members, the more likely there are to be misunderstandings and conflict. Nurses are often called on to act as mediators when conflicts arise or to provide support to an elderly person who feels rejected or misunderstood by his or her children.

Religious or Spiritual Values

Many of today's elderly were raised in an organized church that played an important role in the formulation of their values and beliefs. As a person ages and death nears, the need to make peace with God often

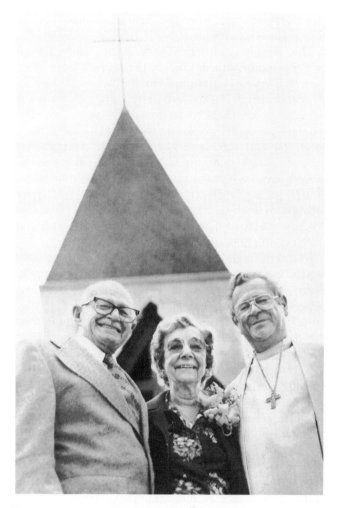

FIG. 19-1 Spiritual guides. (Photograph by Gerald Sundstrom. Courtesy of the American Society on Aging.)

becomes significant. Even people who did not seem to place a high value on religion when they were younger often see a need to seek spiritual guidance when they get older (Fig. 19-1). Spiritual beliefs can be a source of strength to the elderly. People who questioned the existence of a deity may change their minds when faced with the reality of their own deaths. Some never express these needs but will accept spiritual counsel if it is offered. Some continue to reject religious counsel, which is also their right.

Decisions regarding the end of life, including the use of high-technology interventions, living wills, euthanasia, or physician-assisted suicide, are usually based on religious beliefs and value systems. Many elderly wish to have a spiritual advisor available for guidance when serious, often life or death, decisions are made. Decisions that are made on the basis of legitimate religious beliefs must be respected by health care providers, even when their beliefs and values are different. Survival may be less important to an elderly person than the violation of long-held beliefs. Coherent elderly people have the right to make informed choices and have them respected.

The percentage of active, participating church members is significantly higher in the elderly population than in the younger population. Regular church attendance, although highly valued by many elderly, is less common today than it was even a few years ago. This may in part be due to transportation problems or safety concerns that make with regular church attendance difficult. Many elderly persons experience severe distress when they are no longer able to attend church regularly due to illness, hospitalization, or relocation to an institutional setting. Many fear that they are not meeting their spiritual obligations and that they may be denied salvation because of this.

Changes in church structure and the current trend toward cooperation among churches trouble many elderly persons who were taught the value of their own beliefs and are suspicious of religions other than their own. The interdenominational or nondenominational services that are provided in many institutional settings are often rejected by the elderly as heresy.

The elderly may have developed a closeness to a specific spiritual adviser and may be uncomfortable if this person is unavailable. Spiritual counseling often explores intimate secrets and fears. Elderly persons may be unwilling to interact with a stranger, even if this person is a qualified minister. Increased participation of women in the ministry upsets some elderly people who feel that only men were intended to be spiritual advisers. A female chaplain, no matter how qualified, may be rejected by an elderly person who holds these views.

Many elderly persist in older religious practices, which have changed over time. For example, many elderly Catholics will not eat meat on Fridays, even though Catholic law now allows meat eating on Fridays throughout most of the year. Many elderly Jews continue to value orthodox dietary and hygiene practices, even though most younger Jews have accepted less rigid standards. If the person has persisted in these practices over a lifetime, change is highly unlikely. In these cases, nurses and the health care system must be flexible enough to enable these persons to maintain their beliefs and yet also maintain adequate hygiene and nutrition.

Religious rituals are important in many faiths. Prayers, chanting, posturing, cleansing, anointing, and other ritual behaviors are part of the practices of many religions and are used as affirmations of faith. Objects such as icons, menorahs, rosaries, amulets, medals, and holy water are visual symbols of belief that provide comfort and reassurance. A number of books including the Bible, Koran, Torah, Vedas, and Book of Mormon are very important to the practices of their

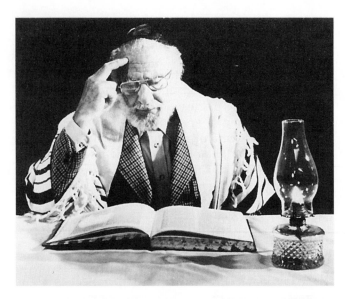

FIG. 19-2 Tradition in thought. (Photograph by Aaron Katz. Courtesy of the American Society on Aging.)

respective religions (Fig. 19-2). Many elderly find great comfort in these texts, often memorizing large segments. Elderly who may be unable to read because of the changes associated with aging or illness find comfort in the mere presence of these valued tenets of their faith. Often the family or spiritual support person will provide these symbols and texts if the elderly person or nurse requests them. Some religious-sponsored institutions provide them routinely.

Individuals with strong religious values and practices often prefer to be hospitalized or live in institutional settings operated by their preferred religious denomination, if these are available in the community.

NURSING PROCESS

VALUE/BELIEF ALTERATION
Assessment of Values and Beliefs

- What is the person's cultural background?
- Does the person have any specific cultural or religious beliefs related to health?
- Is religion or God a significant factor in the person's life?
- Does the person attend religious services regularly?
- What is the person's religious denomination, sect, church, etc?
- Does the person have a preferred spiritual counselor? Does he or she see this person regularly?
- Is the person interested in talking to a priest, minister, or rabbi?

Risk Factors Related to Problems with Values and Beliefs in the Elderly

- Major life stressors such as severe illness or impending death
- A recent significant loss or change in role
- Values and/or beliefs different from those of caregivers or the dominant cultural values
- Removal from a familiar spiritual support system

- What religious books or symbols are meaningful to the person?
- Has aging or illness had an impact on the person's beliefs, values, or spiritual practices?

See Box 19-1 for a list of risk factors for alterations in values and beliefs in the elderly.

Nursing Diagnosis

Spiritual distress

Nursing Goals/Outcomes

The nursing goals for elderly individuals suffering from spiritual distress are (1) to identify and verbalize sources of value conflicts; (2) to specify the spiritual assistance desired; (3) to discuss values and beliefs regarding spiritual practices; and (4) to express feelings of spiritual comfort.

Nursing Interventions

The following nursing interventions should take place in hospitals or extended-care facilities:

1. **Determine whether there are special spiritual practices and/or restrictions.** Nurses should identify the unique spiritual needs of the elderly. Depending on the religion, denomination, or sect within a larger group, specific religious beliefs and practices can vary widely. Many articles and texts identify the major beliefs and practices of the major denominations, but each person or his or her family should clarify the individual's interpretation of and compliance with these. This is particularly important if the religion requires or prohibits certain diets or health behaviors. Every effort should be made to allow the elderly to continue practices and rituals as long as they do not interfere with health maintenance. If there is a conflict between spiritual values or practices and health needs, it is wise to consult with an authority of the specific church to identify acceptable strategies or compromises. Failure to take the elderly person's spiritual beliefs into consideration can result in anger, despondency, and noncompliance with the plan of care.

2. **Identify significant persons who provide spiritual support.** Most religions recognize certain persons as spiritual leaders or guides. These leaders help others to learn and practice the beliefs of the specific faith. Priests, rabbis, ministers, deacons, and religious sisters are commonly recognized as spiritual counselors or chaplains in institutional settings. These individuals are the recognized authorities who are trained to provide counsel to their own members and often to members of different faiths. Many elderly persons have a special closeness to a specific spiritual counselor whom they trust and will appreciate a call or visit from their regular pastor or minister, particularly when hospitalized or in danger of death. Nurses can contact these individuals or can request that the family initiate contact. This task should not be put off as nonessential because many people gain as much sustenance from spiritual counsel as they do from medical treatment.

3. **Determine whether there is any way nurses can aid the elderly in meeting their spiritual needs.** Nurses should do an assessment to determine whether any assistance is required to enable the elderly to meet their spiritual needs. Nurses are often asked to assist the elderly in spiritual practices by contacting spiritual advisers, providing spiritual articles, or facilitating religious rituals.

4. **Determine spiritual articles that have meaning to the person, and obtain these if possible.** Objects that are symbolic of faith should be located so that they can be seen or touched by the elderly; they should not be hidden or put away in a drawer. All religious items should be shown due respect by caregivers. Even if the caregiver is of a different faith, it is important to recognize and respect the symbols of a another person's religion.

5. **Provide opportunities for spiritual guidance with due respect for privacy.** Because spiritual practices often include the sharing of private thoughts and fears, the elderly should be given opportunities to be alone to pray or meditate if desired. A chapel or quiet room free from distractions is desirable. If the person wishes to meet with a spiritual adviser or to perform religious rituals, he or she should have the opportunity to do so. This may require planning so that no interruptions (e.g., cares or treatments) interfere with the religious activity.

6. **Encourage contact with a spiritual counselor in times of crisis.** In times of spiritual crisis, such as the loss of a loved one or imminent death, privacy is particularly important. Severe grief can result in

NURSING CARE PLAN

VALUE-BELIEF

Mr. Quinn, age 78, has attended church regularly and has expressed strong belief in a "merciful God." A week ago, he learned from his doctor that he has terminal cancer and has about 3 months to live. After talking to the doctor, he went to the chapel and cried. Since then he has spent a great deal of time in his room reading his Bible. He frequently verbalizes statements questioning the value of prayer, and states that "God hasn't shown me any mercy, but I probably have to suffer for all I've done wrong in my life."

NURSING DIAGNOSIS

Spiritual distress

DEFINING CHARACTERISTICS

- Withdrawal
- Verbalization of hopelessness and abandonment by God
- Verbalization of feelings of guilt

GOALS/OUTCOMES

Mr. Quinn will recognize that illness places stress on belief system and will express feelings of spiritual comfort.

NURSING INTERVENTIONS

1. Listen to Mr. Quinn's concerns and feelings in a nonjudgmental manner.
2. Request a visit from the hospital chaplain (if desired, contact personal minister).
3. Provide privacy for spiritual counseling and sacraments.
4. Keep the Bible and a prayer book readily available.
5. Assist Mr. Quinn to the chapel as requested.

EVALUATION

Mr. Quinn visits the chapel daily and has a weekly visit with his minister. After each visit he appears more calm, stating that "I still don't know why this is happening to me, but I'll just have to put my trust in God." You will continue the plan of care.

---

questioning of spiritual values. Contact with a spiritual counselor can help the elderly work through feelings of anger, resentment, or ambivalence toward their spirituality. The spiritual counselor can provide support to dying persons and can assist the families in their time of grief. Special care should be taken to arrange for spiritual rituals related to death such as confession, communion, or anointing. Before preparing the body after death, nurses should be aware of the acceptable practices within specific religions.

The following interventions should take place in the home:

1. **Make arrangements that allow the elderly to maintain religious practices.** Arrange for transportation to church or temple. Many churches can find rides for members who cannot walk or drive. If even this is not possible because of severe health problems or immobility, most spiritual advisers are willing to visit in the home if they are notified that a member desires their services.

2. **Use any appropriate interventions that are used in the institutional setting.**

A nursing care plan for spiritual distress is presented on this page.

SUMMARY

Everyone's values and beliefs are unique. They are a product of the individual's culture, education, religion, and society. These values and beliefs form the basis of the elderly person's choices, perceptions, and behaviors. The values and beliefs held by the elderly may significantly differ from those held by younger individuals. If not identified, these differences can result in misunderstandings, confusion, and conflict between the elderly and their families or younger health care providers. Nurses can reduce problems related to differences in values and beliefs by openly communicating with the elderly and by gaining more in-depth information regarding social, spiritual, and cultural diversity.

READINGS AND REFERENCES

Mickley JR, Carson V, Soeken KL: Religion and adult mental health: state of the science in nursing, *Issues Mental Health Nurs* 16:345, 1995.

O'Connell LJ: The role of religion in health-related decision making for elderly patients, *Generations* 18:27, 1994.

SEXUALITY AND AGING

LEARNING OBJECTIVES

1. Describe how sexuality changes with aging.
2. Discuss the effects of illness on sexual functioning.
3. Describe methods for assessing sexual functioning.
4. Identify the elderly persons who are most at risk for experiencing problems related to sexuality.
5. Identify selected nursing diagnoses related to sexuality.
6. Describe nursing interventions that are appropriate for elderly individuals experiencing problems with sexuality.

Sexuality is a part of life and does not cease to exist simply because a person ages. Although society may sometimes prefer to think of the elderly as asexual, this is not the case. Individuals who had an active sex life in younger years are likely to continue to do so as they age. Many elderly continue to have sexually satisfying lives well into old age.

Most women cease reproducing before 50 years of age, but medical research is pushing the limits in this area. Headlines are made when women in their late fifties—and even one woman 63 years of age—successfully give birth to a healthy child. One may question the reasons for and the ethics of considering childbearing at an advanced age, but the fact remains it is possible. Men remain able to father children well into their sixties and seventies without medical assistance. Although uncommon, fathering children at 80 and 90 years of age does occur. Although the ability to reproduce diminishes with age and the frequency and form of sexual activity are likely to change, the need for sexual affection does not disappear with aging.

Sexual touching, fondling, and intercourse remain a part of the lives of many active elderly people. Sexual thoughts and feelings are normal as people age (Fig. 20-1). Studies reveal that close to 40% of married couples over 60 years of age have sexual intercourse at least once a week, and almost half of these couples have sex more frequently. A study of the sexual interests and behavior of persons over age 80 reveals that a significant percentage (63% of men and 30% of women) continue to participate in sexual activity.

Physical changes related to aging, changing health status, and loss of a sex partner all impact on the sexual practices of the elderly. Normal physiologic changes in sexual function may raise concerns for the aging. Elderly women experience changes related to altered hormone levels. When estrogen production decreases, the tissues of the vagina become thinner and less elastic and secrete less natural lubrication. These changes may result in discomfort or pain during intercourse. Hormonal replacement and the use of artificial lubricants can minimize these problems. Estrogen replacement has the additional benefits of reducing osteoporosis and lowering the risk of heart disease in postmenopausal women. Sexual response time generally slows with aging, but the ability to achieve orgasm remains throughout life.

Elderly men experience a delayed reaction to sexual stimuli. They require a longer time to achieve an erection, and the erection is often less firm than at a younger age. Male orgasm takes longer to achieve and is shorter in duration than at a younger age. There is a less forceful ejaculation and smaller volume of seminal fluid released. Loss of erection occurs quickly after orgasm. The time between orgasms generally increases, and orgasm may not occur with every episode of sexual intercourse.

Illness of one or both partners is a common reason for decreased sexual function. Many disease processes interfere with normal sexual function, as do many of the medications taken to treat illness. Diabetes is likely to contribute to impotence in men, even at a young age. If control of the disease does not lead to restoration of function, various devices and procedures are available to help diabetic men achieve erection. New medications such as Viagra may hold some promise for individuals suffering from impotence. Joint pain due to arthritis can interfere with sexual activity. Antiinflammatory medications that reduce pain can also decrease sexual desire. Cardiac problems are likely to interfere with normal sexual activity, although this is more out of fear than from actual danger. The actual risk of death due to sexual intercourse is low, but elderly persons who have experienced a heart attack should discuss their concerns with a physician. Stroke need not prevent sexual activity. Sex is not likely to cause another stroke, although modification in position or use of assistive devices may be needed to compensate for any residual weakness or paralysis. Neither hysterectomy (removal of the

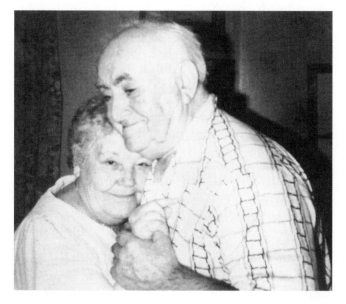

FIG. 20-1 Love and affection are important to the elderly. (Courtesy of American Society on Aging)

uterus) nor mastectomy (removal of a breast) changes sexual functioning, although loss of these organs may make the woman feel like less of a woman or fear that she will be viewed that way. Counseling may be required to help women with these concerns. Prostatectomy (removal of excess prostate tissue) does not normally cause problems with achieving an erection because newer surgical techniques do not cause the nerve damage that was common in the past.

Alcohol and medications affect sexual function in the elderly. Excessive alcohol intake results in delayed orgasm in women and loss of the ability to achieve or maintain an erection in men. Digitalis, diuretics, antihypertensives, tranquilizers, and antidepressants are likely to cause problems with the sex lives of both men and women. Adjustment of the medication or the dosage may help resolve the problem. Interestingly, some antiparkinsonian medications actually enhance sexual desire but not necessarily the ability to perform sexually.

One of the most common reasons for decreased sexual activity in the elderly is loss of the sex partner. Single elderly women experience more of a problem than do single men. According to the Census Bureau, single women over 65 years of age outnumber single men of the same age by 4:1. By age 85 there are 100 single women for every 39 single men. This presents good odds for men interested in relationships but poor odds for women. Single elderly women are often also constrained by social norms. When most of today's elderly grew up, men were expected to initiate contact. Based on this role definition, many elderly women are reluctant to show interest in men, let alone sexual interest. Pursuing a man is not considered socially acceptable.

Most elderly think of sex within the context of marriage. Marriage among senior citizens garners many different responses, particularly from the families of the elderly. Some families are accepting and recognize the need for the elderly to find affection and meaning in later life. Others feel that marriage at a late age is somehow unacceptable. Children often fear that the marriage is a slap in the face of the deceased parent. Many fear that remarriage will displace them from their parent's affection or affect their inheritance. It should be the right of the alert elderly person to determine what is best for him or herself. Hopefully, family and friends will be supportive of the decision.

Marriage is not always an option. Some elderly people, particularly widows, stand to lose a great deal if they remarry. Pensions, insurance benefits, and other financial concerns may be contingent on the person's remaining single. For this reason, some elderly people choose to live together without marrying, which can be a difficult decision for both the elderly

and their families. Longstanding moral or religious values may result in guilt on the part of elderly persons who can see no alternative, and families may have a great deal of difficulty accepting this lifestyle.

Sexuality is a difficult area to address at any age. Young people may not be comfortable with the thought of sexual activity among seniors, believing that it is somehow offensive or abnormal. Even health care professionals may be unaware of or uncomfortable about addressing the sexual needs of the elderly. This situation is not helped by the fact that the elderly are often reluctant to discuss their own sexuality. Fear, shame, or embarrassment over what younger persons may think causes many elderly people to hide their sexual interests and activity even from health care professionals. Physicians, nurses, and others who care for the elderly must be nonjudgmental and sensitive to their values and attitudes. Caregivers need to indicate a willingness to listen and allow adequate time to discuss any concerns that arise.

Other concerns must also be addressed with regard to sexual activity in the elderly. The elderly are often not considered when discussing sexually transmitted diseases, yet 10% of AIDS cases occur in people over 50 years of age. HIV is commonly overlooked because the elderly are not considered to be at risk.

Sexual orientation must also be addressed. For personal or social reasons, persons who have concealed their sexual orientation in younger years may be more comfortable expressing it as they age. Health care providers must be careful to recognize the sexual needs and concerns of elderly lesbians and homosexuals.

Community-dwelling elderly generally have privacy to conduct their sex lives without interference. They are free to touch, hold, and have sex whenever they choose. However, institutional placement of one or both partners can interfere with sexual expression. Obtaining adequate privacy may be difficult, even for married couples who reside in the same institution, particularly if regular medical or nursing care is necessary.

In the past displays of sexual affection were discouraged among the elderly. Fortunately, attitudes are changing as health care providers grow in awareness. Some facilities have policies that indicate respect for the elderly resident's right to keep sexually explicit materials. Touching, handholding, and cuddling are encouraged. Unmarried elderly are allowed to form whatever relationships they desire. A closed door must be respected when privacy for intimacy is desired. Special judgments are necessary when either person suffers from cognitive impairment. When there is any sign of disinterest or resistance to sexual advances, the behavior is not permitted. It is important that institutions protect vulnerable elderly from *un-*

desired physical contact, but mutually agreeable physical contact should remain a right of the elderly.

NURSING PROCESS

SEXUAL DYSFUNCTION

Assessment of Sexuality and the Reproductive System

- Does the person have any discharge or drainage from the genitals?
- If the person is sexually active, does he or she complain of any difficulty or discomfort during sexual activity?
- Does the person have any diseases or disabilities that interfere with sexual activity?
- Does the person take any medications that may interfere with sexual activity?
- What level of sexual activity does the person desire?
- Are there any real or perceived barriers to sexual activity?

See Box 20-1 for a list of risk factors for problems with sexuality in the elderly.

Nursing Diagnosis

Sexual dysfunction

Nursing Goals/Outcomes

The nursing goals for elderly persons with sexual dysfunction are (1) to verbalize feelings about sexual identity; (2) to discuss concerns regarding sexuality; and (3) to describe the effects of aging and illness on sexual functioning.

Nursing Interventions

The following nursing interventions should take place in hospitals, extended-care facilities, and at home:

BOX 20-1

Risk Factors Related to Sexual Dysfunction in the Elderly

- Loss of partner
- Problems with physical mobility
- Institutional setting
- Physical illness or a reaction to therapeutic medications

---

1. **Encourage verbalization of concerns.** Many elderly do not feel comfortable talking about sex to anyone, particularly a younger person. Without undue prying into the elderly person's privacy, nurses should communicate a willingness to discuss any concerns the elderly have, including those that deal with sexuality. Nurses should allow adequate time and provide a private place for these discussions.
2. **Provide privacy.** Alert elderly who wish to court or visit should have the opportunity to do so without interference from nursing staff. Private areas should be available for "dating" interactions. Elderly residents of extended-care facilities should have the opportunity for conjugal visits in the institution or at home if they so desire. Nurses should ensure that these visits meet all federal and state regulations that pertain to residents' rights. Privacy during these visits must be carefully respected.
3. **Protect the sexual dignity of confused elderly.** Individuals who are confused may display sexually inappropriate behaviors (e.g., exposing themselves in public, masturbating, and making inappropriate sexual advances to nursing staff). Undressing in public can be decreased by modifying clothing. For men, elastic-waist pants can replace pants with zippers. For women, buttonless or back-opening tops and slacks instead of skirts can help reduce exposure. Masturbation is common and is not abnormal. Distraction is often effective at reducing the incidence of public masturbation. If distraction is not effective, the person should be taken to his or her room and provided with privacy. Restraints should not be applied to prevent masturbation. If a confused elderly person makes inappropriate sexual advances, nurses should attempt to distract the individual and, if necessary, stop care temporarily. Confused individuals do not realize that their behavior is inappropriate. Nurses should be careful not to overreact to the behavior because this can precipitate violent or verbally abusive episodes.

A nursing care plan for altered sexuality patterns is presented on p. 312.

SUMMARY

Sexuality is an area that is often minimized or ignored in the elderly. Health problems, loss of a partner, and the normal physiologic changes of aging all impact sexual practices. Although these changes affect the type and frequency of sexual activity, many individuals maintain an active interest in sex into old age. Nurses and other younger health care providers must recognize that the elderly are still sexual beings. They continue to have sexual needs, and they have the right to meet those needs without age bias.

NURSING CARE PLAN

SEXUALITY-REPRODUCTION

Mr. Silver, age 89, has a history of hypertension and diabetes. Mrs. Silver, age 87, has severe osteoarthritis and congestive heart failure. Both are residents of Pine Grove Care Center. They have been married for 67 years. Because of space constraints, they have been assigned to separate rooms. Mr. Silver spends a great deal of time at Mrs. Silver's bedside, where he holds her hand and talks to her. Both often verbalize the wish to hold and touch more intimately. They both state, "I wish we just had some privacy around here."

NURSING DIAGNOSIS

Altered sexuality patterns

DEFINING CHARACTERISTICS

- Lack of privacy
- Separation from significant other
- Altered body function related to age and disease processes

GOAL/OUTCOME

Mr. and Mrs. Silver will identify methods for satisfying their need for sexual expression.

NURSING INTERVENTIONS

1. Allow opportunities for both parties to verbalize their feelings about continuing sexual contact.
2. Attempt to arrange for a shared room if this is agreeable to both parties.
3. Develop a method, such as a "Do Not Disturb" sign, for ensuring private time, while recognizing the need for access in case of emergency.
4. Assist with hygiene needs so that both parties are physically clean and attractive.
5. Verbalize an understanding of the continued need for physical closeness throughout life.

EVALUATION

Mr. and Mrs. Silver are observed spending time privately in her room with door closed. After these visits, Mr. Silver states that "it feels good just to touch, share a kiss, and be together quietly for a while. It isn't how I thought we'd end up, but it's better than nothing." You will continue the plan of care.

READINGS AND REFERENCES

Attitudes toward elderly sexuality vary widely, *The Brown University Long-Term Care Quality Letter* 6:7, 1994.

Bower HT: Allowing for same sex preference, *J Gerontol Nurs* 21:5, 1995.

Drench ME, Losee RH: Sexuality and sexual capacities of elderly people, *Rehabil Nurs* 21:118, 1996.

Garden FH, Schramm DM: The effects of aging and chronic illness on sexual function in older adults, *Physical Med Rehabil* 9:463, 1995.

Haffner D: Love and sex after 60: how physical changes affect intimate expression, *Geriatrics* 49:20, 1994.

National Institute on Aging Web site: *Sexuality in later life*, http.//www.agepage.com/sex.html, 1997.

Richardson JP: Sexuality in the nursing home patient, *Am Fam Physician* 51:121, 1995.

Shelton DL: Six myths about sex and the elderly, *Am Med News* 39:20, 1996.

appendix A

LABORATORY VALUES FOR THE ELDERLY

Laboratory Values for the Elderly

Test	Normal value	Standard reference ranges*	Implications and deviations†
Hematology			
Hemoglobin	Slight decrease	Men: 14.0–18.0 g/dl Women: 12.0–16.0 g/dl	
Hematocrit	Slight decrease	Men: 40%–54% Women: 38%–47%	
White blood cells	Slight decrease	4.3–11.0 × 10^3/mm³	
Erythrocyte sedimentation rate (ESR)			
Minivess method	Slight increase	Men: 0–20 mm Women: 0–20 mm	
Differential lymphocytes			
Neutrophils	Unchanged	46%–82%	Increase: Diabetes mellitus Gout Rheumatoid arthritis Stress Bacterial infections Thyroiditis Hemolytic anemia Rheumatic fever Carcinoma Acute hemorrhage Cushing's disease Increased corticosteroids Lead poisoning Pancreatitis Decrease: Vitamin B_{12} deficiency Acute viral infection Folic acid deficiency Bone marrow damage
Lymphocytes	Increased B cells Decreased T cells	11%–45%	
Monocytes	Increased	2.0%–10.0%	Increase: Tuberculosis Subacute bacterial endocarditis
Eosinophils	Increase or decrease	0%–4.0%	Increase: Parasitosis Allergy Colitis Collagen disease Eosinophilic granulomatosis Eosinophilic leukemia
Basophils	Unchanged	0%–2.0%	Increase: Polycythemia vera Myelofibrosis Decrease: Anaphylactic reaction

Laboratory Values for the Elderly—cont'd

Test	Normal value	Standard reference ranges*	Implications and deviations†
Serum chemistry			

Iron‡	Decrease 50%–75% of young adult value at about 71–80 years of age	Men: 49–181 µg/dl
		Women: 37–170 µg/dl
			Increase:
			  Pernicious anemia
			  Hemolytic anemia
			  Hemochromatosis
			  Hepatitis
			Decrease:
			  Iron-deficiency anemia

Vitamin B₁₂‡	Decrease 60%–80% of young adult value at about 70+ years of age	179–1132 pg/ml	
Folate‡	Unchanged	3.1–12.4 ng/ml	
Thyroid			
Thyroxine (T₄)	Slight functional decrease	4.5–12.0 µg/dl	
Triiodothyronine (T₃)	Men: decrease after 70 years of age	86–181 mg/dl	
	Women: decrease around 70–80 years of age	0.49–4.67 µg/ml	
Thyroid-stimulating hormone (TSH)			
Blood chemistry			

Blood urea nitrogen (BUN)	Slight increase	Men: 9–20 mg/dl
		Women: 7–17 mg/dl
			Increase:
			  Dehydration
			  Gastrointestinal hemorrhage
			  Intestinal obstruction
			  Renal disease
			  Acute glomerulonephritis
			  Prostatic hypertrophy
			  Burns
			  High protein intake
			  Mercury poisoning
			  Protein catabolism
			Decrease:
			  Cirrhosis
			  Liver disease
			  Low-protein intake
			  Starvation

Creatinine	Slight increase	Men: 0.8–1.5 mg/dl
		Women: 0.7–1.2 mg/dl
			Increase:
			  Renal dysfunction
			  Chronic glomerulonephritis
			  Tetanus
			  Typhoid fever
			  Salmonella infection

Continued

Laboratory Values for the Elderly—cont'd

Test	Normal value	Standard reference ranges*	Implications and deviations†
Potassium	Age-related increase after sixth decade of life	3.6–5.0 mEq/L	Decrease: Anemia Muscular atrophy Leukemia Renal failure Increase: Addison's disease Bronchial asthma Renal disease Tissue breakdown Trauma Anuria Decrease: Steroid therapy Vomiting Cirrhosis Diarrhea Diuretic therapy Diabetic acidosis Cushing's disease Intravenous therapy
Glucose	Increase	70–110 mg/dl	Increase: Diabetes mellitus Emotional stress Hyperthyroidism Infections Thiazide therapy Increased intracranial pressure Pituitary disorders Decrease: Hyperinsulinism Hypothyroidism Starvation
Fasting blood sugar	Minimal increase		
1-hour postprandial blood sugar	Increase by 10 mg/dl per decade after 30 years of age		
2-hour postprandial blood sugar	Increase to 100+/mg/dl after 40 years of age		
Creatine phosphokinase (CPK)	May not be elevated	Men: 55–170 U/L Women: 30–135 U/L	
Alkaline phosphatase	Increase	38–126 U/L	
Lactic dehydrogenase	1–1.5 times higher, especially in women	313–618 U/L	

Laboratory Values for the Elderly—cont'd

Test	Normal value	Standard reference ranges*	Implications and deviations†
Serum glutamic pyruvic transaminase (SGPT) or alanine transaminase (ALT)	Unchanged	Men: 21–72 IU/L Women: 9–52 IU/L	
Serum glutamic oxaloacetic transaminase (SGOT) or aspartate transaminase (AST)	Unchanged	Men: 17–59 IU/L Women: 14–36 IU/L	
Total protein Serum albumin	Decrease	6.3–8.2 g/dl 3.9–5.0 g/dl	
Cholesterol (total)	Gradual increase with age	200 mg/dl	Increase: Chronic renal disease Hypothyroidism Diabetes mellitus Liver disease Pancreatic dysfunction Decrease: Fasting state Tuberculosis Hypermetabolic states Hyperthyroidism Intestinal obstruction Liver disease Malnutrition Pernicious anemia Hemolytic anemia
High-density lipoprotein (HDL)	Women consistently higher than men, then difference disappears§	>35 mg/dl	
Triglycerides	Increase	35–160 mg/dl	
Calcium	Men: decrease Women: increase	8.4–10.2 mg/dl	
Phosphorus	Men: decrease Women: increase	2.5–4.5 mg/dl	
Uric acid	Men increase more than women	3.5–8.5 mg/dl	Increase: Thiazide diuretic therapy Pneumonia Multiple myeloma Leukemia High salicylate intake Gout
	Women over 44 years of age	2.5–7.5 mg/dl	

Continued

Laboratory Values for the Elderly—cont'd

Test	Normal value	Standard reference ranges*	Implications and deviations†
			Fasting Chronic renal failure Chronic lymphocytic granulocytic leukemia Decrease: Allopurinol therapy
Urinalysis			
Protein	Slight increase	Negative	
Glucose	Unchanged	Negative	
Specific gravity	Decrease	1.005–1.030 o. d. (refractometer)	
Creatinine clearance			
Men	Decrease	85–125 ml/min	Decrease:
Women	Decrease	75–115 ml/min	Renal disease
Arterial blood gases			

Partial pressure of arterial carbon dioxide (Pco_2)	Increase or decrease	34–46 mm Hg	Increase:
			  Metabolic alkalosis
			  Respiratory acidosis
			Decrease:
			  Metabolic acidosis
			  Respiratory alkalosis

Partial pressure of arterial oxygen (Po_2)	Decrease	85–95 mm Hg	Increase:
			  Administration of pure oxygen
			Decrease:
			  Circulatory disorders
			  Decreased hemoglobin
			  Decreased oxygen supply
			  High altitudes
			  Poor oxygen uptake and utilization
			  Respiratory exchange problems

*Standard reference ranges used at St. Francis Hospital Laboratory, Beech Grove, Ind., 1996.

†The deviations list is not all-inclusive but is a helpful guide for many of the frequent deviations seen in the elderly. Modified from Eliopoulos C: *Health assessment of the older adult.* Reading, Mass., 1990, Addison-Wesley; and Eliopoulos A: *A guide to the nursing of the aging,* Baltimore, 1987, Williams & Wilkins.

‡Must be differentiated between normal age changes and anemia.

§Garner B: Guide to changing lab values in the elderly, *Geriatr Nurs* 10(3):144, 1989.

RESOURCES

Administration on Aging
Department of Health and Human
  Services
330 Independence Avenue SW
Washington, DC 20201
(202) 619-0724
FAX (202) 619-3759
Internet aoa—esec@
  bangate.aoa.dhhs.gov
http://www.aoa.dhhs.gov

Aging Network Services
Suite 907
4400 East-West Highway
Bethesda, MD 20814
(301) 657-4329

Alzheimer's Association
Suite 1000
919 North Michigan Avenue
Chicago, IL 60611
(312) 335-8700
FAX (312) 335-1110
TTY (312) 335-8882
Internet http:/www.alz.org

Alzheimer's Disease Education and
  Referral Center
PO Box 8250
Silver Spring, MD 20907-8250
(301) 495-3311
FAX (301) 495-3334
Internet adear@alzheimers.org

American Association of
  Cardiovascular and Pulmonary
  Rehabilitation
Suite 201
7611 Elmwood Avenue
Middleton, WI 53562
(608) 831-6989
FAX (608) 831-5122

American Association for Geriatric
  Psychiatry
Seventh Floor
7910 Woodmont Avenue
Bethesda, MD 20814-3004
(301) 654-7850
FAX (301) 654-4137
Internet aagpgpa@aol.com

American Brain Tumor Association
Suite 146
2720 River Road
Des Plaines, IL 60018
(847) 827-9910
FAX (847) 827-9918
Internet abta@aol.com

American Federation for Aging
  Research
18th Floor
1414 Avenue of the Americas
New York, NY 10019
(212) 752-2327
FAX (212) 832-2298
Internet amsedaging@aol.com

American Geriatrics Society
Suite 300
770 Lexington Avenue
New York, NY 10021
(212) 308-1414
FAX (212) 832-8646
E-Mail:
  info.amger@americangeriatrics.org
http://www.americangeriatrics.org

American Lung Association
1740 Broadway
New York, NY 10019-4374
(212) 315-8700
FAX (212) 265-5642

American Psychiatric Association
1400 K Street NW
Washington, DC 20005
(202) 682-6220

American Health Assistance
  Foundation
Suite 140
15825 Shady Grove Road
Rockville, MD 20850
(301) 948-3244
FAX (301) 258-9454
Internet http://www.ahaf.org

American Society on Aging
Suite 511
833 Market Street
San Francisco, CA 94103
(415) 974-9600
FAX (415) 974-0300
http://www.healthanswers.com/oac/
  asa/
E-mail: info@asa.asaging.org

Association for Adult Development
  and Aging
5999 Stevenson Avenue
Alexandria, VA 22304
(703) 823-9800
FAX (703) 823-0252

Better Hearing Institute
PO Box 1840
Washington, DC 20013
(703) 642-0580

Beverly Foundation
44 South Mentor Avenue
Pasadena, CA 91106
(818) 792-2292

Brookdale Center on Aging
425 East 25th Street
New York, NY 10010
(212) 481-4426
FAX (212) 481-5069

Catholic Golden Age
430 Penn Avenue
Scranton, PA 18503
(717) 342-3294

Clearinghouse on Abuse and Neglect
  of the Elderly
College of Human Resources
University of Delaware
Newark, DE 19716
(302) 831-3525

Disabled American Veterans
807 Maine Avenue SW
Washington, DC 20024
(202) 554-3501

Eldercare Initiative in Consumer Law
National Consumer Law Center, Inc.
Suite 400
18 Tremont Street
Boston, MA 02108
(617) 523-8010
FAX (617) 523-7398
E-mail: aoa@nclc.org
http://www.consumerlaw.org/

Elderhostel
75 Federal Street
Boston, MA 02110-1941
(617) 426-7788

Health Insurance Association of
  America
Suite 600E
555 13th Street NW
Washington, DC 20004
(202) 824-1600

Meeting the Special Concerns of
  Hispanic Older Women
National Hispanic Council on Aging
2713 Ontario Road NW
Washington, DC 20009
(202) 265-1288
FAX (202) 745-2522

National Association of Area Agencies
on Aging
Suite 100
1112 16th Street NW
Washington, DC 20036-4823
(202) 296-8130
FAX (202) 296-8134

National Clearinghouse for Legal
Services, Inc.
Second Floor
205 West Monroe Street
Chicago, IL 60606-5013
(312) 263-3830
FAX (312) 263-3846
Internet ncls@interaccess.com

National Diabetes Information
Clearinghouse
1 Information Way
Bethesda, MD 20892-3560
(301) 654-3327
Internet ndic@aerie.com
http://www.niddk.nih.gov

National Eldercare Legal Assistance
Project
National Senior Citizens
Law Center
Suite 700
1815 H Street NW
Washington, DC 20006
(202) 887-5280
FAX (202) 785-6792

National Indian Council on Aging
City Centre
Suite 510W
6400 Uptown Boulevard NE
Albuquerque, NM 87110
(505) 888-3302
FAX (505) 888-3276

National Institute of Neurological
Disorders and Stroke
Information Office
Building 31, Room 8A06
31 Center Drive MSC 2540
Bethesda, MD 20892-2540
(301) 496-5751

National Institute on Aging
Public Information Office
Building 31, Room 5C27
31 Center Drive MSC 2292
Bethesda, MD 20892-2292
(301) 496-1752
FAX (301) 496-1072

National Interfaith Coalition on Aging
National Council on the Aging
Suite 200
409 3rd Street SW
Washington, DC 20024
(202) 479-1200

National Long-Term Care Resource
Center
Institute for Health Services Research
University of Minnesota School of
Public Health
420 Delaware SE
Box 197 Mayo
Minneapolis, MN 55455
(612) 624-5171
FAX (612) 624-5434

National Policy and Resource Center
on Nutrition and Aging
Department of Dietetics and Nutrition
Florida International University
University Park, OE200
Miami, FL 33199
(305) 348-1517
FAX (305) 348-1518
TTY (800) 955-8771
Internet nutrelder@solix.flu.edu
http://www.fiu.edu//nutreldr

National Senior Sports Association
Suite 204
301 North Harrison Street
Princeton, NJ 08540
(609) 466-0022
FAX (609) 466-9366

National Women's Health Network
Suite 400
514 10th Street NW
Washington, DC 20004
(202) 347-1140
FAX (202) 347-1168

Organization of Chinese Americans
Room 707
1001 Connecticut Avenue NW
Washington, DC 20036
(202) 223-5500
FAX (202) 296-0540
Internet oca@ari.net

President's Council on Physical
Fitness and Sports
Suite 250
701 Pennsylvania Avenue NW
Washington, DC 20004
(202) 272-3421
FAX (202) 504-2064

United Parkinson Foundation
833 West Washington Boulevard
Chicago, IL 60607
(312) 664-2344
FAX (312) 664-2344

STUDENT ACTIVITIES

Chapter 1

1. Describe three types of aging:

a.

b.

c.

2. An abnormal fear of aging or elderly persons is called

_____. An extreme example of

this fear is called _____. When

this fear results in differing treatment of the elderly,

_____ exists.

3. The statistical study of human populations is referred

to as _____. The measurements

obtained from these studies are commonly called

_____.

4. Vital statistics include records of:

a.

b.

c.

d.

e.

f.

5. The most significant demographic group is called the

_____. These individuals

were born between _____ and _____. This

group is significant because it makes up

_____ of all Americans today.

6. Today's over 65 population comprises _____% of

the population. By 2030 it is projected that this group

will comprise over _____% of the population.

7. More than 75% of the elderly population lives in

_____ areas.

8. The major sources of income for the elderly include:

a.

b.

c.

d.

9. Approximately _____% of the elderly live inde-

pendently; _____% live in modified housing set-

tings; and only _____% are institutionalized.

10. Alternative forms of housing for the elderly include:

a.

b.

c.

d.

11. The government program that provides health care

for the elderly is called _____.

Inpatient hospital care is covered by

_____ of this plan, whereas

_____% of the costs for physician services are

covered by _____. Supplemental

financial assistance is available for the most needy

elderly through Title 19, which is known as

_____.

12. Two legal documents used to guide families and

health care providers regarding the type and amount

of health care desired by the elderly are:

a.

b.

13. Identify some of the stressors that affect members of

the "sandwich" generation.

a.

b.

c

14. The most significant change affecting the elderly and

their children is the loss of _____.

15. Signs of self-neglect include:

a.

b.

c.

d.

e.

f.

g.

16. Failure to provide necessary care is called _____. Deliberate harm or mistreatment of another person is called _____.

17. Different forms of abuse include:

a.

b.

c.

18. The proper term to describe desertion of a dependent elderly person is _____.

19. _____ care is one method of providing release time for family caregivers to meet their own needs.

Chapter 2

Matching: Match the theory in column 1 with the description in column 2.

Column 1 (theories)

1. ___ programmed

2. ___ run out of program

3. ___ gene

4. ___ error

5. ___ free radical

6. ___ crosslink

7. ___ wear and tear

8. ___ immunologic

9. ___ somatic mutation

Column 2 (description)

a. cells wear out due to internal and external stressors

b. errors in protein synthesis result in biologic decline

c. cellular DNA or tissue interacts with free radicals, decreasing the body's ability to replace itself

d. harmful genes limit the lifespan

e. the body's "time clock" runs out

f. the immune system loses the ability to distinguish self

g. the limited amount of genetic material is used up

h. DNA is damaged by exposure to the environment

i. substances produced during medabolism are not eliminated, resulting in cell damage

10. The withdrawal from society that is observed in some elderly people is called _____.

11. According to Havighurst, the major task of aging is to maintain _____. Failure to achieve this task results in _____ or _____.

Chapter 3

Integumentary System

1. With aging, the _____ becomes increasingly fragile and subject to damage.

2. Clusters of _____ cause "age spots." The medical term for these is _____.

3. Loss of _____ results in wrinkles.

4. Dry skin, or _____, is likely to result in itching, or _____.

5. Common skin disorders in the elderly include:

    a.

    b.

    c.

    d.

    e.

    f.

6. Loss of subcutaneous _____ tissue can reduce the ability of the elderly to regulate body temperature, leading to an increased risk for _____.

Musculoskeletal System

7. Aging bones tend to show loss of the mineral _____.

8. Shrinkage of intervertebral disks leads to a condition called _____, which results in a hunchback appearance.

9. Muscle mass and tone typically _____ with age, but this effect can be reduced by regular _____.

10. Excessive loss of calcium results in _____, which is characterized by _____, _____, _____ bones that are susceptible to _____.

11. Three forms of arthritis that are seen in the aging population are _____, _____, and _____.

Respiratory System

12. The _____ and _____ of the chest cavity change with aging.

13. Common respiratory disorders observed with aging include:

    a.

    b.

    c.

    d.

    e.

Cardiovascular System

14. Changes in the blood vessels with aging increase the risk of low blood pressure with position changes. This is called _____.

15. Chest pain caused by reduced blood flow to the heart muscle is known as _____.

16. Heart _____ become less pliant with age, resulting in _____ sealing of the valves during heartbeat.

17. Loss of heart pumping effectiveness, called _____ or _____, is a common cardiac problem in the elderly. This condition can be characterized as _____ or _____.

18. Cardiomegaly, or _____ of the heart, is commonly observed with congestive heart failure.

19. Arteriosclerosis results in loss of _____ in the blood vessels.

20. Plaque formation is enhanced by lifestyle factors that include:

    a.

    b.

    c.

21. Hypertension affects more than _____% of individuals over 65 years of age.

Hematopoietic and Lymph Systems

22. Blood values for erythrocytes, leukocytes, and platelets generally remain _____ with aging.

23. Changes in T cells result in a _____ immune response leading to modified signs of _____ .

24. Changes in the signs of infection seen with aging include:

a.

b.

Gastrointestinal System

25. A protrusion of the stomach into the thoracic cavity, known as a _____ , is commonly seen with aging. Gastroesophageal reflux disease, or _____ , results in movement of stomach contents into the _____ , increasing the risk of _____ .

26. Drugs that increase the risk of ulcer formation in the elderly include:

a.

b.

c.

27. Weakness of the intestinal mucosa leads to the formation of _____ .

28. The incidence of colon cancer peaks between _____ and _____ years of age.

Urinary System

29. The kidneys lose about _____ of their efficiency by age 70, resulting in less _____ urine.

30. Many elderly experience the urge to urinate when only _____ ml of urine is present in the bladder.

31. Urinary retention increases the risk of _____ in the elderly. Elderly men with _____ are at risk for this problem.

Nervous System

32. Motor responses take _____ to occur in the elderly. This can result in a slowing of simple everyday activities such as _____ and _____ .

33. A decreased level of the neurotransmitter _____ results in Parkinson's disease.

34. Common symptoms of Parkinson's disease include:

a.

b.

c.

d.

e.

35. Drugs commonly used to treat Parkinson's disease include:

a.

b.

c.

d.

36. _____ is a general term used to describe a permanent or progressive organic mental disorder. A common form of this disorder seen in individuals over 60 years of age is _____ disease.

37. Behavior changes seen with dementia include:

a.

b.

c.

d.

e.

38. A cerebrovascular accident to the right side in the brain will affect the _____ side of the body. One occurring in the left side of the brain will affect the _____ side of the body.

39. Farsightedness that occurs with aging is called

_____ .

40. Changes in the aging eye make it difficult to see in

_____ or _____

environments. A severe form of this problem can

cause _____ .

41. Fluid secretion in the eyes decreases with aging,

resulting in decreased _____

production leading to _____,

_____, or _____

eyes.

42. A clouding of the lens, called _____,

is common with aging. By age 85, _____ % of the

elderly develop this condition.

43. Glaucoma is characterized by increased

_____ pressure, which will cause

_____ if not treated.

44. Hearing changes with aging are likely to result in loss

of the _____-pitched frequencies.

This condition, called _____, is

more commonly observed in _____ .

45. The elderly often comment on changes in the taste

of food. This may be caused by decreased sensory

_____ or may be a side effect of

_____ .

Endocrine System

46. Decreased amounts of thyroid-stimulating hor-

mone can lead to a decrease in the basal

_____ rate.

47. Altered function of the β cells of the pancreas leads

to a disease called _____ . The

incidence of this disorder _____

with each decade of life. Approximately _____ %

of persons over 70 years of age have altered glu-

cose metabolism.

48. Classic signs and symptoms of diabetes mellitus

include:

a.

b.

c.

49. Reduced thyroid function results in decreased

_____ function.

50. Signs and symptoms of hypothyroidism that are often

mistaken as signs of aging include:

a.

b.

c.

d.

e.

Chapter 4

1. It is estimated that _____ % of the elderly live with some chronic health condition.

2. Health promotion is (more/less) expensive than treatment of health problems.

3. Recommended health practices for the elderly include:

   a.

   b.

   c.

   d.

   e.

   f.

   g.

4. Medic alert devices are most important for individuals who have _____, _____, or _____.

5. Elderly persons with _____, _____ and _____ limitations in addition to those who have lost their _____ due to grief or hopelessness are at increased risk for alterations in health maintenance.

6. A person is said to be _____ when he or she fails to follow through with recommended health practices.

7. When a person does not follow through with recommended health practices, it is most important to determine the _____ for noncompliance.

8. Nurses must remain _____ when working with noncompliant individuals.

Chapter 5

1. Effective communication requires a climate of mutual respect and understanding which is known as _____ .

2. _____ is the willingness to attempt to understand the unique world of others.

3. When communicating with others, particularly the elderly, nurses must pay special attention to _____ changes, _____ changes, _____ , and _____ .

4. Nonverbal methods of communication include:

   a.

   b.

   c.

   d.

   e.

   f.

   g.

   h.

   i.

   j.

   k.

5. It is most appropriate to address elderly persons using their _____ . Baby talk names are _____ and _____ to the elderly.

6. When attempting to obtain specific information quickly, it is most appropriate to use _____ questions.

7. _____ questions help to clarify feelings and fears and establish an empathetic climate.

8. Inconsistent information or contradictions may require some form of _____ questions. These should be used _____ and _____ because they can easily _____ the other person.

Chapter 6

1. The energy available in food is measured in units called _____.

2. The amount of calories needed for each individual is based on _____, _____, _____, _____, _____, _____, and _____.

3. Changes in the percentage of body fat and muscle lead to changes in the basal _____ rate.

4. The elderly should consume foods that are high in _____ but low in _____.

5. Foods rich in _____ are needed for tissue repair and healing.

6. Vitamins are a possible source of _____, which are suspected to be of value in blocking free radicals.

7. Vitamin B_{12} deficiency can affect the nervous system, causing changes in _____, _____, and _____.

8. Vitamin E appears to play a role in maintaining function of the _____ system.

9. Anemia in the elderly is commonly a result of inadequate intake of the mineral _____, which can be found in foods such as _____, _____, _____, and _____.

10. Ingestion of vitamin _____ enhances the absorption of iron.

11. Elderly persons are likely to consume excessive amounts of _____, which contains the mineral _____, to compensate for a diminished sense of taste.

12. Potassium deficiency, or _____, is commonly a problem for elderly persons who are taking _____ or _____ medications.

13. Good sources of potassium are _____, _____, _____, and _____.

14. The most common symptom of potassium deficiency is _____.

15. Elderly adults have (more/less) body fluid than do younger adults. Most older adults require between _____ and _____ ml of fluid per day.

16. The nutritional status of the elderly is affected by _____, _____, _____, and _____ factors.

Chapter 7

1. The elderly must be cautious when taking medication because medications can alter their ability to perform normal _____, result in _____ changes, and in the worst cases can be life-_____ .

2. The study of how the elderly respond to medications is called _____ .

3. Drug absorption is affected by decreased gastric _____, _____, and _____ .

4. Water-soluble drugs are likely to be present in (*lower/higher*) concentrations in the bloodstream of the elderly, increasing the risk for _____ .

5. Fat-soluble drugs are likely to become _____ in fatty tissues, resulting in (*low/high*) blood levels. These drugs are released slowly, resulting in _____ drug effects.

6. The likelihood of drug _____ is increased in malnourished elderly.

7. Drug metabolism is affected by altered _____ function.

8. Response to medication is (*more/less*) predictable in the elderly.

9. _____ is the term used to describe the use of multiple medications by the elderly.

10. Factors that contribute to excessive use of medications by the elderly include:
    a.
    b.
    c.
    d.

11. Cognitive problems that contribute to drug errors among the elderly include the lack of:
    a.
    b.
    c.

12. The elderly must be aware that drugs purchased without a prescription, or _____ (OTC) medications, can _____ with other medications.

13. Before administering any medication, nurses must know why the person is receiving the medication. Nurses must also know the _____ of administration, the therapeutic _____, the therapeutic _____, the _____ effects, and signs of _____ .

14. The "rights" of medication administration include the right:
    a.
    b.
    c.
    d.
    e.
    f.
    g.

15. _____ is a major nursing responsibility when an elderly person will be self-medicating.

16. For safety, medications used to promote sleep should not be kept _____ .

Chapter 8

1. Screenings are conducted to _____ elderly persons with significant findings and to _____ them to appropriate resources.

2. All of the information collected about an individual is called _____. This information can be _____ or _____.

3. _____ information is gathered using the senses. Examples of this type of information include _____, _____, _____ and _____. _____ information must be provided by the person being assessed. Examples of this include _____, _____, _____, and _____.

4. List some factors to consider when preparing the environment for an interview with an elderly person.
   a.
   b.
   c.
   d.
   e.

5. Identify ways to establish rapport with the elderly.
   a.
   b.
   c.
   d.
   e.
   f.

6. Commonly used assessment techniques include:
   a.
   b.
   c.
   d.

7. Temperature can be assessed by which routes? Identify the advantages /disadvantages of each.
   a.
   b.
   c.
   d.

8. When taking peripheral pulses nurses should be careful to start with the most _____ pulse and compare pulses on each _____.

9. A decreased _____ rate may be an early indication of infection.

10. Too wide a blood pressure cuff can result in falsely (low/high) readings. A cuff that is too narrow can result in falsely (low/high) readings.

11. Postural changes in blood pressure can result in a condition called _____, with symptoms of _____ or _____. When checking for this condition, blood pressure is first assessed with the patient _____, then _____, then _____.

12. A federally developed assessment tool for extended-care facilities is called the _____, which is abbreviated MDS. This tool has special focus assessments called _____, or RAPS.

Chapter 9

1. Elderly persons make up 11% of the population but account for _____ % of accidental deaths.

2. The four most common causes of accidental death among the elderly are:
   a.
   b.
   c.
   d.

3. Changes in the senses of _____ and _____ increase the risk of accident and injury in the elderly.

4. Risk for falls is increased due to physiologic factors including:
   a.
   b.
   c.
   d.
   e.
   f.
   g.

5. Cardiovascular changes, particularly those that result in postural hypotension, increase the risk of _____ and _____, both of which can lead to falls.

6. Classifications of medications that can contribute to falls include:
   a.
   b.
   c.
   d.
   e.
   f.

7. Emotional factors that increase the risk for injury include _____, _____, and _____.

8. Increasing the base of physical support can improve stability and help to prevent falls. Devices that increase the base of support for the elderly include _____ and _____.

9. Motor vehicle accidents are the _____ most common cause of accidental death among the elderly.

10. Due to changes in thermoregulation, the elderly are at increased risk for both _____ and _____.

11. Medications such as _____ and anti-_____ drugs increase the risk of hyperthermia.

12. It is wise for the elderly to take precautions, particularly when dealing with _____ or going to new _____. This is unfortunate because fear of _____ can make elderly persons prisoners in their own _____.

Chapter 10

1. Inadequate nutrition and fluid intake can result in serious problems such as _____ and _____ . They can also contribute to the development of _____ and _____ .

2. Factors that contribute to inadequate nutrition intake include:

   a.

   b.

   c.

   d.

   e.

   f.

   g.

   h.

3. Weight changes are usually due to changes in the balance between _____ intake and _____ expenditure.

4. Inadequate intake of iron is likely to affect laboratory values for _____ . Common forms of anemia observed in the elderly include _____ , _____ , and _____ .

5. Electrolyte imbalances in the elderly frequently involve:

   a.

   b.

   c.

6. Inadequate nutritional intake is likely to contribute to tissue _____ and slow tissue _____ .

7. Aging results in decreased production of _____ , which can interfere with normal swallowing and lead to changes in _____ sensation.

8. When an individual is on a _____ -restricted diet, beverages such as cola should be restricted.

9. Individuals with diverticuli should avoid corn with _____ .

10. Symptoms of a fluid volume deficit include:

    a.

    b.

    c.

    d.

    e.

    f.

    g.

    h.

    i.

    j.

11. Symptoms of fluid volume excess include:

    a.

    b.

    c.

    d.

    e.

    f.

    g.

    h.

    i.

12. Difficulty swallowing is properly termed _____ .

13. A person who has diminished gag or swallow reflexes is at increased risk for _____ .

14. _____ position is used for individuals receiving tube feedings because in this position _____ helps keep the solution in the stomach.

Chapter 11

1. Traumatic injuries to aging skin are common because the epidermal layer is _____ and there is less _____ padding.

2. Decreased _____ secretions contribute to dryness, which affects between _____% and _____% of those over 65 years of age.

3. Dry skin is likely to result in itching, or _____, which further increases the risk of tissue damage and _____.

4. Common causes of rashes and skin irritation include:
   a.
   b.
   c.

5. The risk for pressure ulcers is increased in older adults who suffer from:
   a.
   b.
   c.
   d.
   e.

6. Common pressure points for individuals who spend extended periods of time sitting include:
   a.
   b.
   c.
   d.
   e.

7. Common foot problems in the elderly include:
   a.
   b.
   c.
   d.
   e.
   f.
   g.
   h.
   i.

8. In order to prevent excessive skin dryness in the elderly, nurses can:
   a.
   b.
   c.

9. To reduce shearing forces the head of the bed should be elevated no more than _____°. Care should be used to reduce _____ when moving or transferring the elderly.

10. Special mattresses are used to decrease pressure over bony prominences. These devices work because they _____ over a larger area.

11. The nutrients _____ and _____ are particularly important for tissue repair.

12. High levels of bacteria in the mouth contribute to _____, _____, and _____ disease.

13. Dryness of the mouth, or _____, can be caused by age-related changes, _____, _____, or _____.

14. Oral mucous membranes can be affected by deficiencies of:
    a.
    b.
    c.

15. Special attention should be paid to the gingiva of individuals receiving medication for _____ or other _____ disorders.

Chapter 12

1. The two major body systems involved in elimination of waste products are the _____ and _____ systems. The _____ plays a minor role in waste removal.

2. Elimination is affected by:

   a.

   b.

   c.

   d.

   e.

   f.

3. Most adults defecate every _____ to _____ days.

4. Most adults experience the urge to urinate when the bladder contains _____ ml of urine. Elderly individuals may experience this urge when only _____ ml is present.

5. Common elimination problems of the elderly include:

   a.

   b.

   c.

6. Factors that contribute to constipation include:

   a.

   b.

   c.

   d.

   e.

   f.

   g.

   h.

   i.

   j.

7. Medications that contribute to constipation include

   a.

   b.

   c.

   d.

   e.

   f.

   g.

   h.

   i.

8. A _____ is a hardened mass of feces that usually results from unrelieved _____. This problem should be suspected in individuals who do not have bowel movements for _____ days or when only _____ stool is passed without any formed material.

9. Common symptoms associated with severe constipation include:

   a.

   b.

   c.

   d.

   e.

10. Digital examination should be used with caution on any elderly person who has a history of a _____ condition because such manipulation can result in a decreased _____, _____, or even loss of _____.

11. Caution must be used to administer adequate _____ to patients receiving a psyllium-based bulk former or complications including _____ or _____ may occur.

12. High-fiber foods include:

a.

b.

c.

d.

13. Fluid intake of _____ ml daily will help reduce the risk of constipation.

14. Elderly persons with diarrhea are at risk for fluid volume _____. Fluids high in _____ are recommended to replace those lost through diarrhea.

15. Signs and symptoms of fluid volume deficit include:

a.

b.

c.

d.

16. Incontinence of bladder and/or bowel is likely to result in:

a.

b.

c.

17. Urinary retention in the elderly is commonly a result of:

a.

b.

c.

d.

e.

f.

g.

18. Signs and symptoms of urinary retention include:

a.

b.

c.

d.

e.

f.

19. Types of urinary incontinence include:

a.

b.

c.

d.

e.

20. Indwelling catheters should only be used when the _____ to the person outweigh the _____. Because urinary retention or _____ incontinence may occur after an indwelling catheter is removed, urinary _____ should be monitored closely.

Chapter 13

1. Activity requires interaction of the _____, _____, _____, and _____ systems.

2. Activity and _____ patterns established at a young age usually continue into older age, although there is typically a decrease in the _____, _____, and _____ of older persons.

3. Physical activity helps to maintain _____ mobility and _____ tone.

4. _____ motor skills tend to remain intact longer than do _____ motor skills.

5. _____ exercises help to maintain joint mobility.

6. Consultation with a _____ or _____ therapist can help identify appropriate activities for an elderly person. These therapists can also recommend _____ devices designed to help the elderly maintain optimal activity.

7. Exercise periods of _____ to _____ minutes at least _____ times per week are recommended for the elderly.

8. Assessment of _____ provides a good indication of the ability of elderly persons to tolerate activity.

9. _____ often results in inadequate reserves of glucose, _____, and _____. Inadequate supplies of these nutrients can contribute to a reduced ability to perform _____ due to muscle _____ and decreased oxygen transport related to _____.

10. Emotional disorders, including _____, _____, and _____, can lead to decreased participation in normal activity.

11. Use of restraints should be _____ because by definition these devices limit _____ and cause joints and muscles to lose function. These changes ultimately increase the risk for _____.

12. _____ range-of-motion exercises will help keep joints flexible but do little to maintain muscle strength. _____ range-of-motion or other types of exercise are needed to tone and strengthen muscles.

13. When an individual has one-sided weakness, assistive devices should be positioned on the _____ side.

14. Excessive respiratory secretions can reduce _____ intake and _____ the ability to participate in activity. The most appropriate nursing diagnosis for an individual who is unable to clear secretions is ineffective _____.

15. Approaches designed to deal with excessive secretions include:

    a.

    b.

    c.

    d.

    e.

16. Medications that may aid individuals with excessive secretions include:

    a.

    b.

    c.

17. Analgesics and sedatives may make activity easier but should be used with caution because they can affect the _____ and _____ of respiration and can increase _____ risks.

18. Self-care deficits are often devastating to the elderly because they lead to _____ and loss of _____, thereby affecting self- _____ .

19. Elderly persons with self-care deficits should be _____ to perform as much self-care as possible. _____ will help maintain motivation.

20. The elderly should be encouraged to select diversional activities that they find _____ .

21. A rehabilitation perspective credits elderly persons with _____ and _____ potential.

22. The long-term goal of rehabilitation is to help older adults achieve and maintain maximum _____ , _____ , and _____ health.

Chapter 14

1. Common behaviors connected to sleep deprivation include:

   a.

   b.

   c.

   d.

   e.

   f.

   g.

   h.

2. As many as _____ of independent-living elderly and _____ of institutionalized elderly are estimated to have sleep disturbances.

3. Sleep is under the influence of chemicals produced within the _____ system.

4. Deepest sleep occurs in stage _____ of non-rapid eye movement (NREM) sleep.

5. Dreaming occurs during the _____ stage of sleep.

6. The average elderly person sleeps (*more/less*) than does the average younger adult.

7. Insomnia affects three phases of sleep and is categorized as:

   a.

   b.

   c.

8. Common factors that affect sleep include:

   a.

   b.

   c.

   d.

   e.

Chapter 15

1. The term perception includes:

   a.

   b.

   c.

2. The term *cognition* includes:

   a.

   b.

   c.

   d.

3. Both perception and cognition rely on effective functioning of the _____ system, particularly sensory input from the senses of _____, _____, _____, _____, and _____.

4. Any disorder that affects the _____ is likely to affect perception and cognition.

5. Older individuals are likely to use _____ intelligence to make judgments. This form of intelligence is based on _____ and _____ gained over a lifetime.

6. The correct medical term for loss of the ability to understand or express oneself using language is _____ or _____. This should not be confused with _____, which is difficulty swallowing.

7. Intelligence does not normally _____ with aging, although responses tend to be _____ and more _____.

8. The _____-term memory of older persons tends to be affected more by aging than does _____-term memory.

9. _____ misperception should be ruled out before _____ disorders are suspected.

10. Confusion is defined as a mental state characterized by disorientation regarding _____, _____, or _____.

11. Confusion is categorized as:

    a.

    b.

    c.

12. Delirium can be caused by:

    a.

    b.

    c.

    d.

    e.

    f.

    g.

    h.

    i.

    j.

    k.

    l.

13. Acute delirium has a sudden onset measured in terms of _____ or _____.

14. Symptoms of acute delirium include:

    a.

    b.

    c.

    d.

    e.

    f.

    g.

    h.

15. Older adults suffering from acute delirium typically do not respond to _____ approaches because the problem has _____ causes.

16. Dementia has a _____, _____ onset.

17. Disease conditions that result in dementia include:

a.

b.

c.

d.

e.

f.

g.

h.

i.

j.

18. Common behaviors observed with dementia include:

a.

b.

c.

d.

e.

f.

19. Behaviors associated with dementia often _____ late in the day. This is referred to as _____ syndrome.

20. Dementia affects up to _____% of the community-dwelling aging population. Estimates place the incidence of dementia in individuals over age 85 at _____%.

21. _____ of care is important when caring for individuals with dementia. Physical and chemical _____ should be avoided because they can make behavior _____.

22. Psychotropic medication should be kept at the _____ dose for the _____ period of time.

23. The elderly are at _____ risk for pain connected with disease processes. _____ or _____ pain can result in behavior changes.

24. Behavior changes observed with pain include:

a.

b.

c.

Chapter 16

1. Self-identity is formed from the _____ and _____ a person holds of him- or herself. It originates in personal _____, life _____, and _____ with others.

2. People with good self-identity usually have strong _____ and a sense of _____ over their lives.

3. _____ feedback from others helps older persons maintain high self-esteem.

4. Nurses can assess a person's self-esteem level by observing:
   a.
   b.
   c.
   d.
   e.

5. Both _____ and _____ have a negative impact on self-image and self-esteem.

6. Placement in an _____ setting can contribute to loss of self-esteem by stripping the elderly of their personal _____ and diminishing the amount of _____ the elderly have over their lives.

7. Institutionalized elderly persons typically experience feelings of _____ or _____, which further diminish self-worth.

8. Nursing diagnoses that address loss of self-image and self-worth include:
   a.
   b.
   c.

9. Loss of physical health and/or deforming injuries are likely to affect an older person's body _____.

10. Nurses should encourage _____, or life review, to help the elderly person find _____ and _____ in their lives. This process can also help the elderly identify their _____ and effective _____ strategies they have used in the past.

11. Common fears experienced by the elderly include those of:
   a.
   b.
   c.
   d.
   e.
   f.
   g.
   h.
   i.

12. A person experiencing fear or anxiety can manifest physical symptoms such as:
   a.
   b.
   c.
   d.
   e.
   f.
   g.
   h.

13. Physiologic stimulation caused by fear or increased anxiety is particularly dangerous to elderly people who have a history of diseases of the _____, _____, _____, or _____ system.

14. Hopelessness can lead an elderly person to engage in self-_____ behaviors, the most serious of which is _____.

15. Competent elderly persons often demonstrate a desire to retain control when they exercise the right to _____ treatments or procedures.

16. Methods of dealing with refusals include:

a.

b.

c.

d.

17. If elderly persons continue to object to or refuse care, nurses should:

a.

b.

c.

Chapter 17

1. People tend to establish their identities and describe themselves based on the _____ they play in life.

2. Roles are _____ and are given value by the _____ in which a person lives. Roles confer _____ and carry various _____ that are communicated through _____, _____, and _____ .

3. A _____ society has clear role expectations for all members. In a complex or _____ society, roles are not as clear; therefore, role _____ and societal _____ are more likely to occur.

4. Aging often results in the _____ of familiar roles. These losses are likely to result in feelings of _____ .

5. Typical life events that affect role identity include:

   a.
   b.
   c.
   d.
   e.

6. Stages of grieving include:

   a.
   b.
   c.
   d.

7. Dysfunctional grief can result in _____, _____, _____, and _____ changes.

8. A series of losses can lead to social _____ and impaired social _____ .

9. An elderly person with adult children may have difficulty accepting change in the _____–_____ roles and relationships. This may lead to a nursing diagnosis of alteration in _____ . This problem is particularly common when the elderly parent is _____ on the child for physical or financial support.

Chapter 18

1. Persons experience stress whenever they are faced with a _____ or _____ threat or a _____ or life-threatening change.

2. Stressors include external physical threats such as _____, _____, or _____; external emotional threats such as changes in _____ or social _____; and internal threats such as disturbing _____ or feelings.

3. Stress level is determined by the person's _____ of an event. Because stress is _____, several minor events can have the same impact as a single _____ event.

4. A very high stress rating for the elderly is given to the _____ of a spouse.

5. The general _____ syndrome, proposed by _____, describes the physical response to stress. According to this theory, both the sympathetic and parasympathetic portions of the _____ nervous system are involved.

6. Physiologic signs of stress include:

   a.

   b.

   c.

   d.

   e.

   f.

   g.

7. Cognitive changes that are evident with severe stress include:

   a.

   b.

   c.

8. Emotional changes that are evident with severe stress include:

   a.

   b.

   c.

   d.

   e.

   f.

9. Behavioral changes that are evident with severe stress include:

   a.

   b.

   c.

   d.

   e.

   f.

10. Stress is closely related to the development of both _____ and _____ illness.

11. _____ strategies help people deal with stress. These strategies include _____, _____, _____, and _____.

12. Approaches that help decrease stress include:

    a.

    b.

    c.

    d.

13. Many of the stressors seen with aging are connected to _____ or _____. One specific problem related to loss or change of residence is called _____ stress.

Chapter 19

1. A person's values and beliefs have their origins in

   _____ , _____ ,

   _____ , and _____ .

2. Most values and belief patterns are established

   _____ in life.

3. _____ and _____

   are likely to occur when people with differing values

   and experience interact.

4. In order to work effectively with a variety of people

   nurses must be willing to try to _____

   and _____ with the other person.

5. Nonjudgmental interaction requires a high level

   of _____ and excellent

   _____ skills.

6. Common values and beliefs of today's elderly population include:

   a.

   b.

   c.

   d.

7. Religious _____ and

   _____ are very important to many

   elderly persons. Many wish to have

   _____ of religious significance

   available for comfort and _____ .

8. Nurses must be careful to demonstrate

   _____ for the religious beliefs of the

   elderly and to offer to contact a _____

   counselor.

Chapter 20

1. Sexual _____, _____, and _____ remain part of the lives of active elderly persons.

2. The major reason for lack of sexual activity is the _____ or _____ of a spouse.

3. Elderly women experience decreased vaginal _____ due to hormone changes. The tissues of the vagina become _____ and less _____.

4. Elderly men experience a _____ re-action to sexual stimuli and take _____ to achieve an erection.

5. Medications likely to cause difficulty with sexual function include:

   a.

   b.

   c.

   d.

   e.

6. Many elderly person's refrain from sexual activity due to _____ of causing their partner _____ or worsening an existing _____.

7. Elderly individuals who reside in institutional settings should be provided with _____ so they can conduct sexual activity without disturbance.

8. Vulnerable elderly should be protected from _____ sexual contact.

STUDENT ACTIVITIES ANSWERS

Chapter 1

1. chronologic, physiologic, functional
2. gerontophobia, ageism, age discrimination
3. demographics, vital statistics
4. a. births
   b. deaths
   c. age at death
   d. marriages
   e. race
   f. income
5. baby boomers, 1946, 1964, one third
6. 12, 21
7. metropolitan
8. a. social security
   b. pensions
   c. income
   d. asset income
9. 68, 27, 5
10. a. independent/assisted living
    b. life-lease facilities
    c. group homes
    d. community-based residential facilities
11. Medicare, Part A, 80, Part B, Medicaid
12. a. durable power of attorney for health care
    b. living will
13. a. work
    b. dependent children
    c. assisting aging parents
14. independence
15. a. inability to maintain activities of daily living
    b. inability to obtain food and fluids
    c. poor hygiene practices
    d. changes in mental functioning
    e. inability to maintain personal finances
    f. failure to keep important appointments
    g. life-threatening acts
16. neglect, abuse
17. a. physical
    b. emotional
    c. financial
18. abandonment
19. Respite

Chapter 2

1. e
2. g
3. d
4. b
5. i
6. c
7. a
8. f
9. h
10. disengagement
11. integrity, anger, despair

Chapter 3

1. skin
2. melanocytes, senile lentigo
3. elastin
4. xerosis, pruritis
5. a. seborrheic keratosis
   b. cutaneous papilloma
   c. senile purpura
   d. rosacea
   e. contact or allergic dermatitis
   f. seborrheic dermatitis
6. adipose, hypothermia
7. calcium
8. kyphosis
9. decrease, exercise
10. osteoporosis, porous, brittle, fragile, fracture
11. osteoarthritis, rheumatoid arthritis, gouty arthritis
12. size, shape
13. a. emphysema
    b. chronic bronchitis
    c. influenza
    d. pneumonia
    e. lung cancer
14. orthostatic hypotension
15. angina pectoris
16. valves, incomplete
17. congestive heart failure, CHF, acute, chronic
18. enlargement
19. elasticity
20. a. obesity
    b. high cholesterol diet
    c. smoking
21. 50
22. within normal limits
23. decreased, infection
24. a. no early elevation in temperature
    b. absence or diminished report of pain or discomfort
25. hiatal hernia, GERD, esophagus, aspiration
26. a. aspirin
    b. iron supplements
    c. nonsteroidal antiinflammatory drugs (NSAIDs)
27. diverticuli
28. 60, 75
29. one third, concentrated
30. 100
31. urinary tract infection, benign prostatic hyperplasia
32. longer, walking, talking
33. dopamine
34. a. tremors
    b. masklike expression

c. rigidity
d. shuffling gait
e. loss of balance

35. a. levodopa/carbodopa
   b. amatidine
   c. bromocriptine
   d. anticholinergics
36. Dementia, Alzheimer's
37. a. personality changes
   b. confusion
   c. disorientation
   d. deterioration of mental/intellectual function (memory and judgment)
   e. loss of emotional control
38. left, right
39. presbyopia
40. dim, dark, night blindness
41. tear, dry, burning, itchy
42. cataracts, 46
43. intraoccular, blindness
44. high, presbycusis, men
45. receptors, medications
46. metabolic
47. diabetes mellitus, doubles, 20
48. a. polyuria
   b. polydipsia
   c. polyphagia
49. metabolic
50. a. cold intolerance
   b. dry skin/dry and thin body hair
   c. constipation
   d. depression
   e. lack of energy

Chapter 4

1. 80
2. less
3. a. well-balanced diet
   b. established exercise program
   c. quit smoking
   d. alcohol consumption in moderation
   e. routine immunization
   f. healthy attitude
   g. regular dental and medical visits
4. allergies, chronic health conditions, implanted medical devices.
5. cognitive, physical, financial, motivation
6. noncompliant
7. reasons
8. nonjudgmental

Chapter 5

1. rapport
2. Empathy
3. hearing, vision, fatigue, pain
4. a. symbols
   b. tone of voice
   c. body language
   d. space, distance, and position
   e. gestures
   f. facial expressions
   g. eye contact
   h. pace of communication
   i. time and timing of communication
   j. touch
   k. silence
5. given names, patronizing and demeaning
6. direct
7. Open-ended
8. confronting, carefully, infrequently, upset

Chapter 6

1. calories
2. age, sex, body size, activity level, emotional status, body temperature, environmental temperature
3. metabolic
4. nutritional value, calories
5. protein
6. antioxidants
7. sensation, balance, memory
8. immune
9. iron, eggs, red meat, organ meats, leafy green vegetables
10. C
11. table salt, sodium
12. hypokalemia, diuretic, antihypertensive
13. citrus fruits, milk, bananas, apple juice
14. muscle weakness
15. less, 2000, 3000
16. personal, economic, social, physiologic

Chapter 7

1. functions, behavior, threatening
2. geropharmacology
3. acid, motility, peristalsis
4. higher, toxicity
5. trapped, low, prolonged
6. toxicity
7. liver
8. less
9. Polypharmacy
10. a. multiple disease conditions
   b. the wide availability of prescription and over-the-counter medications

c. changes in the expectations of the elderly
d. changes in the health care delivery system

11. a. literacy skills
b. understanding
c. judgment

12. over-the-counter, interact

13. routes, effects, dosage, side, toxicity

14. a. resident
b. medication
c. amount
d. dosage form
e. route
f. time
g. documentation

15. Teaching

16. at the bedside

Chapter 8

1. identify, refer

2. data, objective, subjective

3. Objective, rashes, temperature changes, lesions, sores, Subjective, pain, dizziness, fear, anxiety

4. a. Reduce noise and other distractions.
b. Provide adequate lighting without glare.
c. Provide privacy.
d. Provide a comfortable room temperature.
e. Provide bathroom facilities nearby.

5. a. Introduce yourself.
b. Address the individual respectfully, using his or her proper name.
c. Explain the reason for the interview.
d. Focus on and speak directly to the elderly person.
e. Focus on the elderly person's priority concerns first.
f. Consider the person holistically.

6. a. inspection
b. palpation
c. auscultation
d. percussion

7. a. oral—accurate/requires cooperation
b. rectal—accurate, does not require patient cooperation/uncomfortable, possibly traumatic physically or emotionally
c. axillary—accurate/time consuming
d. tympanic—quick, does not require cooperation/ may provide inaccurate readings

8. distal, side of the body

9. respiratory

10. low, high

11. orthostatic hypotension, dizziness, faintness, lying, sitting, standing.

12. minimum data set, resident assessment protocols

Chapter 9

1. 23

2. a. falls
b. burns
c. poisoning
d. auto accidents

3. vision, hearing

4. a. altered balance
b. decreased mobility
c. decreased flexibility
d. decreased muscle strength
e. delayed reaction time
f. gait changes
g. difficulty lifting the feet

5. dizziness, fainting

6. a. sedatives
b. hypnotics
c. tranquilizers
d. diuretics
e. antihypertensives
f. antihistamines

7. depression, distraction, preoccupation

8. canes, walkers

9. second

10. hypothermia, hyperthermia

11. diuretics, parkinsonian

12. strangers, places, injury, homes

Chapter 10

1. malnutrition, dehydration, osteoporosis, skin ulcers

2. a. sensory changes
b. cognitive changes
c. weakness
d. activity intolerance
e. loss of interest
f. depression
g. medications
h. food procurement problems

3. calorie, energy

4. hemoglobin, iron deficiency anemia, pernicious anemia, hemorrhagic anemia

5. a. sodium
b. potassium
c. calcium

6. breakdown, healing

7. saliva, taste

8. sodium

9. husks

10. a. dry mucous membranes
b. thirst
c. decreased skin turgor
d. rapid weight loss
e. weakness
f. decreased urine production

g. increased pulse rate

h. orthostatic hypotension

i. increased body temperature

j. elevated hematocrit

11. a. swelling of dependent extremities

b. shortness of breath

c. dyspnea

d. gurgling respiration

e. frothy sputum

f. rapid weight gain

g. decreased hematocrit

h. swollen, taut, shiny skin

i. behavioral changes including restlessness and anxiety

12. dysphagia

13. aspiration

14. Fowler's, gravity

Chapter 11

1. thinner, subcutaneous

2. sebaceous, 75, 85

3. pruritus, infection

4. a. medications

b. communicable diseases

c. chemicals

5. a. compromised circulation

b. restricted mobility

c. altered level of consciousness

d. fecal or urinary incontinence

e. nutritional problems

6. a. scapula

b. sacrum/coccyx

c. ischium

d. posterior knee

e. soles of the feet

7. a. hyperkeratosis of the nails

b. corns

c. calluses

d. bunions

e. ingrown toenails

f. hammertoe

g. gout

h. fungus

i. metatarsalgia

8. a. reduce the frequency of bathing

b. avoid use of drying soaps and rinse skin thoroughly

c. use emollients

9. 30, friction

10. distribute body weight

11. protein, vitamin C

12. tooth decay, halitosis, periodontal

13. xerostomia, inadequate hydration, disease processes, medications

14. a. riboflavin

b. niacin

c. vitamin C

15. epilepsy, seizure

Chapter 12

1. urinary, gastrointestinal, skin

2. a. diet

b. fluid intake

c. activity

d. lifestyle routines

e. illness

f. medications

3. 1, 2

4. 300, 200

5. a. constipation

b. diarrhea

c. incontinence of bladder and/or bowel

6. a. decreased peristalsis

b. decreased abdominal muscle tone

c. inactivity

d. immobility

e. decreased fluid intake

f. inadequate dietary bulk

g. disease processes

h. medications

i. dependence on laxatives

j. environmenal conditions

7. a. narcotic analgesics, particularly those containing codeine

b. anticholinergics, including many tricyclic antidepressants and antipsychotics

c. diuretics

d. iron supplements

e. calcium-channel blockers

f. antacids containing aluminum carbonate or aluminum hydroxide

g. some anticonvulsants

h. some nonsteroidal antiinflammatory agents

i. some antihypertensive agents such as the angiotensin converting enzyme (ACE) inhibitors

8. fecal impaction, constipation, 3, liquid

9. a. cramping

b. rectal pain

c. abdominal distention

d. loss of appetite

e. detection of hardened fecal mass with digital examination

10. cardiac, heart rate, syncope, consciousness

11. water, constipation, bowel obstruction

12. a. cereals

b. whole-grain breads

c. bran

d. fruits and vegetables

13. 2000

14. deficit, electrolytes

15. a. decreased skin turgor
   b. postural hypotension
   c. tachycardia
   d. altered laboratory values
16. a. loss of self-esteem
   b. skin irritation or breakdown
   c. social isolation
17. a. decreased bladder muscle tone
   b. decreased fluid intake
   c. enlargement of the prostate
   d. perineal trauma
   e. neurologic damage
   f. medications
   g. anxiety
18. a. feeling of fullness in the bladder
   b. bladder tenderness or discomfort
   c. restlessness
   d. diaphoresis
   e. absence of voiding or frequent voiding of small amounts
   f. palpable bladder over the symphysis pubis
19. a. stress
   b. urge
   c. overflow
   d. functional
   e. total
20. benefits, risks, urge, output

Chapter 13

1. musculoskeletal, cardiovascular, neurologic, respiratory
2. exercise, speed, coordination, stamina
3. joint, muscle
4. Gross, fine
5. Range-of-motion
6. physical, occupational, assistive
7. 20, 30, three
8. vital signs
9. Malnutrition, protein, iron, activity, atrophy, anemia
10. severe grief, anxiety, depression
11. avoided, mobility, injury
12. Passive, Active
13. stronger
14. oxygen, decrease, airway clearance
15. a. adequate hydration
   b. encouragement of coughing and deep breathing, incentive spirometry
   c. supplemental oxygen as ordered
   d. suction as necessary
   e. medications as ordered
16. a. mucolytics
   b. bronchodilators
   c. expectorants
17. rate, depth, safety
18. dependence, control, esteem

19. encouraged, Positive reinforcement
20. meaningful
21. unused, unrecognized
22. physical, psychosocial, spiritual

Chapter 14

1. a. altered appetite
   b. fatigue
   c. decreased coordination
   d. increased accidents
   e. increased irritability
   f. emotional instability
   g. difficulty with concentration
   h. impaired judgment
2. one half, two thirds
3. central nervous
4. 4
5. non–rapid eye movement (NREM)
6. less
7. a. sleep initiation problems
   b. sleep maintenance problems
   c. terminal insomnia problems
8. a. medical conditions
   b. psychologic factors
   c. medications
   d. behavioral factors
   e. environmental factors

Chapter 15

1. a. collection of information
   b. interpretation of information
   c. recognition of stimuli
2. a. intelligence
   b. memory
   c. language
   d. decision making
3. nervous, vision, hearing, smell, touch, taste
4. cerebral cortex
5. crystallized, knowledge, experience
6. aphasia, dysphasia, dysphagia
7. decrease, slower, cautious
8. short, long
9. Sensory, cognitive
10. time, person, place
11. a. acute confusion, or delirium
   b. idiopathic confusion
   c. dementia
12. a. uncontrolled pain
   b. infection
   c. metabolic disturbances
   d. vitamin deficiencies
   e. uremia
   f. hypoxia
   g. hypercalcemia

h. endocrine imbalances
i. myocardial infarction
j. constipation
k. drug toxicity
l. drug withdrawal
13. minutes, hours
14. a. rapid mood swings
b. disorganized sleep
c. changes in psychomotor activity, including tremors or spasmotic activity
d. rapid speech patterns
e. loss of attention
f. wide variety of cognitive changes
g. emotional instability
h. possible delusions and auditory or visual hallucinations
15. behavioral, physiologic
16. slow, insidious
17. a. Alzheimer's disease
b. multiple infarcts of the cerebral cortex secondary to cerebrovascular accidents
c. drug intoxication
d. Huntington's disease
e. Creutzfeldt-Jakob disease
f. Pick's disease
g. cerebral hypoxia
h. hyperthyroidism
i. subdural hematoma
j. brain tumors
18. a. wandering
b. excessively emotional (catastrophic) reactions
c. combative behaviors
d. suspiciousness
e. hallucinations
f. delusions
19. worsen, sundown
20. 10, 50
21. Continuity, restraints, worse
22. lowest, shortest
23. increased, Chronic, unrelieved
24. a. anger
b. depression
c. isolation

Chapter 16

1. attitudes, perceptions, values, experiences, interactions
2. values, control
3. Positive
4. a. attention to hygiene and grooming
b. body posture
c. amount and type of eye contact
d. tone of voice and speech patterns
e. type and frequency of emotions exhibited
5. aging, illness

6. institutional, possessions, control
7. rejection, isolation
8. a. self-esteem disturbance
b. hopelessness
c. powerlessness
9. image
10. reminiscence, value, meaning, strengths, coping
11. a. pain
b. crime and victimization
c. loss of loved ones
d. disease or injury
e. pain and suffering
f. loss of independence
g. financial destitution
h. loneliness
i. death
12. a. dilated pupils
b. dry mouth
c. trembling
d. increased pulse, blood pressure, and respiratory rate
e. palpitations
f. diaphoresis
g. diarrhea
h. urinary frequency
13. endocrine, cardiovascular, neurologic, respiratory
14. destructive, suicide
15. refuse
16. a. listening to the reasons for refusal or objections
b. providing good explanations and reasons that address the person's concerns
c. modifying approaches or procedures to accommodate elderly persons
d. consulting with other disciplines
17. a. accept the refusal
b. attempt again later
c. document the refusal and approaches used to gain compliance

Chapter 17

1. roles
2. identified, society, status, expectations, behavior, symbols, relationships
3. homogeneous, heterogeneous, confusion, conflict
4. loss, grief
5. a. retirement
b. loss of spouse
c. loss of home and/or possessions
d. loss of health
e. loss of independence
6. a. shock and numbness
b. searching and yearning
c. disorientation
d. reorganization
7. sadness, anger, denial, functional

8. isolation, interaction
9. parent, child, family processes, dependent

Chapter 18

1. real, perceived, significant
2. cold, noise, trauma, roles, relationships, thoughts
3. perception, cumulative, major
4. death
5. adaptation, Selye, autonomic
6. a. pounding or racing heart
   b. decreased peripheral circulation (cold, clammy hands)
   c. increased pulse rate, blood pressure, and respiratory rate
   d. elevated blood glucose level
   e. increased muscle tension
   f. decreased peristalsis
   g. urinary frequency
7. a. loss of ability to notice details
   b. decreased ability to solve problems
   c. difficulty attending to a thought or mental task
8. a. complaints of fatigue or tension
   b. anxiety
   c. irritability
   d. distractibility
   e. anger
   f. depression
9. a. changes in social interaction patterns
   b. diminished ability to perform or complete tasks
   c. increased disorganization of behavior
   d. increased errors in performance of common activities
   e. scattered or disconnected activity patterns
   f. repetitious or ritualistic behaviors
10. mental, physical
11. Coping, confrontation, escape, avoidance, emotional distancing

12. a. moderate physical activity
    b. relaxation techniques such as progressive relaxation, imaging, meditation, biofeedback, and self-hypnosis
    c. developing a social support network
    d. professional help from counselors, ministers, or mental health professionals
13. losses, change, relocation

Chapter 19

1. religion, philosophy, culture, society
2. early
3. Misunderstandings, conflict
4. understand, empathize
5. patience, communication
6. a. importance of work
   b. "waste not, want not"
   c. respect and obedience to elders and authorities
   d. belief in organized religion
7. practices, rituals, objects, reassurance
8. respect, spiritual

Chapter 20

1. touching, fondling, intercourse
2. illness, death
3. lubrication, thinner, elastic
4. delayed, longer
5. a. digitalis
   b. diuretics
   c. antihypertensives
   d. tranquilizers
   e. antidepressants
6. fear, pain, health condition
7. privacy
8. undesired

INDEX